THE ETHICS OF MANAGED CARE

MEDICAL ETHICS

DAVID H. SMITH AND ROBERT M. VEATCH, EDITORS

Volume 24 in series

THE ETHICS OF MANAGED CARE

A Pragmatic Approach

Mary R. Anderlik

INDIANA UNIVERSITY PRESS

Bloomington and Indianapolis

This book is a publication of

Indiana University Press
601 North Morton Street
Bloomington, Indiana 47404-3797 USA

http://iupress.indiana.edu

Telephone orders   800-842-6796
Fax orders   812-855-7931
Orders by email   iuporder@indiana.edu

The paper used in this publication meets the minimum
requirements of American National Standard for Information
Sciences—Permanence of Paper for Printed Library
Materials, ANSI Z39.48-1984.

Manufactured in the United States of America

Library of Congress Cataloging-in-Publication Data
Anderlik, Mary.
The ethics of managed care : a pragmatic approach / Mary Anderlik.
p.   cm. — (Medical ethics series)
Includes bibliographical references and index.
ISBN 0-253-33848-4 (cl : alk. paper)
1. Managed care plans (Medical care)—Moral and ethical aspects.
I. Title.   II. Series.

RA413 .A618 2001
174'.2—dc21
00-054015

1 2 3 4 5   06 05 04 03 02 01

TO MY PARENTS

CONTENTS

Contents

ACKNOWLEDGMENTS

As I began work on my dissertation on managed care in 1995, I had little notion that the dissertation would become a book, or that managed care would become the wild ride of the past several years. I would not have persevered in researching, writing, and rewriting, or in believing that the work mattered, without the constant support of my advisor, Gerald McKenny. I know the dissertation benefited from his careful critiques. If I have found a standpoint on managed care that conveys a "richer and more ordered landscape," it is owing to his influence. Elizabeth Heitman also read carefully and commented wisely. Beyond this, she has been an inspiration to me, an academic so involved in community service that her commitment nearly cost her tenure. H. Tristram Engelhardt kept me honest about limits, a service he performs for many liberals and liberal-communitarians. Through Texas history drills he also ensured that wherever I may wander, I will never forget the Alamo or Mirabeau B. Lamar, first vice-president and second president of the Republic of Texas. The manuscript has changed enough in its post-dissertation phase that none of these splendid teachers and mentors can justly be held accountable for its failings.

A significant change in 1998 was the addition of a section on the virtue of faithfulness. The addition is attributable to time spent with Rebecca Pentz and the members of the Clinical Ethics Committee at The University of Texas M.D. Anderson Cancer Center. There truly are men and women in the healing professions whose work has a quality that I can only call holy. I will never forget Dr. Arthur Forman's defense of "reverence" as a core value of the institution.

I also owe a great debt of gratitude to Robert Sloan and Jane Lyle of Indiana University Press and several anonymous reviewers. The name of the last reviewer, Griffin Trotter, was disclosed to me, and so I can offer a personal thank you for his endorsement and his helpful comments. I also thank Dr. Trotter for greatly enriching my understanding of and appreciation for the thought and character of Josiah Royce. The work of Royce, and Trotter, is inadequately represented in this book, but perhaps that oversight can be remedied in the future.

Words are inadequate to convey what I owe to my parents, Edward and Carol Schlachtenhaufen. Their love and support I take for granted, and what a gift that is. I am sure Reinhold Niebuhr's treatment of common grace resonates so strongly with me because I have received it, in abundance. To the extent that I have been "freed from self-preoccupation" and "enabled to reach out to others"—a difficult achievement in our self-obsessed culture—it has been their doing. If I have become aware of social injustice and the necessity of striving (however imperfectly) for something better, it has been through their teaching.

THE ETHICS OF MANAGED CARE

INTRODUCTION

My interest in managed care has biographical roots. Before deciding to study ethics, I spent three years in the commercial banking transactions group of a corporate law firm. When I arrived, the group was busy documenting loans in connection with leveraged buy-outs of large corporations. When I departed, the group was busy documenting "work outs" of those loans. Many of the deals consummated in the mergers and acquisitions frenzy of the 1980s had soured.

As my original choice of practice reveals, I know the fascination of the market and complex financial transactions. Still, during my tenure as a transactional lawyer, I became skeptical of the existence of a hidden hand that inevitably weaves the social good out of the uncoordinated actions of individuals and the beneficial operation of the profit motive. I observed how incentives operated in the rush to complete dubious year-end deals, so that bankers could collect year-end bonuses.

I noted the difficulty in assigning responsibility for effects that were difficult to locate in terms of individual actors. The suggestion that we lawyers, as mere facilitators of transactions, should ponder and take responsibility for their social consequences seemed inappropriate or naive. It did not help that we were readily replaceable in an increasingly competitive environment. Health care, by contrast, seemed a field where matters of practical concern were routinely considered in moral terms.

I was not mistaken, judging by the amount of moral perturbation over managed care among practitioners and the growing corps of professional medical ethicists. At the same time, two things are now clearer to me. First, health care is not a field insulated from wider social trends. Indeed, it seems that health care is now the favored arena for deal-making. Second, the psychological and sociological phenomena I observed among bankers and lawyers are much in evidence here.

Organizational structures shape conduct. Roles structure responsibility. But in a world increasingly dominated by large organizations, roles and the limits they set to responsibility are problematic. Actions have ramifications that extend beyond the individuals immediately involved, just as transactions among individuals are constrained by distant forces. Finally, it seems, we are becoming aware of the need for a health care ethic that takes account of organizations and the social environment. Unfortunately, the bioethics literature does not yet provide the guidance one would hope for in these areas.

THE REACTION TO MANAGED CARE: MEDICINE VERSUS BUSINESS

Much of the debate over managed care has been dominated by the idea that there is a fundamental dichotomy between medicine and business, leaving the major task as choosing a side. The work of Ruth Macklin and Mark Waymack illustrates this phenomenon.[1]

Macklin charges that managed care is simply a euphemism for turning medical decisions into business decisions, with the further implication that this is an illegitimate conversion. She is particularly disturbed by the gatekeeping role physicians assume under some forms of managed care. Her criticisms of managed care resolve into two chief concerns: that continuity of relationship and communication are being slighted and that commitment to patient welfare is being compromised.

These *are* weighty concerns. But at each point, consideration of a possible range of practices and justifications yields to a singular categorical judgment: "If the current system errs in providing incentives for ever greater numbers of referrals to specialists, the opposite error of providing incentives to primary care physicians not to refer, when it may be appropriate, is at least as bad." "A system in which bureaucrats at a distance make medical decisions and second-guess clinicians is a system that undermines the doctor-patient relationship and the ability of physicians to practice good clinical medicine in the best interests of their patients." Managed care systems are "run by business managers whose main objective is to minimize costs."[2] And so on.

While these judgments may be correct, one could question whether the conversation about the future of health care has advanced very far. Do *all* managed care organizations offer incentives to discourage referrals, regardless of their appropriateness? Do *all* "bureaucrats" work at a distance, and is *all* bureaucratic interference unwarranted, mere "second-guessing"? If many managed care organizations have ethical failings, is the only alternative a more tenacious embrace of the traditional way of operating, even as it becomes less and less viable?

Few would deny that the physician's main objective should be to benefit the patient. The question is what that entails. Do not current social considerations implicitly qualify the meaning of "benefit"? Surely a physician is not required to steal a drug, even if that would benefit a patient. Should she bend a managed care plan's rules, or misrepresent a patient's condition to ensure more favorable treatment? Finally, Macklin, a strong defender of patient autonomy, would argue that the clinician must respect the patient's choices. What, then, to make of the choice of a health plan?

By way of contrast, the opportunity to choose a plan appears to be the thing that matters most to Waymack. Waymack argues, in essence, that we can construct an adequate moral framework using the consumer choice model. He compares forms of health care organization to automobiles. Traditional fee-for-service health insurance is a Mercedes. The health maintenance organization (HMO) is a Ford.

Waymack states that in many a consumer's judgment, the lower costs of the HMO will "more than balance out the restrictions involved with the service." According to Waymack, the kinds of conflicts generated within an HMO context are not a matter for ethical concern if the consumer "has *willingly chosen* to participate in this kind of health plan." He contrasts this "business" ethic, founded upon autonomy, with the traditional physician ethic, founded upon beneficence: "If the consumers buy into the HMO insurance plan, knowing its costs and conditions, it does not seem right to allow them to cry 'foul' when they (through pure misfortune) become the losers. Thus, when the physician acts as a gatekeeper, he or she is in an important sense acting in accord with the *autonomy* exercised by the patient when that health plan was selected."[3] For Waymack, ethical analysis is focused on ensuring informed choice among individual consumers.

Can health care be this completely assimilated to the automobile? Can ethical concern be narrowed to this isolated act of choice by an individual? The difficulties in aligning reality with the demands of the consumer choice model suggest that it ignores too much of the picture.

First, there is evidence that consumers lack choice *and* information. At present, close to 50 percent of all Americans insured through their employers are offered only one health plan.[4] In a large national survey in 1995, 63 percent of respondents claimed they did not have a good understanding of the differences between traditional fee-for-service and managed care plans. Close to 25 percent of those enrolled in managed care plans did not know that their physician choice was restricted. Nearly 30 percent of the respondents lacked confidence in their ability to make a good choice among health plans with the information available to them.[5]

Second, given the rapidly changing nature of medical technology and health care financing and delivery systems, "costs and conditions" can seldom be exhaustively detailed in contracts.[6] Third and finally, many health care professionals resist the idea that they should act as stern enforcers of autonomous choice. We may resist it also, even if we see the potential injustice of allowing people to escape the consequences of their volitional acts. Imagine a world in which an argument that pediatric surgery by a skilled practitioner will save money in the long-run is met by, "If you pay for a Ford, don't expect a Mercedes."[7] Is this really the paradigm we want to govern health care?

For Macklin and Waymack, the range of moral considerations is narrowly circumscribed. According to Macklin, the physician's duty is to benefit the individual patient within the limits set by respect for autonomy; the duty of third party payers and administrators seems to be to avoid interfering.[8] Waymack draws the circle of moral concern even more tightly. The patient must exercise his or her autonomy in choosing a health plan, and accept the consequences. The physician's duty is to respect that autonomy by holding the patient to her choice.

Macklin uses a few anecdotes to illustrate how managed care is linked to violations of moral duties; in his essay Waymack spends even less time coming to grips with the reality of managed care. Given their interests, and space constraints, neither Macklin nor Waymack says much about the range of social values implicated in managed care, the complexity of human motivation, or the influence of organizations on character and conduct.

CONSTRUCTING A NEW ETHIC

The new (renewed) emphasis on controlling costs and demands for greater accountability on the part of health care providers have inspired others in the field to search for a new ethic. Two exemplary efforts in this area are E. Haavi Morreim's *Balancing Act* and Ezekiel Emanuel's *Ends of Human Life*.[9] *Balancing Act* is one of the first serious, book-length treatments of the issues raised for medical ethics by medicine's "new economics."

Morreim takes the evolving arrangements for health care delivery as a given, and asks what kinds of changes we should make in moral and legal standards to align them more closely with contemporary realities. She can adopt this approach because she believes that these arrangements are imperfect but not intolerable, and because she rejects the view that third-party payers and others outside the physician-patient dyad are "intruders." She defines her project as an exercise in moral problem-solving.

For Morreim, this means that one draws on the resources of theoretical normative reasoning only when practically necessary. Her distinctive contribution is a new framework for analyzing physician duties. She argues that in the current environment, we must recognize two new duties. First, physicians have a duty of economic advocacy for patients. Second, physicians have a duty to minimize conflicts of interest that may compromise their loyalty to patients.

These duties create additional burdens for physicians, but Morreim develops them in ways that lighten the load physicians have been made to bear by traditional moral and legal standards carried forward into changed conditions. In the area of economic advocacy, Morreim distinguishes between "gaming the system" and "pressing the system." Shading the truth or lying to secure the desired treatment for one's patients would be an example of the former.

Morreim introduces powerful arguments against gaming, including principles of nonmaleficence, veracity, and justice. She proposes dividing the moral and legal standard of care, which defines physicians' obligations to patients, into two components. The first is a "standard of medical expertise" demanding a similar level of knowledge, skill, and diligence in the care of every patient, and the second is a "standard of resource use" that will vary with the resource arrangements in effect for each patient.

Morreim defends the departure from a unified and universal standard of care on two grounds. First, she argues that we are facing the "new" problem of fiscal scarcity, as well as the familiar problem of commodity scarcity. Commodity scarcity requires us to make decisions about who will get a bed in the intensive care unit when the number of patients who would benefit exceeds the number of available beds. Fiscal scarcity requires us to consider that every dollar spent on the care of this patient is unavailable for other uses, within or outside health care, and that every dollar spent is a cost to someone.

The individual who does not pay as a patient may pay as an employee, when the escalating costs of health benefits result in the loss of other benefits or a job; as a stockholder, when corporate performance is affected by the high cost of employee health benefits; or as a taxpayer, when the bill for Medicare, Medicaid, and other public spending on health care comes due. This argument suggests that even a "patient" might reasonably reject the traditional ethic that makes medical benefit to the individual the exclusive consideration in health care decision making. Second, Morreim argues that a proper conception of autonomy must include taking responsibility for one's choices, including selecting a health plan offering a defined level of benefits.

Freedom is a prerequisite for autonomy, not its central meaning. In an era of resource constraints, says Morreim, "physicians must shift from an ethic of 'use it if it might help,' to 'don't use it *unless* it quite clearly will help.'"[10] The duty to minimize conflicts of interest prompts Morreim to discuss some of the nuances of incentives. She calls upon physicians to be discriminating, not self-denying.

Like Morreim, I define my project as a practical one. Like Morreim, I reject the view that we must preserve traditional standards at all costs, and I resist the narrowing of moral concern to the physician-patient dyad, denuded of context. Unlike Morreim, who focuses on the physician, I will devote considerable attention to organizations. I will ask how the disciplines of psychology and sociology can inform our understanding of and response to the new developments we label managed care. Finally, I will attempt to establish connections between health care, health care ethics and the contemporary debate over the meaning of social values such as democracy and justice.

What Morreim concludes, that the "economic challenges we now face will force us to ask, openly and carefully, just what we prize," and to create a new order in more inclusive fashion, represents one of my central concerns.[11] New pressures may bring new opportunities to reflect openly and carefully on individual and communal ends. They may also bring a cycle of license and reaction.

Morreim's conclusion is Emanuel's beginning. Rather than a work of problem-solving that largely dispenses with theory, *The Ends of Human Life* is a work of political theory that carries a particular political vision into practice. Emanuel's point of departure is the impossibility of addressing the practical questions we face in health care without considering values and goals. He argues for a liberal communitarian social order, in which the primary goal is to nurture democratic deliberation about the shape of the good life.

Emanuel's distinctive contribution is a proposal for the creation of a federated system of community health programs (CHPs) reflecting different conceptions of the good. Emanuel allows that there may be an Adam Smith CHP and a Jeremy Bentham CHP, as well as CHPs that exemplify conceptions of the good more identified with the liberal communitarian vision.

CHPs will be limited to no more than 20,000–25,000 "citizen-members." Basic financing for health care will be handled through vouchers issued to citizens by the federal government. Some CHPs may cater to those who want unlimited access to health care and are willing to pay more to get it, while others may attract members by offering less and rebating some portion of the voucher amount.

State oversight boards, under the purview of a federal board, will regulate the CHPs. The distinctive concept of the good guiding each CHP will be reflected in its policies and mode of operation. As with Morreim's prescription, Emanuel's reflects a particular view of autonomy. Autonomy or freedom is not only the power "to choose and pursue one's individual conception of the good life" but also the power "to shape the social and political structures in which these choices and pursuits occur."[12]

Like Emanuel, I am interested in problems of participation and scale. I, too, believe that we cannot address our present difficulties without considering what we value in life and why, and that this process of sorting out values must be communal. Unlike Emanuel, I cannot envision a tidy pluralism. Emanuel's account is pluralistic in that allowance is made for different conceptions of the good, but the ideal is a unified (although not necessarily homogenous) community with a coherent ethic. For Emanuel, communities are not fractured internally by a plurality of moral commitments and values; nor do persons have difficulty identifying themselves with a single community. Also, Emanuel, like Morreim, focuses on the physician. He has a stake in ranking some occupations, such as the practice of medicine, as "higher" than others.

I will scrutinize the medical profession and the professional ideal more critically. I am also wary of Emanuel's extension of the political model to health care. I note that while Emanuel says a lot about the activity of citizen-members, he leaves the patient role largely untouched. Agency is concentrated in the citizen-member role. (It is significant that Emanuel's paradigm case, chosen to anchor and guide reflection, involves an incompetent patient.) He does not consider possible alterations in the character of the relationship between physician and patient, or the relationships among providers of care.

Finally, the CHPs play a crucial role within Emanuel's proposal for a truly federal health system, but they are considered as settings for civic deliberation and the resolution of quandaries—assignment of decision-making authority, selection of medical interventions, and resource allocation—rather than as organizations with certain generic features. Hence, Emanuel does not address a highly significant problem in the managed care context, the tension between internal and external goods.

This tension does not exist for CHPs because Emanuel's ideal construct sidesteps the problem of fiscal scarcity. The voucher system will supply CHPs with sufficient resources to provide adequate health care to all. Citizen-members will determine how to allocate resources in accordance with their particular conceptions of the good. Insecurity, fear and greed do not come into play at the organizational or individual level.

OVERVIEW

While I can identify points of disagreement with Macklin and Waymack, Morreim and Emanuel, the larger point is that health care is such a complex subject that emphases are bound to differ. This book is my contribution to constructing a pragmatic, organization-centered approach to the ethics of managed care.

In Chapter 1, I try to provide the reader with a sense of the book's main argument, and I introduce two leitmotives that guide my understanding and evaluation of managed care, the social experiment and the problem. Chapter 2 explores some common ways of framing the analysis of managed care, such as "medicine versus business." I argue that opponents of managed care, under the sway of the ideology of medicine, and defenders of managed care, under the sway of the ideology of business, suffer from a similar defect of vision, a kind of myopia.

The social context is obscured, and certain moral considerations are removed from consideration. Much of the reporting on managed care reproduces these limitations. I consider the story of Christine deMeurers, and of Health Net, the managed care organization that refused to pay for a bone marrow transplant to treat deMeurers's advanced breast cancer. Stories of personal tragedy and corporate greed largely define managed care in the popular press. Yet this story is too complex, too full of moral ambiguity to fit neatly within the confines of any simple framework. I suggest that we need a more complex, more *social* ethic to move beyond the limits of standard approaches to managed care. This social ethic must take account of a key problem of modernity: the increasingly manipulative cast of social relations, and the tendency to identify management with manipulation.

In Chapter 3, I draw on the resources of the pragmatic tradition to construct a moral framework with a distinctive method, understanding of social values, moral psychology, and "moral sociology." The method is broad and experimental, linked to the social value of democracy. If the word "manipulation" captures what needs to be avoided, the word "democracy" offers a vision of what is desirable in social relations. It can also inform our thinking about justice.

The discussion of moral psychology develops the concept of character as both stable and vulnerable. That vulnerability directs attention to organizations as aspects of the environment that may influence character. I turn to the pragmatic tradition in the social sciences for the resources to construct criteria to evaluate organizations in general and health care arrangements, in particular.

First, I ask what kinds of character organizations display, and second, what kinds of character traits they form in the persons they affect. I consider the meaning of virtues of integrity and responsiveness in health care organizations. These virtues are important because they address some of the special problems of organizations: the tension between pursuing external goods and maintaining internal goods, the truncation of the time horizon (i.e., the dominance of short-term considerations in decision-making), and the opacity of organizations to those within and without. Focusing on organizations as agencies of character formation highlights those character traits essential to health care. Traits like faithfulness and openness are valuable in themselves and as sources of resistance to a culture of manipulation.

In Chapter 4, I present a "character study" of the Kaiser Permanente Medical Care Program, one of the oldest and best-known managed care organizations. I explore important aspects of the organization, including leadership, financial incentives, guidelines and rationing of services, rationing of time, innovation, community, and (mis)communication. I use Kaiser to show that occasionally, significant individual and communal goods can be realized within the context of managed care. At the same time, the Kaiser study reveals how difficult it is to find the appropriate balance in negotiating the various tensions of organizational life, especially in a time of rapid change.

In Chapter 5, I return to ideology. I argue for a critical reconstruction of the ideologies of business and medicine and a recovery of the ideology of cooperative egalitarianism that so influenced the pioneers of managed care. Reconstruction entails exposing the limits of each perspective while searching for the germs of insight each perspective offers. In exploring the ideology of business more fully I consider the "profit motive," "efficiency" and the benefits and imperfections of markets.

The close relationship between business and bureaucracy merits attention, along with the relationship of organizational scale and complexity to efficiency and to the pathologies of bureaucracy. In exploring the ideology of medicine more fully, I consider the professional ideal, with its great promise and its susceptibility to abuse. I also consider inter-professional conflict.

Finally, in exploring the ideology of cooperative egalitarianism, I lay out its central features and grapple with some of the difficulties in the area of feasibility. I review efforts that illustrate how cooperative egalitarianism might operate in policy making, in setting standards and setting limits, and in the clinical setting. In assessing the implications of the "corporatization" of health care, I reflect on the uses and abuses of the rhetoric of community in the health care field.

In Chapter 6, I consider the practices that most of us think of when we hear of "managed care": financial incentives and gatekeeping, and the exchanges of disclosure and consent that may lend legitimacy to rationing and to other limits imposed by health plans. I argue that some financial arrangements and some forms of gatekeeping promise considerable benefit, while others should be condemned. I argue that while disclosure and consent may be more or less adequate, these will never be sufficient to legitimate limits on health care. We must also have substantive (regulatory) protections and processes of community formation.

Next, I consider the potential of ethicists, ethics committees and various forms of external oversight to move managed care in desirable directions and to discourage abuses. I conclude that each form of regulation has its weaknesses, thus requiring the support of others. I review the evidence concerning health outcomes in order to grasp the benefits and burdens of managed care from the perspective of society's most vulnerable members.

In the conclusion to this book, I look to the future. I argue that managed care as we know it is a transitional phenomenon, an ongoing experiment in remolding values and organizations. In the course of the experiment, many submerged conflicts and tensions are being forced to the surface. I believe the hope for the future is a clearer social vision for health care informed by a more sophisticated understanding of organizations. Drawing on previous chapters, and the work of the "Tavistock Group," I advance seven statements of conviction and commitment to guide those involved in shaping health care's future.

I need to clarify a few more points. First, although I do not wish to minimize the importance of individual and governmental actors, I will focus on organizations in the private sphere. These organizations are constituted by individuals and influenced by the legislative and regulatory environment. It would go contrary to my understanding of pragmatism to attempt an ethics for organizations free of references to individuals and to the larger social order. But in this inquiry, I consider individuals and society primarily as they affect or are affected by organizations.

Second, I do not examine the special problems of managed mental health care.[13] Third, I have limited my inquiry to managed care as it has developed and is developing within the United States. Even with that qualification, there may be confusion about what I mean by "managed care." It is often a good idea to preface an inquiry with some description of the phenomenon under analysis. Accordingly, I will conclude this introduction with a brief historical overview and a definition.

WHAT IS MANAGED CARE?

Although some speak of managed care as if it were a recent innovation, prepaid health plans offering more or less comprehensive health services have been around for some time. The Sisters of Charity of the Incarnate Word offered a prepaid health plan in 1869. For $.25 a week, or $13.00 a year, a person was assured care at St. Mary's Infirmary in Galveston, Texas.[14]

The standard histories of managed care usually begin around 1929, when Dr. Michael Shadid established a farmers' cooperative health plan in Elk City, Oklahoma. For $50, a family joining the cooperative received a share in a new, state-of-the-art hospital and a discount on all health care. In 1932, the Elk City cooperative implemented a true prepaid health plan. In building on the cooperative idea, Shadid set out to remedy the deficiencies of rural health care. In his autobiographical account, he noted that the high cost of a serious illness put decent comprehensive health care services beyond the reach of many hard-working farming families.

Shadid also observed the connection between poor medical care, especially unnecessary surgeries that often resulted in death, and the combination of severe economic conditions and incentives associated with fee-for-service payment. He was appalled by the neglect of prevention and means of early detection and treatment for serious conditions such as cancer. He argued that solo practice was becoming obsolete as an organizational mode due to advances in technology and knowledge.[15]

Also in 1929, two Los Angeles physicians created a group practice with a prepayment plan and contracted to provide comprehensive health services to approximately two thousand water company employees. The Group Health Association in Washington, D.C. was established in 1937, Kaiser-Permanente Medical Care Programs in 1942, the Group Health Cooperative of Puget Sound and the Health Insurance Plan of Greater New York in 1947, and the Group Health Plan of Minneapolis in 1957. Organized medicine did not welcome these developments. Indeed, many county and state medical societies strenuously opposed the "corporate" practice of medicine. For much of the century, managed care remained a regional phenomenon.[16]

In 1969, amid mounting concern about health care spending—the rhetoric of crisis is nothing new—these prepaid group health plans or "health maintenance organizations" (HMOs) attracted attention as a way of controlling costs. The critical idea was to keep people healthy. Proponents expected "health maintenance strategies" to benefit individuals and society by increasing well-being and productivity, in turn benefiting HMOs and third party payers by providing savings from more expensive sick care. At that juncture, escalating

Introduction

health care costs mainly concerned the federal government. Then as now, the federal government paid for a major portion of health care directly under Medicare and Medicaid (a federal-state partnership), and indirectly through employer tax deductions for health care benefits and the exclusion of these benefits from employee income. In the 1970s, with passage of the Health Maintenance Organization Act of 1973, Congress intended to make HMOs more attractive. But throughout the 1970s and 1980s, HMOs held a rather small, albeit growing, market share.[17]

Health care costs have continued to spiral. In the last decade, large employers, as well as federal and state governments, have become increasingly aggressive in seeking to control them. The moral force behind cost containment comes from trade-offs between health care and other public and private goods. The money society spends on health care cannot be spent on education, housing, and so on. Further, some critics of current spending patterns have argued that health, not health care, should concern us, and that increasing expenditures for health care may not be the best way to decrease morbidity and mortality in a population.[18]

Whatever motivated the turn to managed care, and no doubt the motives are mixed, reducing costs is clearly a major objective in the current wave of health care reform. Many believe managed care achieves the cost-reduction objective; the evidence suggests that some costs are merely shifted to other parts of the system or to informal caregivers.[19]

Whatever the ultimate judgment on the cost issue, managed care has come to dominate health care.[20] And while it would be disingenuous to disregard the cost containment objective, healthcare experts offer reasons other than the potential for controlling costs in favor of managed care. As Shadid noted several decades earlier, traditional fee-for-service payment gives providers incentives to overutilize medical resources. Regional variation among provider practice patterns, without evidence linking treatment intensity to improvements in population health status, nourishes skepticism about physician judgments of medical necessity. And it is not merely a financial matter. Most medical interventions are associated with very real risks to patients. If managed care decreases the use of certain health care services, this is not necessarily a bad thing. In addition, in theory, HMOs provide comprehensive care and devote a greater portion of their resources to prevention.

Managed care comes in many flavors. These include staff-, group-, network-, and independent practice association (IPA)–model HMOs, as well as preferred provider organizations (PPOs) and HMOs with a point-of-service (POS) option.[21] A commonly cited definition of managed care comes from an article by John Iglehart, which appeared in the *New England Journal of Medicine* in 1992:

[A managed care system is one] that integrates the financing and delivery of *appropriate* medical care by means of the following features: contracts with *selected* physicians and hospitals that furnish a *comprehensive* set of health care services to enrolled members, usually for a predetermined, monthly premium; utilization and quality controls that contracting providers agree to accept; financial incentives for patients to use the providers and facilities associated with the plan; and the assumption of some financial risk by doctors, thus fundamentally altering their role from serving as agent for the patient's welfare to balancing the patient's needs against the need for cost control.[22]

This kind of definition commands agreement in the technical literature. But as sociologist David Mechanic and others note, providers and other critics use the term "managed care" promiscuously. Managed care may designate any kind of utilization review, and even more broadly, any form of cost-cutting or cost-consciousness. When I speak of managed care I mean the kind of system described by Iglehart, but I also recognize that the public perception of managed care is shaped by the loose usage of the term.

ONE

Managed Care as Social Experiment and Social Problem

We tend to think of organizations and the problems they raise as newly arrived to health care. Yet even in the days before managed care, physicians and patients experienced the power of incentives structured by organizations, by medical schools, hospitals, professional societies, insurance companies, and government agencies. Discussions of the ethics of medical practice dating back to the Hippocratic corpus in the Western tradition, and the medical ethics movement initiated in the latter part of this century in response to new technologies and popular dissatisfaction with the paternalism of the traditional physician-oriented ethic, remain a valuable legacy. At the same time, the traditional ethic, and the newer ethic of patient autonomy, generally refrain from delving into matters of organization.

At one time, these matters could, for the most part, be ignored. The incentives seemed to work to the benefit of all concerned. The organization of health care on a fee-for-service basis, with relatively generous funding for health care, gave physicians incentives to do as much as possible. Since cost was largely invisible to them, patients had an equivalent incentive to want as much as possible done to or for them. The traditional ethic, and the ethic of patient autonomy, told physicians and patients that it was good and right that they limit their concern to their immediate transactions with one another. If there was a weakness in health care, it was in the failure to extend the luxury of self-concern, and the beneficent attention of a devoted, and well-compensated, physician, to all who might occupy the patient role.

THREE QUESTIONS ABOUT ORGANIZATIONS

The neglect of organizations is no longer benign, if it ever was. In the era of managed care, we can no longer afford to ignore the effects of organizations on conduct and character, or the location of transactions between individuals within a social matrix. Those who cling to the traditional ethic, or the ethic of patient autonomy, are ill-equipped to grasp the problems brought to light, if not created, by managed care. Managed care and related developments have provoked comment from medical ethicists and others, but few have taken up the challenge of constructing an ethic that speaks to organizations. This book is a foray into that largely unexplored territory. Simply put, the argument is that there can be no simple verdict on managed care, no "thumbs up" or "thumbs down" from the moral point of view. The criteria that ought to be employed in evaluation, and the phenomenon itself, are too complex for that. What is relatively straightforward is the wake-up call, the reminder that we neglect organizations at our peril. In particular, we stand in need of answers to three questions: 1) How do organizations affect us? 2) What is their moral status? 3) How might they be evaluated in moral terms?

As one might expect, the answers are not easy. *That* said, the evidence does suggest that certain structures associated with managed care, and certain managed care organizations, have accomplished much that is praiseworthy, in terms of individual and social benefit. *That* said, no structure or organization represents moral perfection, and the future of managed care in any form is in doubt. We cannot and should not look to managed care or any other system of health care for salvation. What we may achieve through diligent investigation and reflection is a more realistic appraisal of the situation, and ultimately a more responsible use of the power we have to shape the organizations that shape us.

HOW TO THINK ABOUT MANAGED CARE: A PRELIMINARY EXERCISE

We can think about managed care in a number of ways. I would suggest that we begin by considering managed care as social experiment and as social problem, as a kind of heuristic or preparatory mental exercise.

Managed Care as Social Experiment

At a rudimentary level, an experiment is an effort to understand relations of cause and effect through a trial. The paradigm I wish to invoke is not, however, the randomized, controlled clinical trial we are familiar with in health care. A trial or experiment in the sense I intend is an ordinary occurrence. Consider a young boy who hits (or hugs) his little sister, and then stands back to see what happens and so decides his future course of action. What I describe with this boy, who may become a delinquent or saint, according to the reaction of his little sister (and his reaction to her reaction, and any interventions by parents, and so on), is not only an experiment, but a social one. Relationships with others are at stake.

Because relationships are so central to my conception of the social experiment, it must be distinguished from another perspective that might fall under that label. According to the view I reject, those whose expertise or privilege removes them from the common lot are authorized to gamble with the lives of less expert or less privileged others. A social experiment in the sense I wish to call up is guided by strong moral commitments; hence my example of a child's testing of limits is not fully adequate. Such an experiment must be regulated so that, among other things, the vulnerable are protected from harm, rights are respected and obligations honored, and those who take the lead in its unfolding are not insulated from its effects.

Managed Care as Social Problem

What is happening with managed care is obviously on a different scale from what happens with the children. Relationships among millions of people are implicated, and these relationships are mediated by organizations. Owing to this difference of scale and complexity, we may fail to make the connection between what we do and what we see transpiring. We feel for the patient-heros and heroines of the news reports on managed care and desire the punishment of the villainous executives of the managed care plans. Yet, we continue to enroll in those very same plans because we believe we have no other option, or because we like their promises of more comprehensive benefits at lower cost. We may even buy or hold stock in them.

But in truth, the "we" does not simply mark the introduction of large numbers of affected individuals. It is also a reminder of the importance of collective deliberation and action. It should prompt us to examine our organizational and social affiliations and responsibilities. Managed care prods us to acknowledge certain social tensions and value conflicts, and so becomes a problem. From this standpoint, we ask questions about organizations. From this standpoint, we ask about the moral costs and benefits of organizational structures and practices associated with managed care and their appropriate regulation.

CONSTRUCTING A FRAMEWORK FOR ANALYSIS

In keeping with the three questions I posed at the beginning of the chapter, this book is an inquiry into managed care as a problem of organizations. This chapter is intended as a guide or roadmap for that inquiry. I spoke earlier of constructing an ethic for organizations. To resume the building metaphor, the constructive project must be preceded by a deconstructive one. The burden of the next chapter is to get rid of the hope for a simple verdict on managed care. Adherents of the ideologies of medicine and business offer the easy answers—easy, that is, if one is willing to accept some dubious assumptions about human psychology, ignore the organizational dimension, and limit the range of moral concerns. Those who are adept in the analysis of managed care as a problem of choice, resource allocation, or conflict of interest offer what is almost as appealing, manageability—if one is willing to suppress the sense that something is lost when a great social drama is transformed into a series of technical exercises.

The deconstructive project aims to clear away some unsatisfactory approaches to the problem of managed care, but it also lays the groundwork for a more adequate approach through the identification of avenues for further inquiry. In particular, it suggests that a more adequate approach must display considerable sociological sophistication. It will have to cross disciplinary boundaries, involving what Albert Hirschman refers to as "trespassing."

Identifying the Perils

Among contemporary ethicists and moral philosophers, Alasdair MacIntyre has ventured the farthest down this path. MacIntyre argues that, within the culture of modernity, management has become manipulation. To the extent that managed care practices are manipulative and foster manipulation, they pose a very great danger, the danger that we will come to regard one another as objects.

We should strenuously oppose such a transformation of human relations. MacIntyre also fastens on the tension between the *internal* goods of practices such as the satisfaction derived from excellent performance and *external* goods such as money and power as a central organizational problem. Here the appropriate response is not opposition, but the maintenance of a balance between these two kinds of goods. Finally, MacIntyre identifies certain generic features of corporate life that tend to work against the moral life: truncation of the time horizon, role fragmentation, and organizational opacity. We must counter each of these tendencies through an appropriate organizational response.

Identifying the Resources

MacIntyre maps many of the critical issues, but his social vision is not generous. One may appropriate his insights without accepting his contempt for all things modern. The early modern intellectual movement known as pragmatism has many features that recommend it for a project of this nature. Pragmatism is best understood not as a complete philosophical or moral system, but as a promising approach to engaged social criticism. Pragmatism provides a warrant for a broad empiricism (and a context for the view of managed care as problem and experiment). The method of moral inquiry and deliberation suggested by pragmatism is practice-oriented, and therefore well-suited for an inquiry into managed care with a view to evaluation.

Certain figures within the pragmatic tradition also provide the resources for a more social ethic, contructed around a compelling vision of democracy and community. If manipulation is the negative value, democracy and community are positive values, ways of describing what we might aspire to in our relations with one another. At the same time, the pragmatic tradition hints at the difficulties that accompany the use of these themes, such as the denial of difference. Difference must not only be acknowledged; it must be affirmed.

The pragmatic tradition supplies a moral psychology that is consonant with the findings of recent research into human development and at odds with the atomism implicit in the ideologies of medicine and business. Character is formed through transactions with the environment; it is both stable and vulnerable. This aspect of psychology is a link to sociology. The importance of organizations derives from their role as environments that form (or deform) character. How do organizations affect us? By shaping who we are and how we interact with one another.

Moving Organizations to the Center

Without imagining an organization as some kind of suprapersonal being, one can recognize that being or acting within an organization differs from being or acting alone. The moral status of organizations follows from the role organizations play in shaping right and wrong action and generating good and bad consequences. What is the moral status of organizations? Organizations are bearers of the kind and degree of moral responsibility appropriate to the nature and extent of their involvement in wrongdoing and harm. (This statement will acquire some flesh in the course of the exposition.) Organizations can also display certain virtues that result in significant goods for the individuals immediately affected, and for society as a whole.

Key organizational virtues include integrity and responsiveness. These two virtues assume prominence because they speak to some of the morally problematic features of organizations previously alluded to: the tendency of organizations to constrict time, responsibility, and vision; the manager's resort to manipulation to further organizational goals, given the complexity of other means of motivating large groups; the difficulty of maintaining the appropriate balance between internal and external goods; and the vulnerability of organizations to influence from the external environment (and vice versa).

Beyond this, we must consider organizations as agencies affecting character formation. An important aspect of evaluating organizations, then, is assessing the effects of particular organizational arrangements or structures on character and on the quality of social relationships. Of particular relevance to health care, organizations may nourish or destroy the potential in individuals for faithfulness, openness, and truthfulness.

We need to carry this discussion into case or character studies of particular managed care organizations. For this effort, I have selected the Kaiser Permanente Medical Care Program. Kaiser is a good object for study, in part, because it differs from most other managed care organizations (a not-for-profit, group-model HMO with a long history, in an "industry" dominated by for-profit, independent practice association model HMOs of recent origin), and in part, because it is just like them (negotiating the tensions and conflicts that beset all organizations, and organizations involved in the financing and delivery of health care to an unusual degree). The case does not merely illustrate the framework but tests its power to illuminate our experience with managed care organizations. The case also exposes the tension between statistical rationalism and what I label "encounter personalism," a tension that is becoming ever more significant in health care.

Exploring the Role of Ideology

If managed care organizations are unique, that uniqueness comes from the intensity of the tensions and conflicts that arise in some form for all organizations. If health care is unique, that uniqueness comes from the particularly delicate negotiation required among ideologies. Ideologies are open to criticism as instruments of distortion, self-delusion and social oppression, but we cannot dispense with ideologies altogether. We need ideologies as clusters of symbols and practices that help us to order and organize organizational fields. Managed care is a synthesis of the ideologies associated with business and medicine, markets, and the professional guild, and also, although we often forget it, the co-operative operated according to egalitarian principles. An adequate response to managed care requires a reconstruction of the ideologies of business and medicine and a recovery of the ideology of cooperative egalitarianism.

In connection with the ideology of business, it is necessary to scrutinize the notion of a "profit motive" and claims to "efficiency"—concepts frequently bandied about but seldom analyzed, to see if they make any sense, or where their sense might lie. Invocations of the profit motive hide more than they explain. Efficiency is meaningless unless it is linked to specific ends and practices; any claim to efficiency should be followed by the question, "more efficient in achieving *what*?" Profitability (or solvency) certainly matters. Profit is a test of performance and basic social usefulness, but within a pragmatic world view, it is not an end. Money is a motivator, but so is meaning, and the latter may be the more powerful.

Markets have desirable features, but even classical economists recognize their imperfections. Moralists have the task of drawing attention to the interdependence markets trade on and tend to obscure. And business must own up to its entanglement with bureaucracy. Bureaucracy is not inherently evil; indeed it has commendable features. Unfortunately, it also has pathologies, which are most evident where manipulation of financial incentives is joined with heavy-handed imposition of bureaucratic controls.

Scale is another organizational dimension to consider. Organizations, with their strengths and weaknesses, are not new in health care, and organization is certainly not unique to managed care. On the other hand, the organizations involved in the managed care revolution tend to be corporate behemoths, matched within health care only by the large, for-profit hospital chains. Efficiency claims frequently trade on assumptions about the economic benefits of increasing size. Yet the problems associated with organizations generically considered seem to increase with size, and the prospect of a society dominated by giant corporations alarmed some early pragmatists, just as it alarms contemporary democratic theorists. Where the large scale organization promises substantial gains in productive efficiency, we need to think about ways to ameliorate the ill-effects. We also need to be open to the idea that what drives organizational growth in many cases is not productive efficiency, but success in manipulating the external environment.

Given concerns about the cogency of the business ideology and the manipulative cast of management, the professional ideology has much to commend it, if it can be recast along more democratic lines and reformed through the judicious incorporation of elements derived from the other ideologies.

There is much that is good in the ideology of medicine and in professionalism generally, but there is also a tendency to overreach. The challenge is to retain the good, while introducing greater accountability. The hope is that physicians will come to accept some measure of external scrutiny. The hope is that physicians will relinquish a perfectionism that harms patients in refusing to acknowledge the potential for harm. The hope is that physicians will recognize competence and dedication to patient well-being in other practitioners, and receive lay participation as a contribution rather than an affront. The hope is that physicians will accept some sacrifice of financial reward in order to preserve internal goods such as pride in the quality of one's work, the respect of colleagues, and the (deserved) trust and gratitude of patients. Fears concerning the potential for abuse of medical authority are justified, but the cure may be worse than the disease: the physician who is deprived of power, who can truly do no harm, is also a physician who can do very little to help.

We often overlook the ideology of cooperative egalitarianism, which informed many of the early experiments in managed care. Although there are serious difficulties in constructing and sustaining social arrangements guided solely by this ideology, difficulties we must take seriously, there are many ways in which recovering it might change thinking and alter structures. Cooperative egalitarianism invites us to play with themes of cooperation and equity. It provides action guides such as "those affected by a problem should participate in its resolution," "favor structures that build cooperation over structures that place persons in relationships where some command and others obey," and "consider the plight of the most vulnerable."

We may, however, learn more about the contours of cooperative egalitarianism from examples than from theoretical explication. Stories give some hint of the rewards and frustrations and opportunities for transformation that arise when actual people go to work on actual problems. In managed care, experimentation with more cooperative structures is possible in areas such as standard setting, limit setting, and clinical practice. Cooperative egalitarianism can also inform our response to corporate giganticism, by bringing forward the idea and ideal of community.

APPLYING THE FRAMEWORK

If I can support each of the preceding points with evidence and argument, I will have the beginnings of a moral framework for evaluating managed care, ready to apply. It will consist of an awareness of the dangers of management as manipulation and the power of organizations to deform human beings and limit moral vision, and an awareness of the freedom to be found in community and the possible virtues of organizations. Of course, this formulation is highly misleading, since construction and evaluation proceed together, while application involves further elaborating the framework. Nevertheless, what has been, primarily, an argument for a certain framework will become, primarily, an argument condemning some practices of managed care organizations, at least in some incarnations, while embracing others.

We need to review specific practices linked to managed care such as financial incentives and gatekeeping, weighing proposals for regulation. We must also consider consent-based legitimations of rationing, and various agencies of internal and external oversight such as ethicists and ethics committees, the media, legislatures, regulators, and judges. A final area of concern meriting closer examination is the effect of managed care on the quality of health care, and more especially, the quality of care for the most vulnerable members of society. From this analysis we should arrive at a number of complex verdicts and a deepened understanding of the pragmatists' insistence upon the significance of change. The practices are constantly evolving.

Today's managed care differs noticeably from the managed care of five years ago. At some point, we will have a phenomenon or set of phenomena so different from what we have now that our terminology will have to change. Change does not make the task of evaluation an exercise in futility, although change can certainly complicate the task and frustrate those carrying it out. Rather, change lends urgency to the task. The pragmatist proceeds in the hope that through analysis and evaluation we can guide, if not manage, at least some of the processes of change, and hence contribute to the flourishing of organizations more compatible with our aspirations than with our fears.

TWO

Managed Care and the Medicine-Business Polemic

"Managed care" is a euphemism for transforming medical decision making
into business decisions.

—Ruth Macklin, *Enemies of Patients*

[J]ust as, when our own resources are not infinite, we may willingly choose
the sturdy Ford over the crafted and polished Mercedes with the real leather
interior, the compact disk stereo and anti-locking brakes, so we may willingly choose the inexpensive but serviceable HMO over the more generous
fee-for-service plan.

—Mark Waymack, "Health Care as a Business"

For Ruth Macklin and others, managed care is a tool of interests hostile to
medicine. Given the prevalence of the view that managed care aligns with the
"business" side of a fundamental dichotomy between medicine and business,
we cannot simply ignore this construction of the problem. Neither ought we to
accept this construction uncritically.

I will begin with two portraits, renderings of the way in which many participants in medicine and business portray themselves and, to a large extent,
one another. I label these portraits "ideologies," because they state a certain
worldview and because they are used to defend certain prerogatives. The explicit or implicit threat is that any departure from the dictates of the ideology
is dangerous.

I readily concede that the portraits are caricatures. Few express belief in
the ideology of business or medicine without qualification, and it is doubtful
whether even their behavior is totally consistent with belief. Still, these particular caricatures have shaped much of the debate over managed care. Polemics in
which one caricature is opposed to the other dominate discussion, curtailing
reflection and deflecting attention away from projects such as the development
of a health care ethic addressed to organizations.

THE MEDICINE-BUSINESS POLEMIC

The Ideology of Medicine

Central to the ideology of Western medicine is an ethos of disinterested philanthropy. The distinctive features of medicine usually cited by practitioners include the special vulnerability of the patient and the noble character demanded of the physician. Physicians also lay claim to a specialized moral and technical vocabulary, arising out of a certain interpretation of the Hippocratic tradition.

The ethical physician acts primarily, if not exclusively, for the benefit of the immediate patient. At the outset, the individual physician bears the burden and privilege, at least initially, of determining where that benefit lies. Politics, and economic and social organization, are peripheral concerns, except to the extent that they seem to interfere with what is, in fact, the preferred form of organization, the autonomous practitioner within an autonomous profession. Fee-for-service payment and solo practice are favored precisely because they seem to secure autonomy and render underlying organization invisible to practicing physicians.

Organized medicine has promoted the image of medicine as philanthropy and defended the autonomy of the profession and the individual physician in its codes of ethics and policy statements. A statement on managed care by the Council on Ethical and Judicial Affairs of the American Medical Association (AMA) stresses the primacy of the physician in the health care system as the one who advocates for the patient, and the primacy of the patient's interest in the motivational structure of the physician: "Without the commitment that physicians place patients' interests *first* and act as agents for their patients *alone,* there is no assurance that the patient's health and well-being will be protected."[1]

The theme of devotion to patient welfare has long been intertwined with claims for professional independence. The first Code of Ethics of the AMA, dating from 1847, makes the private conscience of the individual practitioner the final court of appeal: "A Physician should not only be ever ready to obey the calls of the sick, but his mind ought also to be imbued with the greatness of his mission, and the responsibility he habitually incurs in its discharge. Those obligations are the more deep and enduring, because there is no tribunal other than his own conscience, to adjudge penalties for carelessness or neglect."[2]

In a study of physicians in a prepaid group practice dating from the 1970s, sociologist Eliot Freidson found that "[c]hecking up was associated with 'kindergarten teaching,' 'dossiers,' and even gestapo and 'Big Brother.' . . . 'Thou shalt trust physicians' was the basic commandment, justified by a particular conception of physicians as special people especially deserving of trust." Even those physicians, who had chosen a group practice, stressed independence and self-sufficiency: "Most of the physicians emphasized, above all other sources of motivation to perform well, the physician himself as an individual, believing that he performs more or less independently of the situation he is in and, particularly, independently of the social pressures connected with that situation. Like his basic medical training, his basic character was seen as a more or less permanent and only minimally changeable part of him. . . . The physician was visualized as someone who is guided only by his unchangeable inner needs."[3]

The Ideology of Business

In contrast to medicine, business makes no bones about being an interested activity. Moreover, interest is equated with self-interest, which is identified with material self-interest for the individual and profit-maximization for the firm. Business also has its own specialized technical (managerial) vocabulary, one that increasingly intrudes into the health care field or "industry." The moral claims of business are reflected less in a specialized moral vocabulary than in claims to efficiency. The proof of performance, production targets met or dollars saved, seems to render words superfluous.

Beyond this, the business person exhibits a cheerful amorality. Indeed, the business person incurs something like moral disapproval if he or she allows moral concern to influence the firm's operation and thus usurps the role of the market in achieving the maximal satisfaction of interests. Chief among these are the interests of consumers expressed in purchasing decisions. The corporation is the natural milieu of the business type, but reflecting on the moral significance of organizations and the broader social background is as unlikely for the business person as it is for the solo practitioner of medicine.

The classical business ideology is reflected in the work of Milton Friedman. Friedman's essay, "The Social Responsibility of Business Is to Increase Its Profits,"[4] offers a spirited defense of this image of the business person and its propriety. Friedman is a thorough nominalist. He begins by declaring that only individual persons can have responsibilities. In a free enterprise system, the responsibility of corporate executives and managers is to serve the corporation's owners, who are generally in business to make as much money as possible.

An argument for "corporate social responsibility" can only be a claim that executives should act contrary to the interests of their employer(s). Friedman equates social responsibility with the exercise of state power. He believes there is no space between the purely private, the realm of individuals pursuing their own interests, and the state. Friedman sings the virtues of the free market as the great disciplinarian. Private competitive enterprise forces people, including consumers, to be responsible for their choices, which are, by definition, voluntary.

It follows that if one chooses a Ford rather than a Mercedes, one will have to live without the leather interior and the CD player. If one chooses an HMO rather than a fee-for-service plan, one will have to live with some restrictions on care. The executives of Ford or the HMO are obligated to satisfy the terms of any contract they have made, and that is all the consumer is entitled to. After all, what have business people done in crafting their products, but cater to the preferences of consumers?

In a study of the moral world of corporate managers, Robert Jackall found that managers were adept at developing an armor that enabled them, psychologically, to make the "hard choices" that business was said to demand. They were reassured by the ideology, which told them that the proper role of business is "'to give the public what it wants,'" adopting the market "as the final arbiter not of values, which are always arguable, but, more importantly, of tastes, about which there can be no reasonable dispute."[5]

Overcoming Myopia

Although the ideologies of medicine and business are opposed, in the sense that they incorporate different moral ideals (e.g., philanthropy versus egoism, patient benefit versus efficiency), they also have something in common. Critics have labeled both of them "individualistic." Certainly, the physician and the business person take note of the significance of organization and organizations in practice, and each regards at least one organization, the federal government, as immensely powerful and threatening. However, neither has an ideology displaying any sociological sophistication. Yet, the label of individualism does not quite capture what is problematic.[6]

An ethic that neglects the social and organizational levels of analysis is flawed. But an ethic that focused exclusively on some collective interest would be just as unsatisfactory. It would be nonsense to say that such an ethic was individualistic, but not that it was *myopic*, that is, that it excluded a field of possible ethical relevance from consideration.[7] In the ethics shaped by the ideologies of medicine and business, some fields are outside awareness, while others are actively suppressed. Physicians believe they have an obligation to ignore consequences that extend beyond the medical interests of their present patients. Corporate executives believe they have an obligation to ignore consequences that extend beyond the financial interests of the present owners of the business. Under the sway of ideology, neither physicians nor corporate executives seem aware of the degree to which their roles are socially constituted.

Even if we adopt a more subtle method of characterizing the narrowness in the medical and business ideologies, we still risk oversimplifying matters. Neither medicine nor business is monolithic. Moving beyond acknowledging that essential diversity, we may be led to question whether there is a physician anywhere who truly subscribes to what Robert Veatch calls the "Hippocratic principle." Is there a physician anywhere who truly believes that her sole responsibility is to the immediate patient considered in isolation, without reference to the patient's family, to other patients or users of the health care system, or to other segments of society, and that the ultimate court of appeal on what will benefit the patient is her own conscience?

If there is, it is unlikely that she will be able to sustain this narrow focus in practice. A business person who conforms to Friedman's ideal of the scrupulous profit-maximizer is a rarity as well. Veatch and Friedman have been criticized for offering up caricatures. And yet, caricatures originate somewhere; they work on the principle of exaggeration rather than pure invention. Ideologies influence even where they do not determine behavior.

Ideology and the Managed Care Debate

The ideologies of medicine and business still shape much of the debate over managed care. Of the seven letters printed following an editorial on managed care in the *New England Journal of Medicine,* two emphasize the dedication to patient benefit that distinguishes physicians from all others and two rail against government interference. Those who cling to the Hippocratic tradition are especially eager to distinguish themselves from corporate interests.

One writer thinks it significant that "insurance company executives take no oath whatsoever, and their 'morality' is purely profit driven."[8] This is the preamble to an argument that physicians adhere to a higher moral standard, but this should not bar vigorous action on their part to secure "fair compensation" for their efforts. His colleague is more of a purist and states, "By agreeing to serve the interests of . . . anybody other than the patient, we are giving up the moral high ground—the singleness of motivation that has generated the trust of our patients and society. When we cooperate with managed-care companies and the managed-care agenda, we are reducing ourselves to the level of businesspeople. . . . It is ultimately individual physicians who must determine what is in the best interest of their patients."[9]

There is little doubt that Friedman's ideas continue to exercise considerable influence. In the first instance, they affect the way in which physicians portray business and business people. They also shape the worldview of some business people who have turned their attention to health care.

A Wall Street investment advisor involved in leveraged buyouts of hospitals and health care companies, commenting on the future of Catholic hospitals, states: "The Catholic mission I don't think is doable right now. Health care is becoming a business. . . . They're not really willing to make the tough choices today's well-managed hospitals have to make. When we acquire hospitals, we can tend to lay off upwards of 30 percent of the workforce and not affect direct patient care at all."[10] He adds that if Catholic hospitals were answerable to shareholders or investors, they would be forced to make the hard choices and would be run more efficiently.[11]

Even those who address current health care trends with a great deal of sophistication seldom question the basic tenets of the ideologies that shape their thinking in complex ways. In a famous exchange of letters, Arnold Relman, Editor-in-Chief Emeritus of the *New England Journal of Medicine*, and Professor Emeritus of Medicine and Social Medicine at Harvard Medical School, and Uwe Reinhardt, James Madison Professor of Political Economy at Princeton University, debate for-profit enterprise in health care and, more generally, the nature and future of health care providers at the dawn of the managed care era.[12]

For Relman, for-profit enterprise introduces a new and corrupting element into health care. For Reinhardt, the motivational structure of for-profit enterprise is not very different from that which has always governed physicians and hospitals. In an extensive discussion, we never get far beyond the issue of whether physicians are disinterested philanthropists or just like other "purveyors of goods and services" who, by and large, pursue their narrow self-interest.

In this face-off, Relman and Reinhardt veer away from considering how character and interests develop in relation to particular organizational and social contexts. They vigorously debate the personal virtue of physicians. The same is true of the commitment to service of not-for-profit hospitals. Attention is diverted away from the significance of the *fragility* of virtue and moral commitment.

We never learn how organizations might nurture vulnerable virtues and moral commitments, whether certain kinds of economic pressures are more likely than others to injure persons and relationships, or when the intelligent structuring of incentives crosses the line and begins to feed and breed a culture of manipulation. Subsequent analysis falls into a similar pattern. Albert Jonsen, among the most insightful practitioners in the field of medical ethics, has called the Relman-Reinhardt exchange "a tremendous debate" poising "economic logic against ethical conscience."[13] Of course, Relman is "ethical conscience," and Reinhardt is "economic logic."

The appeal of dichotomizing frameworks is obviously strong and unlikely to be overcome, especially when the categories offer a simple creed to cling to in a period of complex and unsettling change.[14] Still, one may search for an alternative framework, seeking to sidestep the either/or's that bring premature closure. Defenders of the ideologies of medicine and business wish to force a choice: Are you with us or against us? Are physicians and voluntary hospitals and health systems heroic benefactors of patients and communities, or are they generic purveyors of goods and services?

The social vision that might orient and guide moral reflection is never fully worked out. We are far from adequately accounting for the behavior of physicians, administrators, and consumer-patients. It seems impossible to separate the individual entirely from the social, and managed care renders the atomistic view even more suspect. For managed care is above all a phenomenon of organizations.

THE DEMEURERS CASE

In medical ethics, it is customary to use a case to lend concreteness to the discussion of significant moral issues. I will use the deMeurers case to lend concreteness to my discussion of managed care, and to show how the portrayal of managed care in the popular press incorporates the interpretive framework of the medicine-business dichotomy.

For a number of journalists, the story of Christine deMeurers captured the essence of managed care. The following narrative is based on accounts that have appeared in a widely read weekly magazine, a daily newspaper, and a journalist's book on managed care. The narrative both reflects and reflects upon the characteristic concerns and limitations of the journalistic perspective.[15] That perspective is important because it shapes the public perception of managed care.[16]

From Healthy Enrollee to Desperate Patient

Christine deMeurers and her family belonged to a network model HMO called Health Net. The Health Net plan was the least expensive of the three options offered by deMeurers's employer. Family members appeared to be in good health at enrollment time, and neither deMeurers nor her husband, Alan, paid much attention to the details of the contract they received after they enrolled in the plan. In late August 1992, less than two months after she enrolled in Health Net, deMeurers was diagnosed with breast cancer. Her primary care physician referred her to an oncologist, Mahesh Gupta. She underwent a radical mastectomy, radiation therapy and chemotherapy. Nevertheless, the cancer spread, and she was later classified as having Stage IV metastatic breast cancer.[17]

Given the limits of standard therapies, Gupta referred deMeurers to a specialist for a consultation concerning high dose chemotherapy coupled with a bone marrow transplant.[18] On her sister's recommendation, deMeurers also sought a consultation on her own with another transplant specialist, Roy Jones at the University of Colorado. Following the consultation with Jones, deMeurers decided to pursue a transplant. Although there was no solid scientific evidence establishing that transplants for patients with metastatic breast cancer prolong life or improve the quality of life, many specialists considered transplants to be standard of care, and approximately three out of four insurers were willing to pay for them.[19]

Health Net denied coverage on the grounds that a transplant in deMeurers's case would be experimental and hence excluded under its contract. Many managed care plans cover "medically necessary" services, but not "experimental" treatments and procedures. What is experimental can rarely be specified in detail, given the rapidity with which change occurs in medicine and the lack of consensus among physicians in many areas. Contracts tend to be ambiguous and open to conflicting interpretations. The Health Net contract was especially ambiguous on the subject of bone marrow transplants.[20]

Relationships Begin to Fray

According to the published reports, Gupta agreed to make a referral for a second local evaluation, but later told deMeurers that he was not authorized by Health Net to do so. DeMeurers petitioned for a new oncologist. Her new oncologist, Stanley Schinke, suggested that deMeurers go to the University of California-Los Angeles (UCLA) Medical Center for an evaluation. Thereafter, Sam Ho, Health Net's medical director, allegedly called Schinke to tell him that a transplant was not indicated in a case like deMeurers's.

In the meantime, deMeurers, again acting on her own, sought out John Glaspy, a transplant specialist at UCLA. In press accounts, Glaspy recalls telling deMeurers that transplant was an option, but that he could not wholeheartedly recommend it in her case. The deMeurerses thought they heard encouragement. Alan deMeurers told a reporter, "I remember him saying, 'This is the best course of treatment.'"[21] Although there are a number of possible explanations for the discrepancy, including unreliable reporting or memory, it is equally likely that transplant specialists and others who perform risky procedures are schooled to believe in the value of what they do and communicate that belief to patients and their families,[22] while patients and families grasp hold of what is most hopeful in the presentation of options.

Initially, the deMeurerses did not tell Glaspy or anyone at UCLA of their ties to Health Net. The deMeurerses feared that the UCLA physicians would attempt to dissuade them from proceeding with the transplant, if they knew that the deMeurerses were Health Net members. As it turns out, UCLA had entered into an exclusive multi-million dollar contract with Health Net to provide (Health Net-approved) bone marrow transplants to Health Net members in Southern California. Further, Glaspy had served on the Health Net advisory committee that decided to deny coverage for transplants for patients with deMeurers's type and level of disease, although Glaspy himself had voted in favor of coverage.

As an advisory committee member, Glaspy had pledged to serve as an expert witness on Health Net's behalf in any litigation over the twenty-page policy guide that resulted from the panel's deliberations (the "grid"). At one of the advisory committee meetings, Ho, the Health Net administrator, reportedly justified Health Net's approach to coverage determinations along these lines: "This is not a Utopian society that everybody can be everything to all people and paid for by somebody else. We have fiduciary responsibilities to . . . employers to the tune of about $1.5 billion worth of premiums paid to us every year to manage their health care premium dollars responsibly."[23]

Christine deMeurers appealed the Health Net decision to deny coverage, and was again denied. The deMeurerses personally agreed to pay UCLA $92,000 for a transplant. Their lawyer, Mark Hiepler, prepared to sue Health Net. A *Time* magazine cover story reviewed the fund-raising efforts of relatives and friends in poignant detail. The deMeurerses' eight year-old daughter contributed a sign for a yard sale that said, "MONEY GOES TO A MOTHER WITH CANCER." The $17,000 raised by the yard sale and other events covered the harvesting of deMeurers's bone marrow, the first stage of the transplant process.

According to the *Los Angeles Times*, Glaspy is convinced that deMeurers withheld the name of her HMO from him on her lawyer's instructions. Glaspy eventually learned that deMeurers was a Health Net plan member, and he agreed to sign a declaration in support of her suit against Health Net. Later, at the request of Health Net's lawyers, he signed a declaration in opposition to the suit. The *Los Angeles Times* reports that Glaspy *now* believes he should have located another doctor for deMeurers when he first learned of her relationship to Health Net. At the time, he was concerned that ending their relationship might hinder her treatment.

Intramural Conflicts

Sometime between Glaspy's two declarations in the deMeurers-Health Net litigation, Clifford Ossorio, Health Net's associate medical director, called Glaspy's superior, Dennis Slamon, chief of UCLA's division of hematology/oncology. According to the *Los Angeles Times*, Slamon remembers pointed questions from Ossorio about "why Glaspy was recommending a transplant for a Stage IV patient, despite UCLA's commitment to supporting the grid."[24] Ossorio has contended that he was merely smoothing ruffled feathers at UCLA.

In any event, the call reportedly led to a dispute between Slamon and Glaspy over whether harvesting deMeurers's bone marrow obligated UCLA to pay for the transplant. Slamon considered the harvest a pledge by UCLA to complete the treatment. Glaspy disagreed. He was familiar with cases in which a harvest had been undertaken pending resolution of other issues, and he felt that Slamon did not understand the situation. Moreover, the cost of deMeurers's treatment would come out of his unit's budget.

Slamon prevailed. On September 23, 1993, deMeurers entered UCLA for a bone marrow transplant at UCLA's expense. Since HMOs notoriously do not want their members to receive services they do not offer (it draws attention to their coverage limitations, and it suggests that the services provided are "medically necessary" rather than "experimental"), this alone might have been sufficient to strain UCLA's relationship with Health Net. Further, although the deMeurerses were at first "elated" by the news that UCLA would pay for the transplant, they had grown suspicious. Alan deMeurers told the *Los Angeles Times* that with UCLA paying, "We were worried we'd get compromised care.

How would we know if she was getting the best? There was no standard we could hold them up to."[25]

The End of the Story

Christine deMeurers died on March 10, 1995. After the bone marrow transplant, she enjoyed four apparently disease-free months, falling ill again by the spring of 1994. Before she died, the family took a trip across the country to build memories for the children, and spent an additional Christmas together. Alan deMeurers believes the quality of that family time made all they went through to get the transplant worthwhile. Ho believes that the outcome proves that Health Net was right. In October 1995, an arbitration panel determined that Health Net should have paid for the transplant. It also found that the HMO interfered with the doctor-patient relationship by telephoning Christine deMeurers's doctors. The panel awarded one million dollars and legal costs to Alan deMeurers.

Soon after the decision in the deMeurers case, Health Net changed its policy on bone marrow transplants. If a case falls outside the grid, it is forwarded to an outside agency in Virginia. The agency then forwards the case to three independent experts. If even one independent expert believes that a transplant is warranted, Health Net pays for it. The reporter for the *Los Angeles Times* speculated that Christine deMeurers might consider this a victory. He quoted Alan deMeurers: "After Christy got her transplant from UCLA, the question from Health Net was why were we pursuing the case against them . . . She always replied it was to make it easier for the next person."[26]

In September of 1994, the Federal Employee Health Benefits Program mandated that all its health plans cover bone marrow transplants for advanced breast cancer. A number of states passed laws requiring insurers to cover bone marrow transplants for breast cancer.

The Rest of the Story

The central organizational actor in this tale, Health Net, is a very large corporation. In 1995, as these events transpired, the company, the second largest HMO in California, received two billion dollars in premium payments for 1.2 million "covered lives." Health Net is the kind of HMO that many Americans may be offered as a low-cost option. Health Net is not a "fly-by-night" operator. It converted to for-profit status during the period of deMeurers's struggle with cancer, but it traces its roots to Blue Cross of Southern California. Further, in December 1995, around the time of deMeurers's death, Health Net received a one year accreditation from the National Committee for Quality Assurance (NCQA).[27]

Many media accounts juxtapose stories of personal tragedy with stories of the financial machinations of managed care organizations and their executives.

This is certainly true of accounts of the deMeurers case. At the time of its conversion to for-profit status, Health Net was acquired by a smaller competitor, QualMed. Health Net's chief executive officer, Roger Greaves, and the chief executive officer of QualMed, Malik Hasan, both became executives of the holding company created in the merger, Health Systems International (HSI).

In 1994, Greaves and Hasan ranked third and fourth, respectively, in terms of cash compensation for chief executives in the "HMO industry." Greaves received $8.9 million, while Hasan received $8.8 million.[28] Uwe Reinhardt has suggested that these kinds of figures should not cause general concern. He argues that the cash filling the coffers of managed care organizations, and lining the pockets of managed care executives, comes from the socially beneficial activity of "putting the squeeze" on providers and drug companies.[29]

Peter Boland, a managed care consultant, is less sanguine about the social benefits of the transfer of funds from health care providers to managed care organizations. Boland looks at how HMOs are using money, aside from rewarding executives. He asserts that the dominant strategy in the industry is to buy market share, "to grow as quickly as possible through external acquisition, rather than pumping money back into the company to achieve higher levels of patient satisfaction and performance."[30]

In 1995, HSI announced plans to merge with WellPoint Health Networks to create the nation's second-largest for-profit managed care company. WellPoint, a subsidiary of Blue Cross of California, planned to acquire HSI for stock worth $1.89 billion. The deal would have increased the value of Greaves's stockholdings from $300,000 to $31.8 million. Hasan would have held shares worth $175.9 million as a result of the deal. Unfortunately for Greaves, Hasan, and the other stockholders, the merger with WellPoint collapsed in December of 1995.[31] The failed transaction cost HSI $20.2 million. To preserve its profit margin, the company reduced payments to providers and froze salaries across the board, "even for senior managers."[32]

Another HSI transaction in 1995, while less rich, may have been nearly as significant. The Connecticut State Medical Society's M.D. Health Plan was considered one of the success stories in physician attempts to mount a professional challenge to aggressive, multi-state managed care organizations. Society members raised $7 million to start the plan and marketed it with the slogan: "WE DON'T WANT ANYTHING TO COME BETWEEN YOU AND YOUR PHYSICIAN."

The plan negotiated a discounted fee schedule with participating physicians, rather than relying on a gatekeeping system to reduce costs. The plan became Connecticut's second-largest HMO. It also showed the lowest profits and the smallest percentage of premiums going toward administrative expenses. The plan eventually attracted the attention of HSI, which purchased it for $101 million. The plan's 1,500 physician shareholders received a $56,000 return on a $3,000 investment. Although the plan's leaders said they needed access to HSI's capital to remain competitive, "[s]ome observers see the deal as evidence that doctors are as likely as anyone else to take the money and run when the opportunity arises."[33]

Economists and financial consultants disagree on the desirability of such corporate behavior purely in terms of economic impact. From a broader social perspective, it seems relevant that Health Net spent little or no money on medical research, and defended the practice by citing fears of engaging in unlawful discrimination by favoring one disease over another, as well as the exigencies of competition. On the other hand, Health Net could point to the California Wellness Foundation, and its $300 million endowment, as its continuing contribution to the social good. When the company converted to for-profit status, it established the foundation to meet the requirements of California law. Critics believe that the sale price was too low, and hence the amount contributed to the foundation was less than it should have been.[34] Be that as it may, the Foundation has launched a number of worthy projects, including a five-year, $24 million "Violence Prevention Initiative."[35]

Malik Hasan, formerly a practicing neurologist, became for a time the public spokesman for for-profit managed care organizations. In an opinion piece in the *New England Journal of Medicine* entitled "Let's End the Nonprofit Charade," he concluded:

> The energy and entrepreneurial spirit that have made America a leader in all aspects of the world economy are doing the same in health care. Investor-owned plans are spearheading this change in the health care system with improved access, a strong emphasis on preventive care, affordability, and demonstrable quality.
>
> The conversion of the remaining nonprofit plans into investor-owned plans will provide funds that can be used for activities outside the scope of the market [e.g., separate not-for-profit institutions established solely as sites for indigent care, medical education, and testing of experimental procedures]. The time has come to enact these changes and allow the marketplace to continue its comprehensive reform of the American health care system—a reform that benefits every American.[36]

Sam Ho, now vice president and corporate medical director of PacifiCare Health Systems, continues to meld concerns about stewardship of resources and distributive justice with a belief in the power of the marketplace and a commitment to many tenets of the business ideology.[37]

TESTING THE IDEOLOGIES OF MEDICINE AND BUSINESS

The ideology of medicine prepares us to see struggles between virtuous physicians and venal executives, with the patient as helpless victim in this battle of titans. The ideology of business prepares us to see virtue in the venality of executives. The patient is (or ought to be) a knowledgeable consumer who regards her needs and wants in relation to health care in the same light as her needs and wants in relation to transportation. No longer a victim, she is, according to the model, the true sovereign. Organizations fit awkwardly within either view. What does a critical assessment of the behavior of the principal actors in the story of Christine deMeurers reveal concerning these two sets of assumptions?

Physicians and Philanthropy

There is some evidence that some physicians failed to display the imperviousness to social pressures required of them by the ideology of medicine. They are not quite the unblemished heroes, even in the media accounts. Hasan and Greaves tend to be portrayed as the villains, profiting from human suffering. However, we can scarcely attribute their venality to the world of "business" in any straightforward fashion. Hasan is a physician, and Greaves spent his early career running a not-for-profit organization. Further, they are not alone in their desire for material gain. Consider the physician-stockholders of the M.D. Health Plan. Is avarice any less avaricious on a smaller scale? The plan's leaders cited increasing capital needs as a reason for selling the enterprise. Is this credible, or are they simply less honest than Greaves and Hasan?

As for the managers, they seem caught in the middle. They stand between patients such as deMeurers and the treatments those patients, advised by specialists, desperately want. They are trapped in the tension between the ideologies of medicine and business. It is unclear whether they are, or ought to be, servants of individual patients, of corporate profits, or something else.

Patients: Victims or Sovereigns?

What of "the patient"? Or rather, what of the patient and her husband and her lawyer? Is deMeurers a victim, reduced by need to abject dependency on her personal physician? She herself is clearly an agent, making the picture of total dependency inadequate. Is she then an independent consumer seeking to satisfy her preferences? This account also fails. All of the people with whom deMeurers interacts help shape her expectations and choices. It is impossible to label her victim or sovereign. She experienced what she and her husband perceived as a betrayal by some of her physicians and by Health Net. But Glaspy also perceives her and her husband as betrayers.

Once deMeurers is recognized as an agent, her character and her choices are subject to ethical scrutiny. Is she selfish or altruistic? Her husband claims she continued her suit against Health Net past the point where it made any difference to her own treatment "to make it easier for the next person." Since litigation is emotionally and physically draining, there was real sacrifice involved. On the other hand, the verdict and the change in Health Net policy that her case helped bring about only make things easier for the next patient with Stage IV metastatic breast cancer or similarly advanced disease who wants a bone marrow transplant of questionable benefit. The policy change may actually make things worse for other patients affected by the redirection of funds to expensive, borderline treatments.

The Intrusiveness of Organizations

Finally, in this story, it seems clear that problems of organization, problems of hierarchy and coordination, affect for-profit managed care organizations *and* academic medical centers, strongholds of "business" and "medicine." This is only to say, once again, that matters are complex and there is a good deal of ambiguity.

Virtue and venality are not distributed as neatly as the medicine-business dichotomy would suggest. Physicians, managers, and patients have complicated motivational structures. It is no simple matter to press oneself into the mold of philanthropist or *homo economicus*. The philanthropist finds it difficult to conform to a code that demands a character impervious to economic considerations and organizational pressures. *Homo economicus* feels compelled to justify his conduct in moral terms.

Behavior exhibits enough diversity to cast doubt on the assumptions behind the medicine-business dichotomy. Further, this diversity suggests something of the range and complexity of the influences to be addressed. Even talk of "pressures" and "influences" may mislead by suggesting too great an exteriority. The organizations we participate in clearly affect our understanding of our own interests and those of others.

PERPLEXITIES AFFECTING OTHER MODES OF ANALYSIS

Not all moral evaluations of managed care are framed in terms of the medicine-business dichotomy. There is another common approach that ignores the polemic, the call to take sides. Instead, a category (or series of categories) guides the selection of material for discussion and provides the standards for evaluation. Proceeding in this mode, the managed care analyst may organize her discussion in terms of choice, conflict of interest, allocation of resources, or another relevant category. The "standard categories" approach may remedy the deficiencies of the medicine-business dichotomy as a framework for analysis. The story of Christine deMeurers can again serve as a test.

"Choice" as Organizing Category

We generally assume that once we identify or elicit patient or consumer choices, little remains to be done. I do not mean to minimize the importance of individual choice. I only wish to caution against mistaking simplifying assumptions, defensible in some contexts, for reality. In some circumstances, it is better to accept choices than to probe them. The competent man who has consistently insisted that he does not wish to be put on a ventilator ought not to be put on one. But many of those who subscribe to an ethical principle of respect for autonomy or self-determination fall into the habit of thinking and talking about the interests, desires, and preferences expressed in choices as if these were fixed and inherent in the individual, rather than being open to influence and development. In some circumstances, we need to probe choices rather than accept them.

CHOICE AND VOLUNTARINESS

Simplifying assumptions are attractive because they yield straightforward judgments. Take choosing a health plan. In the standard analysis focused on the patient or consumer in isolation, the first and perhaps the last question would be whether deMeurers's choice of the Health Net plan was free and informed. The choice *seems* voluntary. After all, no one held a gun to deMeurers's head. Further, deMeurers's employer offered alternative plans, and the family's circumstances were apparently comfortable enough that choice of a higher cost plan would not have been a simple financial impossibility. True, deMeurers's role is rather passive and contained, but that is not out of line with common understanding and practice.[38]

Mainstream medical ethics has been very concerned with decision-making authority, but largely indifferent to more subtle power issues. Only a more controversial interpretation of "voluntary," linked to an argument for some special incapacity in connection with health care decision making, *or* a break with the focus on the individual in isolation, would support belaboring this aspect of the question.

INFORMATION AND THE QUALITY OF CHOICE

On the other hand, one can make a strong argument that the information deMeurers received about Health Net was inadequate to allow her to make an informed choice. (Whether the availability of more adequate information would have affected her decision is a different and separate question.) The deMeurerses did not receive the Health Net contract until *after* they had enrolled in the plan. Further, there is no evidence they received comparative information on the quality of the various plans among which they could choose. The source of this problem with choice is typically identified as industry reluctance to disclose information, and a lack of standardization that impairs comparative judgments when the information is made available. The standard solution is for the government (or a private organization such as the managed care industry's own NCQA) to develop a "report card" for managed care plans that will include information on coverage and quality.

But what if such a report card is too complicated for the ordinary consumer? Can an incorrigibly uninformed choice ever be a truly voluntary choice? One might conjecture that deMeurers's fear of the difficult subject matter explained her failure to demand copies of plan contracts and information on quality prior to enrolling.

I am highlighting the problem of the extreme complexity of advanced technological medicine. Although we generally allude to complexity to establish the inescapable asymmetry between physician and patient, we can extend the point to the asymmetry between plan and member in light of the baroque arrangements for health care delivery characteristic of our fragmented system.

THE QUALITY OF INFORMATION
There are further perplexities along these lines. For example, how does one evaluate quality? Are aggregations of measures of performance for individual physicians within a network sufficient? If differences in quality tend to average out across groups, this approach may offer little basis for comparative judgments. What is "quality," and how does one measure it? Is quality related to technical competence, suggesting criteria such as board certification, or data on morbidity and mortality, or is it broader and more amorphous? Patient satisfaction measures may provide the best indicators of quality of relationship. But how informed are patient opinions? Can patients assess relational goods such as trust if they are in the dark concerning the financial incentives and other pressures that may influence the judgment of their physicians?

Perhaps the focus of quality assessment should be the plan itself. One could generate numbers that provide insight into its policies-in-practice, such as average length of hospitalization. But is a short stay in the hospital bad, or good? Is it good to return patients as quickly as possible to their families, or is that patient dumping? What about data on administrative expenses as a percentage of total expenditures, or executive compensation? Is high compensation bad, or good? Is a multi-million dollar salary evidence of greed achieving and exploiting monopoly power, or is a robust compensation package a well-deserved reward for efficiency and innovation? And how do these various aspects of a plan fit together? Inevitably, difficult judgments are demanded.

EXISTENTIAL CONSTRAINTS ON CHOICE
Having reviewed some of the difficulties that attend an attempt to respond to the problem of limited knowledge among patients or consumers, it is well to note an even stronger and more controversial statement of the problem. Simply put, not only are consumers incapable of judging health care plans on relatively objective terms, e.g., arriving at an adequate understanding of the terms of contracts and making comparative judgments about plans based on assessments of quality, but they are also incapable of judging their own preferences in relation to health care prior to the occurrence of an event that puts them at the mercy of a plan.[39]

The deMeurerses did not attempt to understand the terms of the Health Net contract, until Christine deMeurers was diagnosed with breast cancer. Some would argue that health care is a special good not only in its complexity, but also in its "existential" significance. Many of us would prefer not to reflect on the possibility of becoming seriously ill; thus we may tend to undervalue health care relative to other goods, until we encounter serious illness. On the other hand, we, or our physicians, may expend large amounts of our own or society's resources on health care that offers little or no prospect of benefit, while neglecting education and other important contributors to individual and social well-being.

Yet what to do? If I choose to ignore my mortality, is that not a personal choice? If I cannot seem to forego the purchase of a new television, or five packs of cigarettes a day, even if it means that I am left with insufficient funds to purchase good health insurance, perhaps that is simply a reflection (and revelation) of my personal ordering of preferences. If neither I nor my physicians have a sense of the proper limits of medicine, or a context or forum in which to weigh the claims of health care—or particular types of health care—against other goods, perhaps these are but consequences, regrettable but unavoidable, of our nature as isolated beings and the subjectivity and relativity of all things moral.

But are mortality, the losses that are a part of processes of aging and illness, and anxieties about the future purely private troubles? Are consumption patterns impervious to social influence? Perhaps matters are not so black and white. It may be that some of our problems, and the means of addressing them, are social as well as individual. It may be that in the health care context, we can assist one another with gifts of understanding as well as material resources. One of our most pressing tasks may be the location or creation of settings for mutual aid.

Conflict of Interest

Similar problems arise with the other standard categories of analysis. The conflict of interest concept is a blunt instrument. Where a physician has a direct financial incentive to overtreat or undertreat patients, conflict of interest analysis helps us to see this and to understand that the arrangement is flawed. But the model has limited scope; we cannot apply it indiscriminately without confusion, or harm to relationships, or both.

Consider the transplant specialist's need to believe in her procedure, or the general discomfort with delivering bad news and the general resistance to hearing it. Certainly these are factors to be considered, but are they best understood as interests in conflict with other interests? Things are even more complicated if some interests arise intersubjectively or in relationship and may not be strictly assignable to one person. Such interests would have to be artificially sundered and reconstructed so that they could "conflict" according to the terms of the concept.

Analysis on these terms effectively dissolves the relationship. Normally, patients and physicians do not watch one another with a suspicious eye. It is a sign of something gone wrong when the relationship must be dissected and every aspect picked over for interests and oppositions.

Resource Allocation

Resource allocation fits under the general heading of distributive justice. The knottiest resource allocation problems are related to rationing, defined as withholding potentially beneficial care.[40] It should be clear by now that there is nothing simple about this activity. We need to decide which considerations to admit, which to exclude and how to weigh the various considerations admitted. We need to decide who should decide. Is this a matter for the patient to resolve in the privacy of her own conscience, based on her conception of the right and the good, or according to whatever preferences she happens to have? The physician? A panel of physicians? A panel of physicians and patients and medical ethicists? How firm should the rationing policies be? Will exceptions be made for "squeaky wheels" and particularly affecting cases? The questions, it seems, are endless.

Identifying the Gaps

A careful analysis would provide a much more exhaustive treatment of each of the categories selected for consideration, attempt to tie up the loose ends and render a general verdict. But proceeding in this way simply fails to capture much of what is striking in the deMeurers story: the spread of fear and suspicion through the networks of relationships; the problem of how we give meaning to our experience and especially our suffering; the active-passive character of the involvement of all of the actors, against, for example, the view of the patient as either victim or sovereign chooser; the disconnection between the wheeling and dealing of the top corporate executives and the distress of the patient and her family; and, finally, the "characters" of the institutional actors. In the category-by-category analysis of choice, conflicts of interest, and rationing principles, the large organizations that figure so prominently in the story— Health Net and the UCLA Medical Center—recede into the background.

We cannot make sense of the interactions among organizations and individuals that constitute the narrative by analyzing it with the standard tools. The concepts do not quite fit, or they create a *fragmentary* analysis, when what we seem to require is a moral vision that can encompass the larger wholes.

Reconstructing the Roles

In order to summarize and reflect on some of the issues raised thus far, I believe it will be helpful to focus on roles, and more particularly the roles of manager, clinician, and patient.

THE ROLE OF THE MANAGER

In the stories of personal tragedy that largely define managed care for the press and the public, the role of executive, administrator or manager emerges as particularly problematic. Reports of greed and insensitivity arouse our indignation. It is important to ask if these traits exhaust the possibilities of the role.

Managers might be responsible for putting in place systems to help clinicians and to contribute to the control of cost and performance in the interests of fairness. They might be charged with assuring that standards of quality are consistently met, yet take professionalism and human relationships seriously. They cannot let themselves be dominated by force of desire in particular cases without risk of unfairness. But being totally invulnerable to the plight of those affected by policies and decisions is not the only other option. They might open up the process of setting standards and communicate with, rather than dictate to, providers and plan members. They might provide leadership and vision, exercising power responsibly and with a degree of humility.

Some skepticism concerning technique, and what good management can do, seems warranted. Good management cannot eliminate organizational problems or personal tragedy. Good managers can, however, respond intelligently to problems and do their best to anticipate and prevent them. They can do their very best to ensure that the manner in which they perform their role serves to lessen, rather than intensify, suffering. The story of Christine deMeurers is more illustrative of the dangers than the contributions of the managerial role, and this is true despite the fact that the managers we encounter are physicians, and hence cannot be dismissed as mere "clerks" or "accountants."

THE ROLE OF THE CLINICIAN

The response of the physicians (and other clinicians) to managers and to the new order in medicine is a separate but related issue. There is a sense that the appropriate response will include "seeing both sides." Clinicians must acknowledge the weight of concerns about justice and the legitimacy of administrative demands for consistency and accountability. They must also display the virtue of faithfulness in their relationships with patients. They must insist that their own patients have special claims on them and legitimately demand responsiveness to their particular needs and desires.

Yet one cannot simply veer erratically between the two poles of moral obligation. The solution to this problem will be bound up with making moral sense of the managerial role. The ability of clinicians to honor appropriately the first set of concerns is linked to the ability of managers to honor the second. Open and honest communication will be essential to the process of creating the conditions for mutual respect.

THE ROLE OF THE PATIENT

The patient is the third member of the triad. We can ask how justice might become a concern of plan member-patients as well as managers and physicians. Ideally, this "consciousness-raising" would occur before persons are most truly patients, in the midst of a health crisis. Ideally, it would occur through involving members in policy making for the health plan and through reforming the health care system to enable patients to participate more fully in their own care.

We are all aware of the scarcity of resources. But because we are not involved in determining how scarce resources are allocated, restrictions that affect us personally are likely to seem arbitrary and unfair. We know that we are, in some sense, responsible for our own health, but we tend to consider health care as something to be done *to us or for us.* Involving plan members in policy making and nurturing their sense of responsibility and self-efficacy in relation to health is not simple. We need to find a way to talk about participation that marks its importance without straining credulity. Michael Shadid's cooperative and the dream of health care as a truly collaborative enterprise seem to have little to do with contemporary managed care practice, yet these ideals remind us of what we may strive *for* in a world of changing health care organization and medical practice.

The prospects for participation are linked to some large existential questions. Sooner or later, we must come to terms with the tensions in our relationships to others, and our vulnerability to various kinds of loss, physical and mental illness, aging, and death. Are these basic forms of insecurity individual or social problems? If others have something to say about the kind of health care I receive, am I being used as a mere means to their ends? If I draw on the resources of others, am I using them as mere means to my ends? In short, we need a way of understanding our corporate projects in this and other areas.

Allow, for the moment, that social influences are important and that members of a society have responsibilities to one another. The range of possible answers is still very broad. We need a social ethic, but a social ethic can take many forms, and draw on a number of social values.

TOWARD A MORE SOCIAL ETHIC: ALASDAIR MACINTYRE AND "STEREOSCOPIC" SOCIAL CRITICISM

In order to understand managed care, we need to get beyond the medicine-business dichotomy and the ideologies of medicine and business. Both ideologies are myopic. Both neglect the organizational and social dimensions of existence. But if we are not to proceed under the banner of "the Hippocratic tradition" or "the business creed," i.e., traditional medical ethics or traditional business ethics, we must find another source of guidance.

Merely looking at this or that fragment, choice, or conflict of interest, or rationing principles, will not enable us to grasp the interconnections among phenomena. We may need a more systematic approach. But, what kind of system? When one surveys the landscape of contemporary medical ethics, or contemporary ethics for that matter, the tools for such an analysis appear few and far between. If a theorist ventures beyond the physician-patient dyad,[41] she is likely to go directly to questions of national scale, neglecting the space in between.

One of the interesting exceptions is the philosopher Alasdair MacIntyre. MacIntyre gained wide recognition in philosophical circles with the publication of *After Virtue*, an indictment of much in contemporary culture and ethical discourse. MacIntyre gives voice to ideas both radical and traditional, liberal and illiberal. [42] His own sources are diverse, ranging from Aristotle to Aquinas, and from the leading thinkers of the Scottish Enlightenment to Max Weber. It is MacIntyre's sociological awareness that most recommends him here.

To begin with, MacIntyre offers an analysis of "the manager" as one of the emblematic social types of late modernity. According to MacIntyre, the manager in our culture enacts the philosophy of emotivism. The central idea of emotivism is that our views on moral issues are simply expressions of our personal preferences. Any justifications offered for managerial activity are merely ex post facto window-dressing. Hence, emotivism represents the obliteration of the distinction between manipulative and non-manipulative social relations.

MacIntyre believes we are losing our sense of what it means to treat someone as an end rather than a means: "To treat someone else as an end is to offer them what I take to be good reasons for acting in one way rather than another, but to leave it to them to evaluate those reasons. . . . By contrast, to treat someone else as a means is to seek to make him or her an instrument of my purposes by adducing whatever influences or considerations will in fact be effective on this or that occasion."[43] We think that if we manage (or incentivize) properly, we can eliminate the need for trust and moral suasion.

MacIntyre argues that managerial effectiveness is part of a *masquerade* of social control. For, it turns out, we are oppressed by impotence rather than true mastery of the circumstances of human existence. Too much escapes our grasp, and the impossible demand for ever greater mastery gives rise to simulation and dissimulation, creating space for arbitrariness and the operation of fear and greed.

From MacInytre's viewpoint, apart from some grounding in a common moral tradition or view of the good, we inevitably find ourselves caught in this vicious cycle. While many will dispute MacIntyre's prescription, retreat to small enclaves for the creation of a counter-culture, his diagnosis seems accurate. Much managed care writing, and managed care practice, reflects a purely instrumental view of persons, combined with a kind of magical thinking about the power of management.

In addition to a cultural critique, MacIntyre offers a general account of social relations. His "partial account of a core conception of the virtues" is an approach to understanding morality informed by sociology. The account consists of a number of interlocking concepts: practice, internal and external goods, virtue, institution, and tradition.

The concept of practice is near the core of the core conception. MacIntyre defines a practice as "any coherent and complex form of socially established cooperative human activity through which goods internal to that form of activity are realized in the course of trying to achieve those standards of excellence which are appropriate to, and partially definitive of, that form of activity, with the result that human powers to achieve excellence, and human conceptions of the ends and goods involved, are systematically extended."[44] MacIntyre's concept of virtue assumes a social world structured by practices. He considers a virtue to be an acquired quality, the possession and exercise of which enables us to achieve the goods internal to practices.

Although virtues may vary with practices, any practice will require the virtues of justice, courage and honesty. One must be able to recognize what is due to whom, take self-endangering risks, and receive and respond to criticism with careful attention to the facts. Without all three of these virtues in some form, we can neither forge moral relationships nor realize internal goods.

A collective activity oriented only to achieving external goods is not a practice. External goods are things such as money, fame or social status, and certain forms of power that bear no necessary connection to any particular practice. Such goods typically have a "zero sum" structure and create definite winners and losers. For all that, external goods are genuine goods: "Not only are they characteristic objects of human desire, whose allocation is what gives point to the virtues of justice and generosity, but no one can despise them altogether without a certain hypocrisy." Yet achieving external goods will often compete with achieving internal goods—"notoriously the cultivation of truthfulness, justice and courage will often, the world being what it contingently is, bar us from being rich or famous or powerful."[45]

Institutions reproduce the competing allegiances of individuals in relation to internal and external goods at another level. MacIntyre says of institutions that they are "characteristically and necessarily" concerned with external goods. Institutions "are involved in acquiring money and other material goods; they are structured in terms of power and status, and they distribute money, power and status as rewards." This is not a perversion, a fall from some purer state of institutional being, but rather part of what it means to say that external goods are genuine goods. Institutions cannot be otherwise than concerned with external goods "if they are to sustain not only themselves, but also the practices of which they are the bearers."[46]

Of course, practices must also "sustain" or give meaning and moral weight to institutions. The virtues of justice, courage, and truthfulness anchor resistance to the corrupting power of institutions; that is, they anchor resistance to the corrupting power of external goods within institutions, and to the power of corrupt institutions within the social order. But we need to say more:

[I]f institutions do have corrupting power, the making and sustaining of forms of human community—and therefore of institutions—itself has all the characteristics of a practice, and moreover of a practice which stands in a peculiarly close relationship to the exercise of the virtues in two important ways. The exercise of the virtues is itself apt to require a highly determinate attitude to social and political issues; and it is always within some particular community with its own specific institutional forms that we learn or fail to learn to exercise the virtues.[47]

An adequate "moral sociology" will take account of the operation of virtues and vices in determinate social and institutional contexts. An adequate moral theory will note that virtues are fostered by certain social institutions and endangered by others. Such a theory will therefore place the classification of social institutions and the problems of organizations on its agenda.

Practical Reflections: Three Problems of Corporate Life

In a piece on business ethics, MacIntyre suggests that three problems of contemporary corporate life threaten virtue. The first problem has to do with organizational time scale, that is, the frequently lamented "short-term" orientation of United States business. The limits of our powers of prediction, and our reliance on predictions in planning, tend to narrow our focus. Our vision is also constricted by our habit of living in perpetual crisis, giving rise to the conviction that we simply lack the time to take the longer, wider view. Second, MacIntyre focuses on the way organizations may fragment the self. Individuals easily become partitioned into a series of roles. Third is the problem of opacity. MacIntyre writes that when those who interact within or through organizations lose a sense of the whole, "a great deal that individuals do and effect in corporations becomes invisible to them and to others."[48]

Each of these problems is structural, and its intensity will vary across forms of organization. An adequate response must draw on a variety of resources. Precisely because remedies for all three problems require changes in organizational and broader cultural forms, MacIntyre believes that legislation at the federal or state levels or action by business or professional associations is unlikely to have much of an effect. Purely formal measures, such as the adoption of codes of ethics, will also fail to contribute significantly to solutions, although codes may serve other purposes.

Stereoscopic Social Criticism

Jeffrey Stout believes we can use MacIntyre's concepts to construct a kind of social criticism that integrates the various levels of social life, what Stout calls "stereoscopic" social criticism. Stout contrasts stereoscopic social criticism with two common forms of analysis, reductionist sociology and a species of cultural anthropology. He writes:

We know how to describe a clinic or an academic profession in the idiom of reductionist sociology, but somehow we make everything look like a system of external goods in which people are moved only by the desire for status, money, and power.

The standard way of compensating for this deficiency is to concentrate attention narrowly on pursuing internal goods and trying to get descriptions that are "thicker," "warmer," or "less dry" than the other approach can provide. This is done by showing "empathy" for participants in the practice, aiming to "understand" their *mentalité* or "social world," rather than trying to "explain" what they are doing as a "function" or "reflection" of institutional structure.

Each approach has affinities with certain areas of human endeavor. A reductionist sociology fits best with the marketplace and the bureaucracy—areas "where people are for the most part pursuing external goods or merely procedural justice and are not surprised to be told so."[49] We should not be shocked that there is gambling in the casino. At the same time, all institutions pursue external goods and employ certain procedures that aim at fairness.

Further, most institutions of any durability, for-profit firms and government agencies included, involve internal goods and relationships that are not strictly rule-defined. If we have experienced such institutions, we may be dissatisfied with sociological accounts that dismiss these aspects of institutional life too readily.

The anthropological approach may commend itself as a way of remedying these deficiencies, but it also conceals certain things. As the mirror image of reductionist sociology, it simplifies matters by ignoring external goods and other sources of conflict. "It takes a more generous view of human motivation and thus grants to others the kind of charity we normally show to ourselves. It allows us to stave off a merely cynical view of people and thus to affirm our own interpretive practices. Too often, however, it seems simply to be wishing away the realities of power and the power of self-deception."[50]

Stout believes that concepts such as practice and institution, and internal and external goods, are necessary to make sense of the whole. These concepts also structure the interests and research agenda of the stereoscopic social critic. Items worthy of exploration include the following: "the tendency of the capitalist marketplace and large-scale bureaucracies to provide the material conditions that permit social practices to flourish, while at the same time they undermine the moral conditions needed to achieve goods internal to such practices" and "the tendency of professionalization and bureaucratic enforcement of rights, in some instances, to mitigate the bad effects of the marketplace on specific social practices and the people participating in them."[51]

Creating an Agenda

In concluding this chapter, I want to set out a loose set of requirements for an adequate social ethic—adequate, that is, to the range of concerns raised by managed care. I organize those requirements in terms of four fields of moral discourse. They are *method, social values, moral psychology,* and *moral sociology.* Because the fields are interrelated, a problem encountered in one field will likely have reverberations in each of the others.

Method. We need to begin with some understanding of how one ought to approach a question about what to do, or about what kinds of social arrangements are morally desirable. In my usage, "method" is simply a general term to describe such an understanding, one that is less demanding than theory or system. A method is a way of modeling moral reflection.

The model may be one in which we construct and apply a theory, but it need not be. If we feel the pull of diverse and sometimes conflicting considerations when we read a story such as Christine deMeurers's, we will want a method that does justice to that multiplicity. We should recognize that these kinds of stories, and our responses to them, provide an important but insufficient basis for judging a phenomenon as complex as managed care. What we need is a method that will prompt wider investigation and guide reflection, but refrain from prejudging the issue by removing whole areas of experience from consideration.

Social values. We must find some way of evaluating managed care, of understanding which features of managed care are to be approved and which are to be disapproved. This assessment will require us to consider how managed care stands in relation to important social values.

No doubt there are many ways of placing managed care in the context of a broader social vision. The failure to reach agreement on any comprehensive reform of health care in the United States in 1993–1994 testifies to the diversity of viewpoints in this area. Any adequate account must take account of this diversity. At the same time, the tendency to consider what transpires in the political realm as decisive reflects a truncated view of society. We need a reading of social values that captures the qualities of common life that matter to persons who are more than citizens.

Moral psychology. Moral psychology is clearly of great importance to moral understanding and to ethics. An ethical analysis of managed care, with its heavy reliance on incentives and its assumptions about human responses to them, clearly demands an exploration of the nexus between character and conduct. We also need to investigate the other psychological categories used in the managed care debate, such as the "self" in self-interest.

Moral sociology. Moral sociology, unlike moral psychology, is not a term in current use, but rather a marker for a subdiscipline we presently need. Faced with a phenomenon like managed care, we must begin, however inadequately, to make use of sociological insights. At the very least, we must consider the relation between the individual and the social, and we must try to anchor our moral judgments in the appropriate social and institutional contexts.

In particular, I wish to contribute to the correction of a deficiency in much scholarship in the field of medical ethics: the failure to think seriously about organizations. MacIntyre's account of institutions is helpful, but his concepts must be developed and supplemented by the work of social scientists studying the generic features of organizations and by consideration of the peculiar dynamics of managed care organizations.[52]

In subsequent chapters, I will argue that many of the tools for constructing a social ethic for the managed care era can be found through retrieving elements of the pragmatic tradition. The work of philosophers and scholars such as Richard Bernstein, Richard Rorty, Cornel West, and Jeffrey Stout has sparked a resurgence of interest in pragmatism. Pragmatism, at its best, is not unprincipled yielding to expediency, but the creative melding of insights from various sources to address social problems. Pragmatism is the firm refusal of dualisms and simplistic either/or's, although it does not deny the necessity of discrimination and choice. It combines normative commitments with an interest in psychology and sociology.

Managed care has finally succeeded in placing institutional concerns on the agenda for medical ethics, but work in this area is still limited.[53] As we seek guidance, the work of John Dewey and others within the pragmatic tradition is extremely suggestive, and the beauty of the fit seems to have inspired Susan Wolf's heralding of a pragmatic reformation of medical ethics.[54] When the "corporatization" of America is finally experienced as a significant development even in the medical enclave, there may be good reason to draw on the work of those who considered the arrival of "corporate civilization" momentous for ethics.

THREE

An Ethic for an Age of Organizations

One can only see from a certain standpoint, but this fact does not make all standpoints of equal value. A standpoint which is nowhere in particular and from which things are not seen at a special angle is an absurdity. But one may have affection for a standpoint which gives a rich and ordered landscape rather than for one from which things are seen confusedly and meagerly.

—John Dewey, "Context and Thought"

[D]eliberation takes its point of departure not from non-sense, but rather from insufficient sense; and it culminates not in Archimedean vision of a determinate terminus, but rather in conduct's emergence on a path whose sense can be fully ascertained only by following it into the situations toward which it points.

—Timothy Kaufman-Osborn, *Politics/Sense/Experience*

The pragmatic tradition offers inquiry as an alternative to simple reaction to change. It holds out the promise that, through inquiry, we can find a standpoint that affords a richer, more orderly "landscape." The pragmatic method of doing ethics that I develop in this chapter is broad and inclusive. It is experimental in the sense that the implementation and aftermath of moral judgment are as important as the deliberative process leading to judgment; and particular judgments are always open to revision. The method is linked to a democratic vision that focuses on the quality of relationships nurtured by particular social arrangements.

The fracturing of relationships is one of the most troubling aspects of the deMeurers case. Against some communitarians, a pragmatist would assert that our being troubled does not depend on identifying with the communities of identity of the central actors. We face many common problems. This insight is deepened in working through themes of commonality, community, and communication; but there is also an effort to show how these presume and benefit from difference. Subsidiarity, a concept I borrow from Catholic social thought, links democracy to justice. Justice, as informed by subsidiarity, departs from the mainstream in its emphasis on developing capacities, as well as distributing goods and services.

The pragmatic tradition can also serve as a resource in resolving or moving beyond some of the argumentative dead ends in the medicine-business polemic. I will direct my efforts to clarifying the relationship between conduct and character and scrutinizing beliefs about self-interest. Spatial limits circumscribe my ability to treat these topics exhaustively here, so I will tailor the discussion to the problem at hand.

In the medicine-business polemic, the plasticity of human nature emerged as a significant question. The concept of character allows for the formation of relatively stable patterns of conduct. Human beings are not entirely malleable. At the same time, character is pried loose from the grip of consciousness and intention. Human beings do not have the degree of self-control the ideology of medicine requires of physicians or the ideology of business requires of consumers. Further, because selves and interests vary with social forms, self-interest is unreliable as a guide—and questionable as an object of opposition.

It *is* desirable to nurture social affections that have the power to broaden and transform interests. Unfortunately, these sentiments cannot eliminate the insecurity created by freedom and finitude. Reinhold Niebuhr has argued that this insecurity poses a powerful barrier to intelligent social reform. Still, insecurity is itself social as well as individual, and we may lessen or intensify it through social action. The latter is a truth expressed in Niebuhr's notion of "common grace."

Finally, the pragmatic tradition prompts us to consider organizations as moral agents with their own distinctive character. The concept of character, applied to an organization, refers to the commitments and opportunities the organization supports or forecloses, as well as its particular combination of virtues and failings. Organizations can only act through persons, but persons act differently depending upon the kind of organization they inhabit. The organizational virtue of integrity requires vigilance vis-à-vis the risk of organizational surrender and careful negotiation of the tension between internal and external goods. The organizational virtue of responsiveness requires us to attend to factors that tend to narrow the range of interests and values to which organizations respond.

Organizations not only display character, they form the character of the individuals they touch. Health care organizations have the opportunity to nurture (or stunt) the growth of individual qualities like faithfulness, openness, and truthfulness, and thus affect the dimensions of the corporate problems of role fragmentation and organizational opacity and the cultural problem of manipulation.

My object in this chapter is not to lay the groundwork for a new philosophy or social theory, but rather to lay out some of the tools for a stereoscopic social criticism tailored to managed care. I will be making two kinds of claims. First,

I will argue that unless we consider certain features of the moral and social landscape, we will misdirect our activity. If we adopt a method of doing ethics that does not account for the full range of considerations, we ensure that our actions will lead to consequences that are unexpected and find us unprepared. And we cannot simply dispense with values, or ignore the role of some subset of values in orienting moral discourse. More strongly, values, or our interpretations of them, shape our definition of what is at stake in any situation.

In the area of moral psychology, we must recognize that character is malleable, and that it also offers some resistance to manipulation. The image of the physician as impervious to influence is untenable, but so is the instrumentalist view of the person as a set of predictable responses to particular stimuli. We ignore the role of organizations in shaping conduct and character at our peril.

Second, I will suggest that certain ways of framing or developing these features are appealing, at least to those with a certain sensibility or range of experience. This strand will emerge most strongly in the section on social values. I present the views of democracy and justice not as self-evident truths, nor as defensible through "superpower" arguments.[1] Although I can support them with reasons, they are more in the realm of emotion than logic.

In the area of moral psychology, claims for normative intersubjectivity—the assignment of moral value to human relationships—are of a similar nature. So is my discussion of the qualities of character that organizations ought to cultivate. Using a pragmatic framework invites the audience to question an interpretation or analysis, asking not only "Does this comport with 'reality'?" but "Does this help us to negotiate our way through this particular problematic situation?" I hope to demonstrate that in each of these areas, a pragmatic approach yields insights that may prove fruitful in practice.

A PRAGMATIC METHOD FOR MORAL INQUIRY

Ethics as Relation-Mapping and Problem-Solving

To begin with, an adequate approach to ethics must be broad enough to capture the concerns of Arnold Relman, editor emeritus of the *New England Journal*, and Princeton health economics professor Uwe Reinhardt. Reinhardt does not simply oppose "economic logic" to "ethical conscience." He argues, among other things, that Relman fails to consider how far actual conduct falls short of the philanthropic ideal and the consequences of this divergence.

It would hardly be helpful to define ethics in a manner that swallows the universe. At the same time, restrictive definitions often reflect attempts to exclude concerns the author does not share. That is, the author uses the definition polemically to dignify her own preoccupations, and to denigrate those of others as non-moral. Hence, there is good reason to favor an inclusive approach, meaning the conditions for admission of claims and concerns should be weak. Here, ethics denotes making an inquiry with a view toward rendering judgment of right or wrong, good or bad, with an emphasis on the *relations among* phenomena. Indeed, I would refer to this version of pragmatic ethics as "relation-mapping."

Pragmatic ethics attends to consequences. However, it cannot be termed consequentialist because it looks at the whole network of relations bearing on the object of evaluation and not the consequences alone.[2] Assume, for example, that the question is whether I should lie to a patient about a cancer diagnosis. If I am a consequentialist, I may consider the pain or pleasure, happiness or unhappiness that may result from the lie, as compared to truthful disclosure of the diagnosis. If I am inclined to be comprehensive, I will include the social impact of a lie in the calculus, e.g., the extent to which necessary social trust may be eroded by the accretion of such instances. It seems strained, however, to frame my exploration of the rationale for the rule against lying, as a prelude to judgment about this instance, as a yet broader version of consequentialist analysis.

Reflecting on the *considerations* that underlie a rule in determining if, when, and how to use it to guide conduct is different from evaluating the consequences that will likely follow in determining whether to observe or break the rule.[3] Further, in a relational, as opposed to consequentialist, analysis, my purposes, motivations, and reasons for acting will become relevant, independent of the results my action produces.

Beyond this, it is possible to describe consequentialist and deontological approaches to ethics as complementary rather than opposed. For example, Robert Nozick, a prominent deontologist, offers the maxim "among those acts available to you that don't violate constraints C, act so as to maximize goal G" as a way of bringing side-constraints and end-states together.[4] The same is true of rule-based and virtue-based approaches to ethics. In a book titled *Towards Justice and Virtue,* Onora O'Neill shows how rules and virtues are tailored to distinct areas of the moral terrain, the distinction reflecting the different kinds of vulnerabilities addressed. Rules, especially principles of justice, address "characteristic and persistent vulnerabilities," while virtues address "variable and selective vulnerabilities."[5] The open-ended nature of virtues (and values) is adapted to the kind of moral work they do.

A pragmatic ethics influenced by John Dewey will focus on problems. In general, it is reasonable to assert that the occasion for moral reflection is a problem, either a conflict of values or obligations experienced as unsettling, or an unsettling of received views due to change. Only then does a portion of "customary morality," the stock of inherited ideals, concepts, maxims, rules, and so on that we take for granted in daily living, become an object of inquiry.

Managed care poses a problem because we value care *and* efficiency, and because we value health, and health care, very highly, but not to the exclusion of other personal and social goods. Managed care poses a problem because we believe that health care professionals have obligations to individual patients *and* that health plans (and perhaps health care professionals) have obligations to patient populations. The message of the medicine-business polemic is "choose!" The message here is "reflect!" What reflection, or moral deliberation, entails must now be explored in greater depth.

Moral Deliberation

Those influenced by the pragmatic tradition typically model deliberation as a series of steps. Dividing deliberation into distinct steps is somewhat artificial, but inquiry benefits from structure:

1. Develop an initial (provisional) definition of the problem.

In the beginning is the problem, a state of affairs that creates doubt about what should be done. The definition of the problem should be broad enough to include most of the significant relationships, but not so broad as to overwhelm the human capacity to make sense. Storytelling about the problem is important both as an aid to comprehension and as an anchor for inquiry.

2. Gather information about and perspectives on the problem.

The first stage in resolving the problematic situation involves investigating the facts with an eye toward more clearly defining the problem. We should construe the word "facts" broadly, and conceive of the investigator as an engaged, emotionally responsive being rather than as a disembodied intellect. The facts of the situation will include the full complement of social resources that may contribute to understanding, including moral theory, codes and customs, historical and social science research, statutes and judicial decisions, and journalistic reports.

3. Frame the options and rule out certain options as unacceptable.

At some point, it makes sense to set out the range of possible responses to the problem. We can identify *viable* responses by screening out options that fail to advance moral values or that violate moral side-constraints. This screening process involves projecting what each path will entail for the character of an individual or organization or society. The pragmatist will give great weight to values of democracy and community. Other values can be found in (or teased out of) the history and mission of the particular individual or group.

Side-constraints include obligations to demonstrate respect for persons, honor claims of justice, and fulfill commitments. For example, consider injunctions to "tell the truth" and "keep your promises." At the very least, these rules or principles alert us to the severity of the problem posed by managed care.[6] In the deMeurers case, there are allegations that several of the protagonists economized on the truth and failed to keep faith. The distinctive pragmatic contribution is recognizing the importance of creativity in moral reflection. The objective of conducting a pragmatic investigation is not merely to achieve equilibrium or consistency between principles and our considered judgments in particular cases. Although such internal consistency of belief is by no means to be disdained, we may learn and create new things through our engagements with the world and with one another.

4. Interrogate the remaining option(s) as to desirability and feasibility.

The next step is to test each remaining option for its capacity to produce change in accordance with specific purposes. Questions might include: Has this (or something like this) been tried before? With what results? Should these results be taken as definitive for the present, or has the context changed in significant ways? Is a trial possible? What would it look like, and what would the evaluation standards be? If an option seems too idealistic, does this reflect a failure of vision and courage, or does the option bump up against real human limits? If the former, is it possible to identify structures that might fortify and sustain the effort? Finally, we will need to face up to any difficult trade-offs that we must make, while remaining on the lookout for false oppositions.

5. Render judgment and then implement.

Evaluative judgment emerges within the process of projecting and interrogating, as the various elements "come together."[7] In this sense, judgment is holistic or holographic.[8] At the same time, we may employ a more analytical style in revisiting a judgment in light of new evidence. The structure of moral deliberation is heterarchical rather than hierarchical.[9] As suggested by Step 4, implementation is not an afterthought. Rather, it becomes a crucial aspect of resolving the problem and requires much forethought and care.

6. Continue the deliberative process through monitoring and evaluation.

Judgments must always be open to revision, which gives pragmatism its experimental cast. Implementing this principle requires care, since pragmatism has been (mis)characterized as a kind of success philosophy.[10] Pragmatism demands willingness to reconsider one's position based on evidence at odds with one's initial view, but it does not sanction yielding up principle in the interests of expediency.

The process of moral deliberation described here is pluralistic in two ways. First, it may not lead to identification of a single most desirable option, given current information and conditions. Second, deliberation is communal. Although an *individual* may adopt the approach outlined above, even then the process is conversational in that reading and writing are understood as forms of engagement with others.

The Importance of Experience

An introduction to pragmatic ethics would be incomplete without mention of the importance of experience. In the work of Dewey and others, experience is not total absorption in some other, nor the impress of external forces on an essentially separated being, but rather a flow of trans-actions. Experience can be put to use because we can affect the environment that affects us.

Pragmatism does not support a sentimental view of immediate or unanalyzed experience.[11] Distance is necessary to problem solving; without it we are likely to feel overwhelmed or immobilized by fear or anxiety. A problem in its immediacy creates a state of confusion, disorientation, frustration, insufficient sense. To define some set of circumstances *as* a problem is already to take charge, to begin to recover a sense of efficacy. On the other hand, neglecting immediate experience can lead to arbitrary intellectualism. Science as well as philosophy can be unempirical in unduly restricting the range of experience it takes to be relevant.

Experience can also refer to practical learning, developing certain aptitudes and skills over a lifetime.[12] We may speak of an experienced physician or nurse, and also of an experienced patient. Stanley Reiser has chronicled how the patient's experience of illness was progressively devalued, as physicians increasingly understood their work in terms set by the natural sciences. Patients became objects of study and sites for the application of technique. This trend began to change when the appropriate use of new technologies became a pressing question, calling not for a better disease classification scheme or technique, but rather for explicit value judgments. Along with developments in the culture at large, such as the civil rights movement, a new awareness that science itself could not provide all the answers set the stage for the "reemergence" of the patient. Reiser makes a number of innovative proposals that draw on the notion of the experienced or expert patient.[13]

Anticipation of Some Objections to Pragmatic Ethics

I must still respond to some of the possible objections to pragmatic ethics. Detractors might castigate pragmatism as a form of scientism, that is, naïve faith in science, or of calculative rationality. If pragmatism is committed to reducing "the other" to an object of manipulation through science or reason, it can scarcely serve as a resource for those concerned about the increasingly manipulative cast of relationships in health care.

PRAGMATISM AS SCIENTISM

Early pragmatists opposed separating thought from experience, and their reservations concerning an abstract and hegemonic philosophy extended to an abstract and hegemonic science.[14] Dewey warned against confusing the method he called "experimentalism" with thoughtless empiricism. Observation must be directed by general ideas, otherwise it falls prey to covert manipulation. The social sciences in particular have the potential to "multiply the agencies by which some human beings manipulate other human beings for their own advantage," and hence must be subject to moral direction.[15]

PRAGMATISM AND CALCULATIVE RATIONALITY

Related to the charge of scientism, pragmatists have been accused of propagating a purely instrumental or calculative rationality. I believe a pragmatist will allow that calculation, the quantification and comparison of benefits and harms, may be helpful, but only where this process can be accomplished without doing violence to distinctions of quality. It is a good idea, then, to arm oneself in advance against the dangers, including neglect of the relationship between means and ends, disjunction between activities and an overarching end or mission, and displacement of moral deliberation by technique.

First, recognizing the power means have to shape and reshape ends, we should make aligning means and ends into a conscious project.[16] Modifying the usual assertion, that the end justifies the means, we might assert that the means "justify" the end, in the sense of showing the end to be right, just and reasonable. Operating an organization dedicated to the spread of democracy on democratic principles, and realizing the promised goods of democracy among its members, provide the best evidence of the practicability and desirability of democracy as an end. We must also appreciate means *as* ends. In the example given, each interaction with a fellow member has an intrinsic value or disvalue, existing alongside whatever value it may have by reason of its consequences in relation to the goal of the overall enterprise.

Second, we must maintain links between activities and mission. We are bound to narrow the field of considerations in carrying out our various responsibilities. The correction demanded is not an effort to keep all considerations in view at all times, but rather a periodic check to ensure that activities remain consistent with and in the service of broader ends or goals. Consider an example from contemporary health care administration. What are the consequences of using the term "medical-loss ratio" to refer to the proportion of premium dollars actually spent on delivering health care and embracing this ratio as a marker for organizational success?

Preventing illness (and attendant upon that, reducing the need for medical services) is highly desirable. Likewise, we should always strive to reduce unnecessary expenditures—waste—through eliminating redundancies, useless medical work, useless paperwork, and so on. At the same time, it is perverse to equate such goals with the goal of minimizing medical services, absolutely. The term medical-loss ratio suggests that providing health care is itself loss, waste.[17] Taken together with other terms currently in vogue, such as the term "covered life" for persons who have entrusted their health care to a plan or provider, the term medical-loss ratio establishes the greatest possible distance between the activities of administrators and the mission of providing appropriate health care.

Third, we must acknowledge the specific limitations of specific techniques. Consider the use of cost-benefit and cost-effectiveness analysis in resource allocation. Cost-benefit analysis is especially controversial because it involves the monetarization of costs and benefits. (In cost-effectiveness analysis, two or more paths to the same benefit are compared. The comparison takes place in monetary terms, but the benefit itself need not be assigned a monetary value.)

Performing a cost-benefit analysis is difficult in health care, where many things that people may either suffer or gain are not typically priced. Frequently, consumers are asked how much they would be willing to pay to avoid some risk (cost) or attain some benefit, or how much they would have to receive to assume some risk (cost) or forego some benefit. The questions are usually hypothetical, which may introduce various forms of bias.[18]

The quality-adjusted life year (QALY) approach—a form of cost-effectiveness analysis in that benefits are not monetarized—is an alternative to the "willingness to pay" approach to valuation. Like the willingness to pay approach, the QALY approach relies on individual preferences elicited through hypothetical questions. Respondents are presented with a series of impairment descriptions and asked to rank them on a 0–1 scale, with death equaling zero. Values can be negative, if the respondent considers a particular impairment worse than death. Unlike the willingness to pay approach, the QALY approach is intended to minimize the effects of economic factors such as income and price on valuations.

Although any valuation of health states is highly controversial, and all of the major approaches are subject to technical difficulties, economists point out that reliably estimating the changes in health that will result from adopting a policy may be even more difficult.[19] Results may differ significantly depending upon the scope of the effects captured, for example, whether broader social costs such as increased caregiving burdens on family members are considered. Yet many still present these methodologies as unproblematic solutions to the problem of resource allocation. This breezy confidence reflects a failure by some health services researchers to attend to the limits of cost-benefit and cost-effectiveness analyses as economic tools.

Further, the economic worldview is itself limited in ways that should be acknowledged.[20] Cost-benefit analysis has been criticized for its failure to give sufficient weight to expectations, or, in the language of justice, rights. Steven Kelman suggests that the methodology may obscure the significance people accord to having a right. It assumes "there is no difference between the price a person would require for *giving up* something to which he has a preexisting right and the price he would pay to *gain* something to which he enjoys no right."[21]

Kelman also criticizes another assumption he considers unwarranted, the assumption that there is no difference between how people value certain things in private individual transactions and how they would wish those same things to be valued in public collective decisions.[22] To repeat, quantifying and comparing benefits and harms may be helpful, but only where this process can be accomplished without doing violence to distinctions of quality.

Contemporary corporate and regulatory culture fosters models of rationality according to which ends are given and unproblematic; their realization is a matter of selection and refinement of technique. Hence, the stress here will be on problematizing goals and broadening responsibility. In the health care field, that means thinking critically about the penetration of practice by accounting terminology, the increasing reliance on cost-benefit and cost-effectiveness analyses, and the turn to incentive schemes to control behavior.

SOCIAL VALUES: DEMOCRACY AND JUSTICE

As defined by Charles Dougherty, a leading scholar of ethics and health policy, a value is a "desired state of affairs."[23] Moral values are values we regard as particularly significant because they are linked to obligation or to our aspiration to transcendence. A social value of the moral variety expresses what is desirable—what ought to be desired—in relationships with others. Dougherty notes that moral values tend to be vague: "The aspirational dimension of values makes them properly indistinct because it links judgment and action to ideal states that can be only partially and imaginatively understood and felt. Therefore, this vagueness in meaning, though sometimes frustrating, is often an important positive dimension of moral values, allowing and even promoting multiple articulations of the idea at hand and thereby offering different directions from which the ideal can be approximated."[24] Principles and rules provide the structure; values introduce dynamism into ethics.

Democracy

Although some might disagree, I would assert that democracy is the social value at the heart of the pragmatist vision. To begin with, democracy informs and is informed by pragmatic modes of inquiry. This is so because inquiry involves having a positive regard for the experience, intelligence, and humanity of others, even and perhaps especially regard for those who hold opposing views. In carrying out the task of inquiry, we are not only searching for solutions to the problems of social life, we are in fact living, socially. We are engaged in an experiment in community life, a social experiment. The adoption and implementation of universal moral respect and reciprocity, and the cultivation of the ability to take the standpoint of the other, are the instrumentalities through which democracy is realized.[25]

Democracy, in its political aspect, may include procedural protections such as universal suffrage, majority rule subject to constitutional constraints, and the panoply of rules and regulations designed to assure impartial governmental administration. But these are less than the whole, even of political democracy. The viability of political democracy is, in any event, linked to the flourishing of "social democracy," a concept that is much broader in scope. Most managed care organizations, for-profit and not-for-profit, are part of civil society, and civil society has special importance for those working in the pragmatic tradition. Pragmatists, especially those influenced by Dewey, have concerned themselves with understanding and cultivating the goods of voluntary association.

DEMOCRACY AS IDEAL AND STANDARD

Democracy suggests a moral ideal and a standard for judging social arrangements, but it precludes any simple solutions to social problems. As Dewey put it: "To 'make others happy' except through liberating their powers and engaging them in activities that enlarge the meaning of life is to harm them and to indulge ourselves under the cover of exercising a special virtue." The "moral measure" for evaluating an existing or proposed arrangement should be its effect on human capacities. The goal is to "foster conditions that widen the horizon of others [e.g., broaden interests and spur creative thought] and give them command of their own powers."[26]

This may be too flexible, too open-ended, to please many moralists. It rules out a simple utilitarian calculus. We cannot dole out happiness, or health, as if it were a commodity. And it would be presumptuous, anti-experimental, and undemocratic to lay down the moral law for all persons, times, and places with too much specificity. But we can exhibit moral concern in contributing to the formation of social institutions that nurture capacities for happiness and health.

The democratic perspective departs from the utilitarian one in another way. Since a distinctively *moral* happiness includes appreciating what is truly desirable, pursuing happiness entails moral deliberation, and not simply solicitation of individual preferences. As Dewey noted in *The Quest for Certainty*, "The fact that something is desired only raises the *question* of its desirability; it does not settle it. Only a child in the degree of his immaturity thinks to settle the question of desirability by reiterated proclamation: 'I want it, I want it.' "[27] Respect for others is not expressed in treating their spontaneous desires as final.

INTERSUBJECTIVITY AND COMMUNITY

The individual and society are often spoken of as separate and opposed entities. We seldom reflect on the evidence of human interdependence, from the infant's absolute dependence, to the dependence of individuality itself on social nurture, to the omnipresence of language. These "facts of life" are so familiar that we miss their import: an individual exists because of and in relations with others. Imagined apart from these relations, one is an individual "only as a stick of wood is, namely, as spatially and numerically separate."[28]

Shared experience, or community, is the apex of the development of associated life, the consummation of the democratic vision.[29] Interacting, a basic feature of existence, becomes elaborated as shared activity, which makes possible the emergence of shared values. This is the stage that defines true community: "Wherever there is conjoint activity whose consequences are appreciated as good by all singular persons who take part in it, and where the realization of the good is such as to effect an energetic desire and effort to sustain it in being just because it is a good shared by all, there is in so far a community."[30]

Community will often be a matter of degree, a partial or temporary achievement. The degree of homogeneity, or unity on matters of belief, is not necessarily a good index of community. Although community cannot exist without some degree of shared experience and shared meanings, "this communality implies also a richness, a complexity of possible perspectives to enter into, not the simplicity of identity."[31] It is consistent with this view to allow for limited communities, composed of persons who might otherwise be moral strangers, formed to address a common problem such as managed care—if working together is experienced as a good and so on—and to recognize community even where there are deep divisions.

Community is bound up with communication, sharing meanings. The communication paradigm can be contrasted with a paradigm of disclosure. The disclosure paradigm focuses on transferring identified pieces of information. A subject is required to receive the information, but the origination point and vehicle of disclosure are largely a matter of indifference.

The communication paradigm shifts the focus to what happens *between* two or more subjects: "To be a recipient of a communication is to have an enlarged and changed experience. One shares in what another has thought and felt and in so far, meagerly or amply, has his own attitude modified. Nor is the one who communicates left unaffected. . . . The experience has to be formulated in order to be communicated. To formulate requires getting outside of it, seeing it as another would see it, considering what points of contact it has with the life of another so that it may be got into such form that he can appreciate its meaning."[32] Both recipient and communicator are changed, and in a genuine conversation the positions are reversible.[33]

Finally, conversation, with its potential for mutual transformation, should be distinguished from interest-group debate, where participants are merely bent on advancing their pre-established interests. In conversation "the ideas of one are corrected and changed by what others say."[34] What is confirmed is not one's prior judgment, which may have been narrow and ill-informed, but rather the capacity to judge wisely.

Democracy and Justice

Justice names the forms of regulation that develop to sustain a community. As O'Neill suggests, principles of justice ought to provide order and protection in areas where vulnerabilities, or needs, are widely shared and persistent. Traditionally, a distinction is made between distributive justice and commutative justice. Since I cannot provide a comprehensive treatment here, I will suggest a definition of distributive justice, sketch one approach to the subject, briefly review some other accounts of distributive justice, and finally, comment on commutative justice.

DISTRIBUTIVE JUSTICE

According to the classical account of Thomas Aquinas, distributive justice refers to the proportionate distribution of common goods, or "what the whole owes the parts."[35] For much of history, Western societies understood the requirements of distributive justice in terms of certain formulas, such as "like cases should be treated alike," i.e., persons should be treated similarly (receive equal shares and so on), unless there are good reasons, relevant to the particular instance of distribution, for treating them differently. The contemporary debate over distributive justice extends to disagreement over the notion of "common goods."

Michael Walzer argues that all goods are *social*, but only some are *common* in the sense that they are to be distributed by the whole. In other words, there are distinct "spheres" of justice.[36] The whole, or the community, provides certain goods to all because community members recognize them as especially significant. Walzer holds that in areas of communal provision, the appropriate principle of distribution is need, meaning that difference in need forms the only proper basis for differential treatment. He observes that in our society health care is understood as a good of special significance, and so should be distributed according to the principle of need. Walzer allows for other goods to be distributed according to principles of mutual agreement (private contract) or desert.

I will rely on Walzer's work in sketching a pragmatic approach to justice in health care. However, I would be remiss if I failed to mention several highly influential theories or accounts of justice: utilitarianism, Rawlsian social contract theory, and Alasdair MacIntyre's Aristotelian communitarianism. The object in this cursory review will be to provide the nonspecialist reader a sense of the range of alternatives and to locate them in relation to Walzer, and to convey to the specialist reader my understanding that the views presented here are contested.

Utilitarianism is among the chief contenders in the arena of moral theory. Although it has been under severe attack in moral philosophy, it remains the taken-for-granted standard for disciplines such as economics and political science. In utilitarian theory, or more properly, theories, the ultimate criterion for the whole of morality is a maximization principle, first enunciated by Jeremy Bentham[37]: one should act so as to secure the greatest happiness for the greatest number. This principle can be worked out in various ways with various implications for the distribution of goods such as health care.

Walzer rejects the search for a single unifying principle for the whole of morality, and so is unsympathetic to utilitarianism in a fundamental way. That said, there may be substantial agreement on the requirements of justice among persons who start from very different moral theories. Utilitarians and Walzerians may be united in their commitment to individual rights (e.g., a right to health care), just as deontologists may join utilitarians in recognizing the force of considerations of general welfare in developing social policy.

John Rawls works from a hypothetical social contract (devised in a thought experiment Rawls terms the "original position") to arrive at two principles of distributive justice. Stated in their most refined form, the two principles are as follows: (1) Each person has an equal right to a fully adequate scheme of basic liberties, which is compatible with a similar scheme of liberties for all. (2) Social and economic inequalities must satisfy two conditions. First, they must be attached to offices and positions open to all under conditions of fair equality of opportunity; and second, they must provide the greatest benefit to society's least advantaged members.[38]

The approach, which Rawls terms "justice as fairness," differs greatly from Walzer's. But again, it is important to understand that very different approaches may converge on specific requirements.[39] For example, if one places health care under the fair equality of opportunity provision of the second principle of justice, the kinds of deliberation called for to work out what is required in practice will be very similar to what goes on in specifying the entailments of a principle of distribution according to need. The two approaches would appear to hold several "unsolved rationing problems" in common.[40]

Finally, in his work on justice, MacIntyre stresses the importance of desert as a principle of distribution within the best type of community, the community dedicated to virtue and excellence and agreed on standards for judging achievement. Again there is some overlap with Walzer's account of distributive justice, but less than complete agreement. While Walzer allows that it is best to distribute certain goods according to the principle of desert, he does not extend the principle to the distribution of basic goods such as health care.

COMMUTATIVE JUSTICE

Rawls treats all significant goods as common goods to be distributed according to the two principles. At the same time, he suggests that justice as fairness is founded upon a basic intuition concerning mutual advantage and an appreciation of the importance of willing cooperation in social life. These are the supports for commutative justice.

Commutative justice is one aspect of the dealings between "private" persons. The sphere of private transactions is contrasted with the sphere of public administration, although private transactions are facilitated by laws and by the availability of public processes for settling disputes. We sometimes term this kind of justice "contractual justice," because it concerns the standards that govern the making and carrying out and breaking of voluntary agreements or contracts.

Some of the moral importance of contractual justice derives from the weight we attach to promise-making and promise-keeping. While some within the law and economics movement wish to remove the moral "taint" from breach of contract, the experience of having one's expectations of others disappointed is typically infused by strong feelings of injustice and betrayal. The weight we attach to a contract varies according to the conditions of its making. Insurance contracts, for example, are commonly regarded as "contracts of adhesion," and the absence of any real opportunity for negotiation on the part of the consumer affects their interpretation.

THE SPRINGS AND LIMITS OF SOCIAL JUSTICE

If one conceives of justice as the development of forms of regulation, moral and legal, to aid in the maintenance of community, justice is both natural and artificial. Although we may end up with a set of very general principles in a highly cosmopolitan society, even those general principles need some emotional nourishment. When we issue the call to social justice, we seldom rely on the force of logic alone.

Philosopher Robert Solomon argues that emotions are the raw material of justice, and that justice is corrupted whenever its emotional connections are denied or obscured: "Justice begins not with Socratic insights but with the promptings of some basic emotions, among them envy, jealousy, and resentment, a sense of being personally cheated or neglected, and the desire to get even—but also, of course, those basic feelings of sharing, compassion, sympathy, and generosity. . . . Whatever one's principles of justice, they are utterly meaningless without that fundamental human sense of caring and the ability to understand and personally care about the well-being of other human beings. . . . "[41] No one emotion need predominate. Allowing for this multiplicity, we can understand why justice has been accounted for in terms of fear or insecurity, mutual advantage, an appreciation of excellence or merit, and sympathy.[42]

Diverse cultures recognize certain vulnerabilities or needs, and related to them, obligations, with such regularity that they are appropriately labeled universal or basic. On the other hand, what justice requires will vary across cultures and communities. And, without giving up the insistence that we have obligations to others, there may be good reasons for marking off some region of personal inviolability from coercion. Doing so will set limits on who and what can be conscripted to achieve social goals. We may disagree about what is encompassed in the region of personal inviolability, but the basic principle is one that we should respect.[43]

DISTRIBUTIVE JUSTICE AND HEALTH CARE

The difficulty comes in weighing all of these considerations in a particular case. Most participants in the managed care debate agree that we cannot neglect the health care needs of our fellows altogether, and that an interpretation of social meanings will guide distribution. (Even the utilitarian must have some way of understanding how and why health care leads to happiness.) Further, we seem agreed that need, related to some incapacity that can be corrected or ameliorated by health care, is the appropriate distributional principle, at least once one has been admitted to the system.

In addition, Walzer persuasively argues that in areas of social provision it is unjust to require people to contribute to goods from which they are excluded (*de facto* if not *de jure*), especially if the result is a transfer of wealth from the poor to the affluent. It is unjust for the comfortable majority to support employer tax deductions for employee health benefits, the exclusion of health benefits from employees' taxable income,[44] and the use of public funds for medical education and research and hospital construction, without giving the remainder of their fellow citizens access to the institutions through which the benefits of such public programs are made available. It is unjust to require a sales clerk, whose corporate employer does not offer health insurance to the majority of its employees, to subsidize the health care of the company's chief executive officer through the taxes she pays.

By reason of their role in distributing a good subject to social provision, heath care organizations have special public responsibilities. Fulfilling these responsibilities is especially pressing in the absence of some form of universal insurance, but concerns about fairness would not disappear even were Medicare-type benefits extended to the entire population. Even in such a scenario, it would be important for organizations to resist the temptation to engage in "cherry-picking" or "cream-skimming," recruiting patients or enrollees selectively according to health status.[45]

Where payment is premised on an even distribution of hard cases, cost-shifting across organizations invites, indeed demands, the kind of heavy-handed regulation that may be in nobody's best interest. Beyond this, the manner in which the principle of distribution according to need will be worked out, and health care services will be organized and delivered, is a matter for communal inquiry and decision.[46]

MOVING BEYOND THE DISTRIBUTIVE PARADIGM: SUBSIDIARITY

That, at least, is where political democracy and political philosophy leave us. Social democracy introduces an additional consideration, one that does not fit neatly within the standard paradigms of distributive justice. The standard paradigms focus on the question of who gets what (division). Social democracy moves beyond that question. The idea is not simply that people should receive their fair share of commodities, or at least enough to meet their basic needs. People should receive help in developing their capacities, including the capacity to supply their own needs to the greatest extent possible.[47] Distribution is viewed from the angle of multiplication: there are multiple centers of power, and goods are dynamic, their production and consumption intertwined in the realization of human capacities.

These sorts of concerns have figured prominently in recent Roman Catholic social thought and are captured in what has become known as the principle of subsidiarity. Pope Pius XI first articulated the principle in response to the kind of corporatism associated with Italian fascism. In *Quadragesimo Anno*, the Pope stated that "Inasmuch as every social activity should, by its very nature, prove a help to members of the social body, it should never destroy or absorb them."[48]

The principle has guided the thinking of the U.S. Catholic bishops on health and health care and the economy.[49]

In an introduction to church teachings concerning health care, Kevin O'Rourke and Philip Boyle state the developed principle clearly and concisely, as follows: "(1) Decision making rests first with the person, then with the lower social levels, and horizontally with functional social units; and (2) The higher social units intervene only to supply the lower units with the goods they cannot achieve by themselves, while at the same time working to make it easier in the future for lower units and individuals to satisfy these needs by their own efforts."[50] From this perspective, self-help and social support are complementary.

The principle of subsidiarity can inform our thinking about justice in at least four ways. First, the relational aspects of basic goods assume greater prominence. Relationships, fellowship and fellow feeling, belonging to a community, and being recognized and respected by others, are recognized as the "primary currency" of justice.[51] An account of basic or primary goods must include satisfying human relationships. At the same time, these goods cannot be separated from other goods. Fulfilling relationships are fostered when other basic needs are met. Homelessness, joblessness, and poor health, or anxieties about any of these conditions, corrode relationships.

Second, we are urged to recognize the connection between process and outcome. Consider two elderly women recovering from strokes of comparable severity. One receives extensive physical therapy and is able to do her own grocery shopping and so on. The other receives minimal physical therapy but is supplied with a home health aide who meets her needs for food and the like. Justice requires that basic needs be provided for, and so it might seem that neither woman has cause for complaint. But justice informed by the principle of subsidiarity requires favoring restorative over maintenance measures.[52] Given that restorative measures are clearly feasible, the woman who is managed as a "head in a bed" can claim that she is being treated unjustly.

Third, while the principle of subsidiarity alone will not support an absolute priority for the least advantaged, the effort to enable all to participate fully in associated life will require greater attention to those without adequate social and material supports for effective freedom and moral equality.[53] It will entail some skepticism of forms of cost-benefit analysis that reinforce existing patterns of discrimination among social groups, e.g., the discounted future earnings approach to the valuation of life. Under the discounted future earnings approach, if one is poorly paid, one's life is worth less; if one is without employment prospects, one's life is literally worthless.[54] The principle of subsidiarity should also caution against patronizing people, either by excluding them from deliberation about what is to be done for them, or by absolving them of responsibility to contribute to the common good.

Fourth, the kind of universalism associated with the principle of subsidiarity is not opposed in principle to special relationships. It does not require that

I abandon a healthy self-regard or special concern for family members, friends, my own patients or clients, or the associations to which I belong. I am, however, required to work for social conditions that will support the flourishing of other persons, families, professional relationships, and associations.

COMMUTATIVE JUSTICE AND HEALTH CARE

Commutative justice requires that health care organizations treat third-party payers, providers, and potential and actual member-patients fairly.[55] In this context, fairness means adopting marketing practices and disclosure policies that make consumer and patient choice meaningful and honoring rather than attempting to weasel out of the terms of contracts, especially concerning responsibilities to members.[56] Health care organizations should avoid erecting barriers of inconvenience to the receipt of covered benefits, recognizing that fear is a cost unjustly imposed on members, and the public at large, when administration is not reliable.

Health care organizations should also do what they can to ensure that practitioners treat patients fairly. For example, practitioners cannot help liking some patients more than others, and contracts seldom command equal liking. But somewhere between treating patients differently (e.g., joking more with Sally than with Jane) and *treating* patients differently (e.g., offering therapeutic options to Sally that are not offered to Jane) lies a kind of favoritism that easily becomes injustice in the context of managed care (e.g., becoming an "economic advocate" for Sally but not for Jane).

Finally, health care organizations should treat employees fairly, by paying a decent wage, instituting due process protections in the case of terminations, and involving practitioners, and the entire range of employees, in at least some aspects of policy creation and governance. Justice may not require any particular level of pay, process, or participation, but the principle of subsidiarity seems to pull in the direction of more participation than we have at present.

MORAL PSYCHOLOGY: CHARACTER AND SELF-INTEREST

Conduct and Character

The occasion for moral reflection is a question about the proper course of conduct, a question of how to act in the face of uncertainty or conflict. At the same time, the agent's character is at stake in any moral situation: we are always asking "who shall I *be?*" as well as "what shall I *do*?" Particular acts strengthen or weaken tendencies to action or habits, and habits constitute character.

PLACING ACTS IN CONTEXT

An act is not an isolated phenomenon. Acts, including acts of choice, have reverberations, often beyond what we intend or foresee. What I choose now, indeed, the nature of the choices I face, is partially determined by what I have done or chosen before. My future choices, and the nature of those choices, are partially determined by all my past and present choices.

When John Glaspy agreed to serve as a consultant for Health Net, he no doubt failed to foresee (or wished not to dwell upon the likelihood of) a serious conflict of obligations down the road. Choices of affiliation are particularly weighty acts, since they open and close whole fields of action. They condition the moral problems we will face, even what we will see as a moral problem, since, in choosing, we reinforce commitments to certain values and neglect others or allow them to disappear altogether. What would at one time have been a problem becomes merely a part of the routine.[57]

IDENTIFYING AND ASSESSING CHARACTER

Judgments about character follow observation. Such judgments are bound to be complex, because the relationships among habits, and between habits and the environment, are complex. Further, important aspects of character are beyond internal control. The observer may detect a pattern to which the self is oblivious. And character is vulnerable; even good character is not proof against misfortune.[58] This vulnerability has a positive side; sometimes the things that just happen prove immensely significant and valuable. Also, although the old saying that suffering builds character is open to challenge, it does contain a grain of truth. Conflict and tension and disappointment are part of the normal process of character formation. Contending with these difficulties can develop strengths or virtues.[59] Finally, character is a historical phenomenon. If you ask me about the character of x, you are inviting a biography—but an open one.[60]

SELF-INTEREST AND SELF-GIVING

This "character" discussion opens up a number of significant questions forced upon us by advocates for and opponents of managed care—advocates who rely on a fortunate egoism, rational and highly amenable to manipulation, and opponents who hope to vanquish the greedy business people causing all the trouble by enlightening their innocent dupes (the public) and creating a groundswell of support for a truly just system. So what of self-interest, and what of the prospects for reforms that depend for their success on a high degree of social awareness and concern, that is, a high degree of self-giving?

SELF-INTEREST

It is not uncommon to find something called "self-interest" credited as the universal motivator. It lurks in the managed care debate, but antagonists seldom examine the concept. Some begin with the view that morality consists in denying the claims of the self (surely a strand in the ideology of medicine). Although self-scrutiny may be in order, this view can be harmful for a number of reasons.

To begin with, when we emphasize the need to control desire rather than the good achieved through keeping desire in check, morality acquires a negative cast. And as feminist social critics point out, women are the usual casualties of the doctrine of self-denial, suffering the resultant deformations of the self. Also, the self denied frequently displays a kind of deviousness in demanding recognition and reward: "The one who is conscious of continually denying himself cannot rid himself of the idea that it ought to be 'made up' to him; that a compensating happiness is due him for what he has sacrificed, somewhat increased, if anything, on account of the unnatural virtue he has displayed."[61] Many physicians no doubt emerge from the multiple deprivations of residency with a sense of entitlement.

Egoism of the kind associated with the ideology of business takes the enemy constructed by the doctrine of self-denial—the affirming, acquisitive, power-seeking self—and makes it the ideal. The survival of the fittest is not only accepted as a law of nature; it is fashioned into a moral law. This is in some ways a healthy reaction to the negativity of self-denial. But to pursue power for power's sake is to fall under the sway of an abstraction. And, although it is in some ways the mirror image of self-denial, self-assertion also demands the sacrifice of certain dispositions or capacities of the self. Friendship and family ties, play and recreation, and community involvement may be slighted in the drive to get or hold on to power.[62]

One group argues that the self must be dispossessed of certain interests and objects, the other that the self's primary interest is in possessing as many objects as possible. In either case, the self and its interests are assumed to exist separately from objects or goods pursued. Adherents of the self-assertion school tend to regard *interests* as fixed drives to possess certain external goods, and as fundamentally asocial, or even anti-social.[63] When we attend to the processes through which the self is continually formed and reformed, we cannot continue to consider interests in this manner. It is truer to experience to picture a self that takes shape through a series of transactions or interactions with the natural and social environment. This view is consistent with findings from studies of infant and child development.[64] At birth we are primed to relate to our environment. From the beginning, we differentiate between persons to whom we relate on terms of mutuality (not, primarily, drive- or need-satisfaction), and objects with which other kinds of relations are appropriate.

If selves vary with their objects, and interests vary with the social environment, then, in matters of self-interest, the crucial questions will concern the nature (or character) of the self served, and the nature (or character) of the social environment.[65] In general, there is a division of labor that makes it both natural and right that our chief responsibilities flow to maintaining ourselves and those with whom we are most intimately involved. At the same time, morality requires us to cultivate the widest possible sphere of attention, concern, and responsiveness.

Instincts are morally neutral: an instinct of sympathy, or acquisitiveness, is open to variable development, and its expression may be socially valuable, or damaging. One can, for example, harm others by seeking to do too many things to them or for them. (This is a special hazard of philanthropy, which posits an identity of interests between benefactor and recipient.) Yet sympathy is less neutral than the other instincts. To paraphrase St. Paul, the greatest of the instincts are the social affections, because they have the power to transform all the others. "When an interest in power is permeated with an affectionate impulse, it is protected from being a tendency to dominate and tyrannize; it becomes an interest in *effectiveness of regard for common ends.*"[66]

The moral life calls for a kind of "disinterested interest" that neither disregards nor inappropriately narrows the concerns of the self, nor denies others their appropriate independence. This is not apathy or lack of interest, but rather interest affected by concern for others. It is the habit of considering the consequences of one's actions for others *as part of what matters to oneself* in any deliberation.

As for acquisitiveness, a long line of philosophers, including Aristotle and John Rawls, regards excessive concern with external goods as a kind of moral failure. These same philosophers regard great wealth as a moral hindrance, without denying the value of material comforts or the necessity of a certain level of material welfare for a moral life. Turn-of-the-century religious reformers feared that wealth would render capitalism's winners insensitive to the common lot, removing any constraints of fellow-feeling that might prevent the deployment of wealth "to distort the structures of the common life for private ends."[67] There is some evidence of a correlation between privilege and insensitivity to the misery of others in the deMeurers case. Roger Greaves and Malik Hasan inhabit a different world from the middle-class deMeurerses, let alone the poor.

In his manifesto against acquisitiveness, British economic historian and social critic R. H. Tawney emphasized the scandal of disproportion, describing the executive's bloated income in terms of the number of families that might support themselves with his salary: "It is true that special talent is worth any price, and that a payment of £10,000 a year to the head of a business with a turnover of millions is economically a bagatelle. But economic considerations are not the only considerations. There is also 'the point of honor.' The truth is that these hundred-family salaries are ungentlemanly."[68] Even allowing for inflation, and translation between currencies, Roger Greaves's $8.9 million salary must qualify as ungentlemanly.

The terminology may be quaint, but there is something attractive about this holdover from a morality of personal honor and social seemliness. There is something unseemly in the contrast between the stinginess some managed care executives display in relation to patient care or provider payments, and their lavish compensation packages. *Wall Street Journal* writer George Anders cleverly labels these executives the "barons of austerity." Anders recounts how one baron, Dan Crowley of Foundation Health, led the industry in 1994 with a compensation package valued at $19 million (a pittance by today's standards). The deal provoked outrage, and the next year Crowley accepted a more modest package. In a speech to a physician group, Crowley conceded, "In this environment, it's doggone piggy to put your face that far in the trough when other people are hurting."[69]

I would distinguish the plea for disinterested interest from a call for continual evaluation of one's conduct to determine whether others are being maximally benefited. Under ordinary conditions, being absorbed in one's work—if it is good work—requires no apology. In health care, the philanthropic ethic and the incentivizing strategy both upset this condition of moral health by forcing the question of who benefits in everyday clinical encounters.

The phrase "good, cost-effective medicine" expresses the hope that legitimate concerns about resource use can be integrated into medicine on terms other than the repeated weighing of "my benefit versus yours." This cannot happen where there are direct financial conflicts of interest between clinician and patient. With the removal of obvious conflicts, we can imagine forms of health care organization adapted to changed conditions, yet permitting practitioners to do good work.

THE LIMITS OF HUMAN FREEDOM AND PROSPECTS FOR SOCIAL REFORM

For Dewey and his heirs, freedom is an interstitial phenomenon *within* nature and culture. This may be an undramatic view, but precisely because nature and culture are not fixed, intelligent social reform becomes a genuine possibility.

For pragmatist theologian and Dewey critic Reinhold Niebuhr, a specifically human freedom is freedom *over* nature and culture. The creature gains an awareness of its creatureliness and its transcendence simultaneously—and becomes hostage to its insecurity. The combination of finitude and freedom, and the insecurity to which it gives rise, confer on human wants and desires a certain inordinateness. This inordinateness of human wants and desires continually confounds the rationalists and upsets the plans of the social reformers. Freedom and our ambivalence towards it, as much as our creatureliness, limit the possibilities for social progress.

History has proved Niebuhr more right than Dewey on the recalcitrance of human beings to moral improvement, and Niebuhr's attribution of this recalcitrance to insecurity created by an awakening to one's finitude is credible. How many moral failures can we trace to either fear or greed? And what underlies these two, but insecurity? Still, our freedom may be more modest and more bound up with nature and culture, for good or ill, than Niebuhr allowed. Insecurity is a social as well as an individual, or purely personal, phenomenon: "Fear of loss of work, dread of the oncoming of old age, create anxiety and eat into self-respect."[70] Social isolation and loneliness intensify fear.

SELF-GIVING AND COMMON GRACE

Even if the tendency to limit my "self" to "*my* self" (over against or in competition with others) is a stronger part of our constitution than we like to admit, it remains true that direct concern for others is a genuine possibility arising in and through developing relationships; that development is itself a vitally important feature of the moral life. In a late work, *Man's Nature and His Communities,* in an essay entitled "Man's Selfhood in Its Self-Seeking and Self-Giving," Niebuhr developed a notion of "common grace" that ventures in that direction.[71] Common grace is "the power of responsibilities and affections to draw the self beyond itself, and thus create the conditions for self-fulfillment, which a consistent drive for self-realization can not accomplish and which always leads to self-defeat."[72] It is grace mediated through parental affection, help from others in a crisis, and the demands of a situation in which we find the strength to help others.

I cannot offer assurance through the perspective presented here that the person of good character will be impervious to economic or social pressures. On the other hand, neither do I offer much comfort to those who would create a system of economic and social pressures so precisely calibrated that conduct is perfectly conformed to the intentions of the designers and character is rendered superfluous.

We cannot afford to ignore incentives, but neither can we afford to rely on incentives alone to achieve our ends. Further, we have reason to guard against the transformations in our relations with others that occur when we get into the habit of regarding them solely as means to our own ends. Niebuhr's notion of common grace provides one way of understanding how true freedom and community might develop together, in complementarity.

MORAL SOCIOLOGY: ORGANIZATIONS

Sociologists often distinguish between organizations, meaning groups or associations that have reached a certain stage of formalization, and institutions as broad social phenomena (e.g., the family, the church). We can also use the concept of institution in a developmental scheme to suggest the formation of a distinctive corporate identity and culture.

Sociologist Philip Selznick, one of the founders of the "institutional school" of organizational theory, uses pragmatist ideas and ideals to study this process. Selznick describes institutionalization as "the emergence of orderly, stable, *socially integrating* patterns out of unstable, loosely organized, or narrowly technical activities." He calls organizations that display such patterns institutions.[73] As a move toward *relative* fixity and permanence, institutionalization carries with it the problem of achieving the appropriate balance between preserving identity and being receptive to change. We can use the concept of community to describe the culmination of the process of institutionalization in a sense of shared history and purpose within an organization, and the development of relations of interdependence with encircling communities.[74]

Some have criticized the institutional school for failing to devote sufficient attention to conflict. Organizational theorist Charles Perrow writes that "there is no 'community' value; there is only the conflict of group interests."[75] This seems half right. There are groups and their interests conflict. By using "community" to refer to an organization or its concerns, we do not magically confer unity on a body of diverse individuals and groups. At the same time, some interests are widely shared and can serve as the basis for alliances across groups, while others are truly community interests, in the sense that they reflect aspirations for the community (or society) as a whole. We can link interests to values that are similarly generous in scope.

It is important to ask whose values and interests are being served by a specific organization or organizational practice. But "community values and interests" should not be removed from the list of possible answers to the question.

Organizational Agency and Responsibility

The ascription of moral agency and responsibility to organizations is the subject of ongoing debate in legal and philosophical circles. The pragmatist's approach is to ask, "What difference does it make?"[76] First, why might one resist this ascription?

Some might argue that applied to organizations rather than to persons, these concepts simply do not make sense. Analogies between persons and social groupings go back at least as far as Plato. Persons and organizations are obviously similar in some ways and different in others. Lacking easy answers, we must look more closely at the particular concepts and what they entail.

What does moral agency suggest with persons? Very generally, some level of competence or ability to effect consequences in accordance with purposes, and some level of accountability. Accountability means that other agents may (rationally) demand an account.

An organization clearly has the ability to bring about consequences in accordance with collective purposes. The organization can only act through persons, but the actions of those persons are shaped by the fact that they act with others, and by tangible and intangible aspects of the organization such as plant, equipment, rules, and policies. People act differently when they act in coordinated fashion: "the attributes, successes, and failures of organizations are phenomena that emerge from the coordination of persons' attributes and . . . explanations of such phenomena require categories of analysis and description beyond the level of the individual."[77]

As for accountability, it would be irrational to demand an account from a tree that happened to shed a branch on your head. The tree isn't going to respond. It would be nonsensical to ascribe moral agency to a tree; there are limits to intelligibility. It would not be irrational to demand an account from a corporation that polluted your town's well.

The corporation can respond, in two ways. It can issue a press release or write you a letter, acting through persons who would not do what they do were it not for their roles in the corporation. It can also change how it operates to avoid further pollution and compensate the town for the harm, or oppositely, it can refuse to change or provide compensation. So the description of organizations as moral agents is not senseless.

If moral agency makes sense, then moral responsibility likely will also. Moral responsibility is usually associated with terms like rationality and respect. In a classic article on business ethics, Kenneth Goodpaster and John Matthews argue that rationality and respect, in organizational terms, would include things like assessing social costs and benefits, justice in distributing goods and services, recognizing basic rights and duties, and being faithful to contracts.[78] Of course, intelligibility is not the only consideration. There may be other reasons to oppose extending these concepts to organizations.

REASONS AGAINST ASCRIBING AGENCY AND RESPONSIBILITY TO ORGANIZATIONS

Some may fear that if we grant organizations moral agency and responsibility, we may also need to credit them with moral rights in competition with individual rights.[79] I consider this fear misplaced. People acting collectively or in association should have moral rights, claims to be free of state interference, and so on. To be effective, these rights must attach to the association. If the community is more than an aggregate of individuals, if the whole is greater than the sum of its parts, then communal goods can only be protected by protecting the community itself. That said, treating an association—at least one that has reached a certain level of formal organization—as a moral agent bearing moral responsibility does not add to its moral rights. The rules, policies, plant, and equipment do not somehow become endowed with moral claims that float free of the people whose cooperative project the organization is.[80]

Another objection might be that if we ascribe moral responsibility to organizations, we will erode individual moral responsibility. People will begin to believe they are less responsible, or people may actually *become* less responsible in the sense that, given the scope of their agency within an organization, we cannot properly blame them for harms or wrongs.

If a manufacturing plant pollutes a town's well due to a series of oversights, minor mistakes, and design failures all down the line, there may be no one individual or group of individuals to blame. If there is an erosion of individual moral responsibility in this sense, it is occurring regardless of our terminology. We must focus on belief, and on the fear that using moral language in relation to organizations will deaden the sense of individual responsibility. I can only stress that this need not happen.

There is no reason why we cannot hold on to individual responsibility while asking how to reform organizations to lessen the risk of malpractice or malfeasance. Opportunities for dual attribution of responsibility arise repeatedly in the context of managed care, where organizational policies may render practitioners more or less likely to make certain kinds of mistakes or to engage in certain kinds of wrongdoing.

REASONS FOR ASCRIBING AGENCY AND RESPONSIBILITY TO ORGANIZATIONS

If all of this is true, what affirmative reasons can we offer for using the language of moral agency and moral responsibility in relation to organizations? We might want to use this language precisely to draw attention to organizational features connected with wrongful conduct, and to effect change. If I say that an HMO such as Health Net is morally responsible for administrative practices that contribute to the suffering of member-patients such as Christine de-Meurers, I am saying no more than that the consequences of actions taken in the name of the organization should be better assessed, that there should be more attention to justice, a fuller recognition of rights and obligations, and a greater conscientiousness in contractual matters—and that the organization must remedy any failures.

Managers should be urged to consider consequences beyond the company's short-term financial performance. Like cases should be treated alike. Doctors and managed care plan managers alike must recognize the rights and obligations attached to the doctor-patient relationship. Managed care plans must promptly honor contractual provisions that appear to promise a benefit to plan members. These corrections will require changes in policies, procedures, hiring practices, reward systems, and the like. In other words, organizational structures, and not merely minds and hearts, will have to be changed.

Understanding Organizational Agency

ORGANIZATIONAL STRUCTURES

In order to understand better the moral agency of organizations, we need to pay more attention to organizational structures. To use the standard terminology, organizations always consist of both "formal" and "informal" structures.[81] Formal structures are the norms and behavior patterns that exist regardless of the characteristics of the individual actors, such as the hierarchy reflected on organizational charts, the organization's decision-making structure, its rules and roles, its system of financial incentives and rewards, and its mission statement and code of ethics. Informal structures reflect the personal characteristics or resources of specific participants. Informal structures include such items as the regular gripe sessions in the break room or the enormous power wielded by the administrative assistant who has made himself the gatekeeper for the CEO.

Theorists may view the informal structure as an impediment to implementing the formal design, or as a corrective for its inadequacies. For example, we may credit informal structures with easing communication, facilitating trust, or sabotaging critical policies. Those who view organizations as natural systems emphasize the limits of formal structures: "No planners are so foresighted or omniscient as to be able to anticipate all the possible contingencies that might confront each position in the organization. Attempts to program in advance the behavior of participants are often misguided, if not foolhardy. Such programming can easily become maladaptive and lead to behaviors both ineffective and inefficient. . . . Further, formal arrangements that curtail individual problem solving and the use of discretion undermine participants' initiative and self-confidence, causing them to become alienated and apathetic."[82]

INTEGRATING FORMAL AND INFORMAL STRUCTURES:
THE EXAMPLE OF CARING

Formal and informal structures may be more or less integrated with one another. In an interesting article relevant to the issue of structural integration, sociologist David Mechanic and colleagues assert that caring can be defined in cognitive, affective, and behavioral terms; that people can learn how to express it; and that medical practice can be organized, administered, and financed in ways that will cultivate and sustain it.[83] They argue that caring is undermined by some common formal and informal structures, including quantitative approaches to cost-containment, specialization, the assignment of nurses to wards rather than to patient panels, and the antagonism and poor communication between physicians and nurses.

Mechanic and his co-authors make two major recommendations. First, they suggest better training and supervision of staff using models developed in the service industries. They find deficiencies in this area across the medical hierarchy, but they are especially struck by the tendency to ignore the training needs of personnel who have patient contact but little power or education. Second, they suggest better reimbursement for cognitive services (talking with patients). Especially in these cost-conscious times, they believe it is essential to stress that caring is the task of the entire organization, meaning each person who has contact with a patient. Consistent caring can become a reality only if staff develop a different understanding of their work; socialization processes, specific policies, and the organization of work will have to be changed.

MEDICAL ETHICS AND THE NEGLECT OF INFORMAL STRUCTURES

Medical ethicists, to the extent that they have been organizationally aware, have tended to focus on mechanisms associated with the formal structure, that is, codes of ethics, and written policies and procedures. Policies concerning topics such as conflicts of interest, marketing, admission, transfer, discharge, billing practices, and relationships with other institutions are now being crafted in response to the inclusion of "organizational ethics" in standards for accreditation. The accreditation manual published by the Joint Commission on Accreditation of Healthcare Organizations suggests that most of these issues can be satisfactorily addressed by adding to the organization's existing code of ethics.[84] Yet we have evidence that codes of ethics, especially codes of ethics that are poorly institutionalized, are mostly irrelevant to practice.[85] Indeed, it is hard to see how they could have much effect, when members of an organization may not know that they exist, likely did not participate in their development, and have little notion of their implications for day-to-day activity. Ethicists must become much more sensitive to organizational complexity.

Organizational Character and its Assessment

The concept of character, like the concept of moral agency, can be used in relation to organizations as well as persons. Character can refer to "the commitments that help to determine the kinds of tasks an organization takes on, the opportunities it creates or closes off, the priorities it sets, and the abuses to which it is prone."[86] Character for an organization resembles character for a person. Both are transactional and historical in nature. Both link being and doing, combine controlled (planned) and uncontrolled (unplanned) elements, and allow for some interpenetrating of elements without demanding unity. Finally, both are highly variable. Every individual has a character, but character differs dramatically across individuals, along dimensions of coherence and goodness. The same is true for organizations.

Goodpaster and Matthews observe that "when we look about us, we can readily see differences in moral responsibility among corporations in much the same way that we see differences among persons. Some corporations have built features into their management incentive systems, board structures, internal control systems, and research agendas that in a person we would call self-control, integrity, and conscientiousness. Some have institutionalized awareness and concern for consumers, employees, and the rest of the public in ways that others clearly have not."[87]

INTEGRITY AND RESPONSIVENESS

Integrity and responsiveness are key aspects of organizational character. They are "virtues" that address two of the morally problematic features of organizations identified by Alasdair MacIntyre: the tendency of those in organizations to lose sight of internal goods in their pursuit of external goods, and the constriction of the time horizon in corporate planning.

Integrity is an inward-looking virtue. It requires the appropriate maintenance of boundaries, of identity. It also looks at the articulation of inwardness, that is, how organizational structures fit together, or fail to do so. Responsiveness is an outward-looking virtue. It requires the appropriate disruption of boundaries, in consideration of the associated or social nature of persons and organizations. It also directs attention to structures—structures that keep an organization open to those it affects within and without, and structures that allow it to adapt to a changed environment.

INTEGRITY AND THE RISK OF ORGANIZATIONAL SURRENDER

Integrity begins with being faithful to self-defined principles. To use integrity as a test of organizational character, one must begin by identifying the organization's mission and principles, and then evaluate the organization's structures and practices against that standard. Integrity implies wholeness, soundness, and coherence, but not, as Selznick says, "coherence of every sort." The coherence sought is moral coherence. Hence, we must distinguish integrity from simple consistency. Consistency "asks too little if it does not require judgment based on the integration of purpose, policy, and implementation; it asks too much because integrity is not sacrificed merely because decisions are highly circumstantial, selective, or for other reasons do not follow a definite pattern."[88]

These distinctions ensure that judging integrity will be no simple matter. It is no accident that proponents of the institutional school favor detailed case studies, or that Selznick himself wrote a well-known case study of the Tennessee Valley Authority (TVA). Selznick chronicled how the TVA's official doctrine or ideology favoring "grass roots" democracy took shape in practice in the ceding of certain areas of its mandate to local agencies. Representatives of local agencies were appointed to key administrative posts within the TVA, assuring that there would be no internal checks to the turn-over of authority and responsibility to their former associates. The local agencies, as might have been expected, tended to favor established interests. In particular, the aid channeled through the TVA actually reinforced existing patterns of racial segregation and economic inequality. As Selznick made clear, all of this occurred without any real villains. Further, the doctrine of grass roots involvement had and has substantial moral and tactical appeal; and not all compromise is anathema to the pragmatist.

Selznick pinpointed a breach in organizational integrity as the key factor that set the course from compromise to capitulation: "This was not a case of simple compromise made by an organization capable of retaining its internal unity. Rather, a split in the character of the agency was created. As a result, the TVA was unable to retain control over the course of the basic compromise. Concessions were demanded and won which may not have been essential if there had been fundamental unity within the organization." *"If there is a practical lesson for leadership here, it is this: if you have to compromise, guard against organizational surrender."*[89]

This warning is not without weight at a time when many mission-guided agencies are tempted to make deals with for-profit companies. As described by their promoters, some of these deals seem too good to be true: ready access to capital and assurances that cherished values will be respected. The deal may be *that* good, but common sense skepticism is often justified.

ACHIEVING BALANCE: INTERNAL AND EXTERNAL GOODS

Still, any organization that neglects capital needs entirely is not long for this world.[90] Although those guiding an organization must be vigilant in guarding against surrendering its integrity, they do not compromise integrity by recognizing money's value in furthering good works. Recall MacIntyre's handling of the distinction between internal and external goods.

Internal goods are intrinsically related to social practices and cannot be separated from the specific activities that constitute a practice. To use an example from medical practice, the exhilaration of arriving at the correct diagnosis following the careful detective work involved in taking a history, ordering appropriate tests, and interpreting the results in light of the history, belongs to just this sequence of activities. It cannot be purchased.

External goods such as money lack an intrinsic connection to any particular activity. Yet they are genuine goods. Without some level of external goods, social practices could not continue. Physicians could not practice medicine apart from social institutions, not just medical schools and hospitals, but all the organizations linked to the financing and material support of medical work. Of course, on occasion, a physician may work with little immediate assistance.

Tension arises because the quest for external goods, initially sought to support particular practices, is constantly threatening to distort or undermine those very practices and damage their internal goods. A vicious cycle can result, in which the loss of internal goods stimulates the quest for external goods. This leads to the further erosion of internal goods, compensated for with yet more external goods, and so on.

Many fear that this cycle is currently in motion in health care. Salaried physicians meet with demands for greater productivity. They must squeeze more and more "patient encounters" into a workday. Genuine conversations with others, patients or colleagues, become out of the question.

Practitioners begin to resent external monitoring and criticism, even when justified. For those compensated through capitation rather than salary, every patient becomes an object of suspicion. The patient is either a potential loss, someone with a serious health problem that will eat into the physician's income, or a potential waste of time, someone with a trivial complaint determined to get the attention she (or her employer or the government) has paid for.

As satisfactions derived from good work and meaningful personal relationships diminish, bonuses and other financial incentives become increasingly significant. But if one is to receive greater financial rewards, one must learn how to manipulate patients and others with greater finesse. One must become adept at "churning," "cherry-picking" or "cream-skimming," and "buffing" and "turfing." Churning involves increasing the revisit rate of existing patients more than is medically necessary; it tends to occur where the reward system emphasizes productivity. At the physician level, "cherry-picking" and "cream-skimming" are labels for culling sick patients from one's practice in order to make one's utilization profile look better. "Buffing" is making this practice appear justifiable, and "turfing" is transferring the sickest patients to other physicians participating in the plan.

The same kinds of processes may operate at the organizational level. As competition becomes fiercer, the object of winning more "covered lives" (taking in more premium dollars), while spending as little as possible on health care, predominates. Everywhere one seems to find confirmation of the Darwinism of Herbert Spencer. Plan marketers court large employers assiduously. The plan puts a quality improvement program in place, since this is a major selling point. But because appearance rather than substance is the concern, plan managers "teach to the test." They work hard to improve quality, but only in the areas specifically covered by the standardized report card. Marketing and administrative costs increase. Since premiums may not increase, plan managers apply additional pressure to physicians to hold down costs and absorb more risk.

A physician may agree to live with more "downside" risk, but only on condition that she receive a greater share in the "upside" profit, if she succeeds in further increasing productivity or shrinking utilization. Here profit-sharing is not a path to greater solidarity or a way of rewarding good work, but rather the instrument for destroying a sense of collegiality and other practice values. The two cycles feed one another. The only possible way out is to step back and to reconsider personal and organizational commitments. The only way to secure fragile goods against displacement is to institutionalize protections.

RESPONSIVENESS AND RESPONSIBILITY
The virtue of responsiveness is a potential counter to the virtue of integrity. Some other factors that may work against integrity lack moral weight. The mad scramble for external goods, and the "successful" operation of the organization on terms inconsistent with its mission and principles, have little moral dignity. The appropriate response is institutionalizing a process of recollection and restraint to restore balance. But concerns about integrity do not absolve an organization of responsibility for addressing new problems, taking account of the effects of new forces in the environment, and considering new claims and expectations. Responsiveness is an aspect of moral responsibility, of thinking of a person or organization as responsible to and for others.

Responsiveness requires that an organization avoid insularity without embracing opportunism, here in the form of "uncontrolled adaptation" or capitulation to pressure.[91] There is an element of integrity in responsiveness, and vice versa. Being responsible means being reliable. Stakeholders, either inside or outside an organization, cannot rely on managers who yield to every pressure or follow every fad. On the other hand, integrity is a hollow virtue if it exists "for itself."

DEFINING THE SCOPE OF RESPONSIBILITY
The assumption that organizations must be either persons or (moral) nullities has been a great barrier to the appropriate regulation of organizations and organizational behavior. I have argued that some responsibilities are organizational rather than individual. Identifying the corporation with one set of individuals, the shareholders, has had an especially pernicious effect on corporate rationality, as what is rational for shareholders, or certain shareholder groups, may not be rational for the organization as a whole or the larger community, e.g., takeover and looting. Such concerns have fueled a debate over the meaning of "corporate social responsibility." In what relation does the corporation stand to the needs and interests of the community?

Opinion ranges from Milton Friedman's pronouncement that the responsibility of business is to increase its profits, to a kind of casual volunteerism, to traditional arts-oriented philanthropy, to proposals for active corporate involvement in bettering life in all segments of the community, including projects such as single-handedly taking responsibility for rehabilitating the hard-core unemployed in a particular region. Selznick argues for a kind of responsibility anchored in identity: "The moral responsibility of the enterprise, like that of the natural person, runs primarily to the control *of its own conduct* (1) in the light of how its activities affect the community, especially those persons, institutions, and values in which it is directly implicated, and (2) in the light of its internal morality, that is, of the ends and means to which it is committed."[92]

RESPONSIVENESS AND REPRESENTATION

To frame the issue in terms of values is to reject the carry-over of interest group democracy from the political to the private sphere. Frequently, institutionalizing responsiveness begins, and ends, with appointing representatives of major constituencies to the board of directors. This sort of group representation may seem to follow from the shift in focus from stockholders to stakeholders, but it can have unfortunate consequences. At its worst, it becomes a kind of tokenism that makes values totally irrelevant, so long as each of the most vocal groups in the community is represented on the decision-making body and hence "has its say." It is a tricky issue, since the tokenism label may be used to challenge every attempt to extend the range of values brought to bear on the operations of an organization, or to close the organization to those who criticize its practices.

What is required is a sense of balance. Persons who do not share the central commitments of the organization ought not to become a part of it. Their efforts are better directed to founding an alternative organization that reflects their own commitments or working to regulate the existing organization if they think its operations are sufficiently harmful. Within the circle of those who largely share the organization's commitments, every effort should be made to gather persons with different life experiences for committees and boards. This will require conscious effort on the part of corporate leaders and some overcoming of resistance, as we tend to surround ourselves with people who are like us. There need be no intent to discriminate, only a normal desire for comfort that has injurious consequences in organizational contexts.

Collecting a diversity of experience ensures that policy discussions will be full and rich, while agreement on basic values and principles ensures that policy debates will not degenerate into unwieldy free-for-alls. The goal is to create space for communication and mutual correction. If deliberation becomes nothing more than a contest of wills, decision-making will become arbitrary or empty, as in the case of decision by failure to decide. Where stalemates are common, those charged with guiding or governing the organization are in effect neutralized.[93]

RESISTING THE CULTURE OF SHORTSIGHTEDNESS

Even if a board is composed of persons who combine commitment to values and principles with awareness of the needs and interests of the community, the organization can go astray if no other steps are taken to institutionalize responsiveness. Many factors narrow the field of concern for managers and their subordinates. MacIntyre, Selznick, and many others have claimed that American management participates in a culture of shortsightedness. A number of developments, including a relative decline in spending on research and development, choice of imitative over innovative product designs, recruitment of leaders from finance and law rather than based on specific knowledge of, and commitment to, production and technology, and a preoccupation with mergers and acquisitions, have tended to reinforce one another.[94] One might also mention mobility within and across organizations. Executives and managers often make decisions that are economically and socially costly in the long run, because they expect to be elsewhere when the costs are incurred.[95]

Only structural changes, such as adjustments to the internal reward system, modification of employee recruitment and retention policies, and retraining of managers, can ameliorate the time horizon problem. Yet it is difficult to see how a single organization, or even a number of organizations acting separately, can hold out against a culture that dominates the "resource system"[96] and is enshrined in significant practices.

These practices may or may not have been intended to orient businesses toward short-term financial results. Some critics point to the influence of modern accounting as a culprit. Developed primarily for external financial reporting, contemporary accounting practices emphasize direct labor costs and short-term returns, structuring thinking in terms of fiscal quarters rather than years or decades.[97] The critics argue, in effect, that a socially destructive restriction of time (and space) has been the unintended by-product of attempts to increase accountability and information flow. What was unintended initially has now been taken up enthusiastically.[98]

INSTITUTIONAL ISOMORPHISM

If such practices are becoming more widespread in health care, does this constitute evidence of a link between short-term thinking and economic efficiency, if not more strictly moral desiderata? Arguably, no. Two scholars of organizations, Paul DiMaggio and Walter Powell, observe that "bureaucratization and other forms of organizational change occur as the result of processes that make organizations more similar, without necessarily making them more efficient." They argue, persuasively, that "[t]he ubiquity of certain kinds of structural arrangements can more likely be credited to the universality of mimetic processes than to any concrete evidence that the adopted models enhance efficiency" and that "[t]o the extent that organizational effectiveness is enhanced, the reason will often be that organizations are rewarded for being similar to other organizations in their fields."[99] Among the factors that predict "isomorphic" change are the centralization of the supply of vital resources, uncertain technology, ambiguous goals, and a scarcity of visible alternative organizational models.[100] These factors clearly operate in health care.

Two points are especially important here. First, the focus on short-term results provides good evidence that such practices are rewarded by "resource suppliers," i.e., Wall Street and government, and not much else. A study of six health plans and three markets, Boston, Los Angeles, and Philadelphia, found informants agreed in their identification of the high-quality plans in their respective areas. However, plans with poor local reputations for quality continued to expand, usually through mergers and acquisitions. Market success was also poorly correlated with performance judged by financial and organizational stability. The researchers concluded that pressures toward consolidation and for-profit status often stimulated the growth of managed care groups with the characteristics of poor-quality HMOs: domination by a large parent company, a mixed model structure resulting from acquisitions and mergers, and a lack of managerial stability. Size allowed these HMOs to strong arm providers and underprice smaller, better performing HMOs, driving them out of business. Indeed, the researchers reported "growing concern that the best-performing and most highly-regarded HMOs may not be the ones that survive."[101]

Consider what happened to managed care giant U.S. Healthcare (since acquired by Aetna, since merged with Prudential Health Care) when it announced plans to increase physician compensation to improve the quality of its networks. The company had managed a medical-loss ratio of just 68 percent in the fourth quarter of 1994; the announcement of the quality improvement initiative came in April of 1995. Within a two-day period following the announcement, U.S. Healthcare's stock price "tumbled," wiping out more than $1 billion in shareholder value.[102] This was a powerful sanction against deviation from the short-term perspective. Although investors merit consideration, even they are not necessarily well-served by companies that bow to this kind of pressure.

Second, even if the short-term focus has unfortunate consequences, moral or economic, and likely both, it will be difficult to alter it absent changes in the attitudes and behavior of investors and administrators of government programs. What, then, can organizations and individuals do? They might define their own goals with greater care, and work to increase the visibility of alternative organizational models, while working to change attitudes and behavior through alliances with like-minded others.

The Pedagogical Role of Organizations

In *A Theory of Justice,* John Rawls initially defines an institution as a system of rules. But he later describes institutions as agencies of character formation or pedagogues.[103] From a pedagogical standpoint, the incentivizer's use of organizational structures to shape behavior in accordance with a simple reward/punishment paradigm is wrongheaded, and dangerous. Hope of reward and fear of punishment are powerful motivators, but actions performed on their account are seldom considered praiseworthy. More importantly, appealing regularly to such motives weakens rather than strengthens the disposition to do what is right.[104]

We can best understand external rewards and sanctions as reinforcements for ethical conduct. Conduct is "ethical" not merely because it conforms to certain norms, but because it expresses or enacts good character. Organizations are valuable and valued not merely for what they produce but for the conduct and character they form and the kinds of social relationships they foster. Organizations should make us aware of the realities of association, awake to the rights of others and the demands they appropriately make upon us. They should foster a sense of obligation to respect those rights and demands, a virtue termed fidelity or faithfulness. They should also cultivate character traits such as openness and truthfulness that may alleviate the problems of role fragmentation and organizational opacity and create conditions more conducive to cooperation than manipulation.[105]

FAITHFULNESS

Human relationships depend on trust. In forming relationships, we commit ourselves to a course of conduct and assume obligations to others. We seek to assure others that we will be faithful in honoring our commitments, and we seek to strengthen ourselves to be faithful. Likewise, we entrust ourselves to others in the hope that they, too, will be faithful.

Relationships create expectations. These expectations are in part socially defined, and in part the result of the unique understandings and agreements of the particular individuals involved. When those we trust act contrary to our expectations, we feel betrayed. Finding faithfulness lacking, we may become faith*less*, experiencing a weakening of our sense of obligation to others, or a loss of the trust that permits us to establish new relationships. The deMeurers case illustrates how organizations may contribute to the erosion of faithfulness. Subjected to certain organizational structures, physicians and patients lose a sense of what they owe one another and fail to meet one another's expectations.[106]

Organizations aiming to create conditions conducive to faithfulness must do at least two things. First, they must value trust and recognize that it is easily destroyed and rebuilt only with great difficulty. Managed care organizations have become the targets of all of the frustrations people experience with the health care system and with large, impersonal bureaucracies. This is unfortunate insofar as it detracts from a balanced assessment and response, but it is scarcely undeserved. Many managed care organizations play on the fear and greed of physicians, thus undermining trust in clinical relationships. They have also failed to honor their own commitments to patients and providers.

Second, organizations that would foster faithfulness must contribute to the clarification of expectations and obligations. Public expectations of the health care system may be unrealistic. It may be that the obligations imposed on physicians must change in light of today's changed conditions. Faithfulness can survive the dispelling of illusions and the recognition of limits. It cannot survive seeming arbitrariness and subterranean maneuvering. Hence, faithfulness is linked to justice and to openness and truthfulness.

OPENNESS

Openness as sensitivity to the other is a mode of resistance to the fragmentation of the self into roles that set up moral blinders. It is important that organizational pressures not harden managers and clinicians to patient needs or cause them to ignore the promptings of their own moral sense.

Consider the case of Dr. Linda Peeno. Peeno was hired by a large managed care organization as a medical reviewer. She received a request to authorize a heart transplant. According to her own account, this is what happened:

> I sat at my desk, contemplating the paper given to me by the nurse, who had reminded me, in her dutiful way, that this was a "very expensive" case. I knew well by now what this euphemism meant: You better find a way to deny this. Medically this case was clear, with no grounds upon which I could issue a denial based on necessity. . . . I was left only with finding a loophole that would justify the denial of payment based on coverage limitations. A few quick calls to the benefit department about contracts in Nevada, and a review of the language in this man's own "certificate of coverage" gave me what I needed. . . . That this man, who I would never know, would fail to get his heart was of less importance to me at that moment than the accolades I would get when word spread that I saved the company several hundred thousand dollars.[107]

There is every reason to believe that Peeno was and is a person of sound character, but within a certain organizational environment she became desensitized.

Openness as sensitivity is nourished when managers are invited and even forced to consider the full human dimensions of what they do. Health care organizations should nurture an awareness in managers, clinicians, and patients of their personal responsibility to each of the "others" with whom they interact *as a person*. Ideally, the proximity of managers to clinicians and patients will support the contact that reminds managers of "what we're here for."[108]

The role of managed care utilization reviewer may render those who inhabit it particularly prone to an impersonality that goes beyond what the task demands. Fellowship with each and every plan member, or affiliated practitioner, may be precluded. This fact of life does not excuse callousness or brutality. Significant decisions should be given a human face, by power of sympathetic imagination and by periodic visits to sites where services are delivered.

TRUTHFULNESS

Organizations cultivate truthfulness by modeling it. At a minimum, health care organizations must communicate honestly when information is requested or disclosure is required. Merely honoring requests for information and meeting legal requirements is not enough, however. Health care organizations should substitute the communication paradigm for the disclosure paradigm wherever possible.

Organizations should open their operations to public view, especially when questions arise about how to handle a problem. The deMeurerses thought they were up against a network of institutions "managing" Christine deMeurers's case through channels that were not visible to them, and they responded by hiding information from health care providers. It is easier to adopt and honor a rule of openness if openness is already standard practice, if the organization does not shield important decisions from the public eye and publishes important policies so that dissenters and critics can have their say. This is also a way of addressing the problem of organizational opacity.[109]

ORGANIZATIONS AS SOURCES OF MORAL CORRUPTION
Niebuhr charged that Dewey and his fellow liberals failed to appreciate the "brutal" character of the behavior of all human groups, what Niebuhr called the "power of collective egoism" in intergroup relations.[110] He assumed that the characters of concrete human beings are radically separate from society, and that the character of collectivities is somehow fixed by the very nature of group dynamics. Rejecting Niebuhr's notion of radical freedom, one can still identify problematic features of groups, but these must be specified with care.

RELENTLESSNESS
Organizational theorist Richard Scott has identified relentlessness as the chief pathology of organizations. He uses the term to capture a number of organizational features, but his main point is that corporate interests are narrower than those of natural persons. Organizations are by no means monolithic, but compared with natural persons, they have relatively specialized purposes and they are (typically) intended and designed to pursue these purposes "unreservedly."[111] Yet, even here, the focus may change over time, escaping the intentions of the organization's founders.

POWER
Scott also believes that in the world of organizations, power is a non-zero sum game. He asserts that "in a social structure containing both natural persons and corporate actors, it is possible for one natural person to lose power [to an organization] without a corresponding gain on the part of another natural person."[112] But then, it is also possible for organizations to benefit natural persons by increasing their power without loss on the part of any natural person. We can accomplish things corporately that we cannot accomplish individually.

It is a mistake to regard power monolithically. We can distinguish among various types of power, with contrast pairs such as persuasive and coercive, emancipatory and manipulative, receptive and active, and shared and individual.[113] Power may liberate as well as oppress. Organizations may play a constructive role in relationships by supporting fluctuating or flagging individual commitments.[114] Organizations may provide the structures through which persons mediate common grace to one another.

The Individual and the Social

Even so, some may be inclined to regard the prospect of "organizations as pedagogues" apprehensively, as totalitarian. Some resistance *is* justified. In this account, justice serves as a brake on corporate power. I consider it important that social life is, and continue to be, pluralistic. In a dynamic universe, the options available for human consideration, judgment, and choice are present in the conflicting patterns in the realm of organizations. According to Dewey, the problem "is to extract the desirable traits of forms of community life which actually exist, and employ them to criticize undesirable features and suggest improvement."[115] Especially in modern, complex societies, a survey of organizations will offer up multiple patterns for organizing social relations.

The hope, at least, is that we can use the differences we discover to serve the cause of social transformation in morally desirable directions.[116] One kernel of truth in the medicine-business dichotomy lies here. Organizations do not confront us as an undifferentiated mass. There are significant differences in structure and purpose among them, related to different kinds of character, relationship, and practice.

Finally, I do not intend to deny the importance of the individual. Neither recognizing the fact of social dependence, nor embracing a social ethic, necessarily leads to rejecting individualism as a belief in the unique capacities and potentialities of each human being. The responsibility of individual actors for their own conduct need not disappear. I intend to make the case that *concentrated* social forces are extremely powerful; under certain conditions, they are irresistible. At the same time, such conditions rarely obtain.

If anything, I wish to stress that individuals are inclined to underestimate their personal power, or the power they could exercise allied with like-minded others, either because exerting power and organizing involves considerable effort, or because they are unwilling to risk some degree of hardship for themselves or their dependents. They exaggerate the effort required or the possible hardship to the point where it seems foolhardy to resist or to work for change. Less cynically, it is also true that sometimes people simply cannot imagine alternatives. One goal in exploring an array of organizations is to expose the range and texture of the alternatives, and to increase the visibility of certain neglected options.

FOUR

Kaiser Permanente
An Organizational Character Study

To my mind, the proper perspective of the social critic is that of the moral pragmatist. The latter does not shrink from symbolism nor does he reject the rhetoric of hope and aspiration. He knows that a steady diet of cynicism and self-doubt can be spiritually corrosive and politically enervating. Therefore he cannot forego ideology. Yet as a pragmatist he seeks never to lose his critical sensibility, never to stop asking whether the end he has in view or the means he uses are governed by truly operative criteria of moral worth. Therefore, he strives to think concretely, to look at real choices and trace their actual consequences. And the consequences he has most in mind are those that redound back on the character of the actor.
—Philip Selznick, Preface, *TVA and the Grass Roots*

If you've seen one HMO, you've seen one HMO.
—popular adage among health care analysts

Heeding Dewey's call to survey the field to "extract the desirable traits of forms of community life which actually exist," I will present a study of the character of one the oldest American managed care organizations, Kaiser Permanente. Such a choice might seem strange, since Kaiser is something of an anomaly—a group model, not-for-profit HMO in a market dominated by managed care organizations that are aggressively for-profit and have looser organizational structures.[1] I would defend the choice of Kaiser on a number of grounds.

First, Kaiser is important precisely as an aberration. By showing what might be, such anomalies destroy the illusion that only one mode of organization is possible. Also, organizations, like individuals, may have influence disproportionate to their size if they display virtues—and create structures or programs —that are capable of inspiring others. There are few Mother Theresas, but many "ordinary people" benefit from her example, even if they fail to emulate her life plan in all respects.

If one reason to study Kaiser is to demonstrate the viability of structures and practices that are different from, and possibly superior to, the norm, another reason is to explore what it has in common with other managed care organizations. In some ways, and to a greater extent than HMOs organized on the cooperative model, Kaiser is an attempt to marry big business and medicine.

Kaiser was formed to prove the worth of the managerial techniques of private industry in health care. Its struggles with the tensions inherent in that project over time are informative for other organizations traveling the same territory, albeit with somewhat altered conditions and objectives.[2] Further, managed care as such is associated with certain tensions. There are the strains created by attempts to control clinical practice through the development and implementation of guidelines and financial incentive plans, and the frustrations engendered by time constraints on communication, as well as the generic organizational tensions identified by MacIntyre and others.

Finally, in surveying the current health care landscape, we must guard against the tendency to think in terms of a static universe. One may assume that organizations are fixed entities within a stable typology. One may assume that the future of health care will be in line with the present, the property of for-profit health plans such as Health Net. Neither assumption is justified.

Organizations are continually evolving, often into strange hybrids that wreak havoc with our typologies. The present constrains the future but does not determine it. Change, even radical change, is possible, especially if there are major changes in the policies of third-party payers, legislators, and regulators. Arguably, federal policy towards HMOs has fostered the rapid growth of for-profit plans with network or independent practice association (IPA) structures over the last several decades.[3]

In sum, I turn to Kaiser to illustrate some of the ways in which managed care might improve health and health care *and* contribute to the development of community. I also turn to Kaiser to illustrate some of the perennial problems of organizations, as well as some of the ethical problems linked to managed health care. The case study method allows us to see, concretely, the force of ethicists' concerns about features of managed care such as reliance on cost-benefit or cost-effectiveness analysis. It also provides insight into the nature of the challenges faced by health care organizations with a sense of mission in a time of rapid change and great uncertainty. Finally, this case study should promote an enhanced appreciation of the dynamic nature of managed care itself.

KAISER PERMANENTE

The Kaiser Permanente Medical Care Program is one of the oldest and largest health maintenance organizations in the United States. Henry J. Kaiser, a prominent industrialist, founded the program in the 1930s to provide health care to workers in remote locations. In the 1940s, the program was opened to the public at large. It consists of the Kaiser Foundation Health Plan, a not-for-profit health plan corporation that enrolls members, manages finances, and maintains membership records, along with its regional subsidiaries; Kaiser Foundation Hospitals, a not-for-profit hospital corporation that owns and operates a number of hospitals and medical offices; and the regionally based Permanente Medical Groups, independent professional corporations composed of physicians who provide medical care to plan members. The corporate family also includes the Kaiser Permanente Center for Health Research, founded in the 1960s to conduct health services research at Kaiser facilities.

Given the current equation of managed care with the triumph of business over medicine in medical practice, it is interesting to note that in earlier rhetorical battles, advocates of managed care in the Kaiser style offered relief from business concerns as a selling point to physicians. For example, Herman Weiner, medical director and chairman of the board of the Southern California Permanente Medical Group in the 1970s, asserted, "We have taken the doctor out of the 'business' of being a doctor—freed him from the worries of paying rent, maintaining equipment, and meeting a payroll—and enabled him to establish doctor-patient relationships uncontaminated by any financial negotiations."[4]

Structurally, Kaiser's distancing of financial and administrative concerns from medical practice is reflected in the separation of the health plan and the hospital foundation from the medical groups. This arrangement is termed "duality of management," i.e., management responsibility resides with the experts in the functional area. Historically, conflict has been managed through a corporate culture that values and rewards the cooperative virtues in managers on both sides.[5] The physicians in a particular region determine leadership of the medical groups through periodic voting.

Kaiser currently boasts approximately 8 million members. Responding to an unprecedented decline in total membership in 1993, the organization instituted an aggressive growth strategy, resulting in a 19 percent membership increase in 1997. Due in part to the side effects of the expansion effort, Kaiser reported a $270 million net loss for 1997, the first net loss in its history. (National revenues for 1997 totaled $14 billion.)[6] The financial picture did not begin improving until the first quarter of 1999.

In the face of competition for patients and financial pressures, Kaiser tried modifying its organizational structure in significant ways. Responding to consumer demand, Kaiser introduced a point-of-service (POS) option that extends coverage to treatment received outside the Kaiser provider network, albeit at reduced levels. Kaiser also attempted to form networks of outside physicians. At the same time, the Permanente medical groups formed a new corporation with its own centralized administrative structure, a corporation that may contract with health plans other than Kaiser.[7] Kaiser has also formed an alliance with Group Health Cooperative of Puget Sound.

David M. Lawrence is the current chairman and chief executive officer of the Plan and Kaiser Foundation Hospitals. Before joining Kaiser, Lawrence served as a county health officer, an academic physician, and a Peace Corps doctor. Lawrence failed to join Greaves and Hasan on the list of managed care's ten highest paid executives for 1993; in 1994, at the time of the deMeureres' battle with Health Net, he earned a relatively modest $600,000.[8] Also in 1994, Lawrence gave an extensive interview to John Iglehart in which he shared his philosophy, and the philosophy of his organization.

An Interview with Kaiser's CEO

Referring, perhaps, to the organization of medical groups by region, Lawrence remarks that, "While we have a national presence, our health plans and physicians are community based, and they respond to local members and community needs."[9] Integration is central to the organization's identity, but this is distinct from centralized ownership and control. A prepaid, capitated payment covers a full range of services, "whether provided in a hospital, a doctor's office, or the patient's home," but these services are coordinated at the regional level.

Lawrence contrasts the Kaiser approach with that of the more common IPA-model HMOs, in which the planning of physicians, hospitals, and home health agencies is not directly tied to the health plan. Concerning Kaiser's not-for-profit status, he says, "The net income we generate is used solely for the benefit of members—to provide facilities, purchase medical technology, and fund health care research and innovations. This amount is planned, based on capital needs, and we make no attempt to maximize earnings." (On the other hand, under pressure from purchasers, Kaiser does attempt to minimize costs.[10])

Lawrence is an articulate spokesman for Kaiser and for its style of managed care. He also has a coherent vision. This becomes apparent in the course of the interview, as Lawrence and Iglehart tackle increasingly knotty issues.

Asked about using financial incentives in a managed care system, with the associated risks of undertreatment, Lawrence admits there are risks, "particularly in organizations in which the profit motive is dominant and understanding of health care delivery is minimal." On the other hand, he sees great opportunities for rationalizing health care delivery and promoting preventive services and early intervention in the disease process. Lawrence then takes issue with the question, for implying that the incentive effects of fee-for-service payment are benign. Lawrence adds that while we need to rely upon the character of health care professionals, government regulation is also necessary to assure that we detect and address the most egregious abuses.

Following up on Lawrence's reference to the profit motive, Iglehart asks if Kaiser really differs from for-profit managed care plans driven by bottom-line considerations. Lawrence responds:

> Absolutely. We are different in several ways. We operate on the social insurance, not the commercial insurance, side of the spectrum. We do not underwrite groups and have no preexisting condition exclusions for groups. We have always offered

to convert to an individual membership, without medical review, members who have lost their group coverage. We were forced by the market to abandon community rating and adopt adjusted community rating, which charges groups based on their past use and demographics. Even so, we placed an upper cap on the amount we charge small groups and individuals under adjusted community rating, and we established a dues subsidy program to subsidize the coverage of low-income persons.

Kaiser has clearly been unwilling to "go it alone" against increasingly severe economic pressures, to the point of institutional suicide. Kaiser is no martyr among organizations. At the same time, its distinctive commitments have shaped its response to market forces and to the environment generally.

Kaiser has tried to mitigate the negative consequences of its adaptation to market conditions. Lawrence's response stresses the ways in which Kaiser is structured to serve interests other than the generation of profit. Yes, Lawrence argues that Kaiser's dedication to social service distinguishes it from its for-profit competitors, and one may rightly be skeptical of such self-serving rhetoric. However, Lawrence anchors his argument in the various ways Kaiser has institutionalized its social commitment through specific policies and practices.

Iglehart also asks about the conflicts between "medicine" and "management," at Kaiser. He refers to battles between medical directors and plan managers over resource allocation. Lawrence replies that viewing the relationship exclusively in conflictual terms does not do justice to Kaiser's approach to allocation decisions. Kaiser's approach—by which Lawrence appears to mean a species of global budgeting and supply side controls[11]—does not eliminate all conflict, but rather creates agreement on broad principles that prevents conflict from escalating into warfare, or a mere contest of forces:

> Our approach—so greatly misunderstood by critics—involves changing the economics and delivery of health care so that it is possible to provide the right care at the right time and place. Management and medicine work together to achieve this kind of efficient, high-quality care with the appropriate consumption of resources. What happens when the quality of medical care is high? Costs go down. So managers and physicians have a common vision. While at times there may be dynamic negotiations between the medical directors and regional managers, this shared vision takes a lot of the unhealthy tension out of the relationship.
>
> From the member's point of view, being in a group-practice HMO means that physicians can truly be patient advocates, because individual clinical decisions do not directly affect physicians' income. Knowing that patients will not be financially burdened also frees physicians to base clinical decisions on what is medically appropriate and to provide care in the setting that best meets the patient's needs.

This presentation is no doubt simplistic. For example, it is hard to see any *straightforward* connection between high quality and low costs. The basic point seems to be that Kaiser has been at least partially successful in creating a system in which administrators and physicians, and physicians and patients, have reason to trust one another. There may still be conflict, but conflicts emerge against a background of agreement on certain shared principles and priorities.

The Ethics of Managed Care

Asked about the prospects for "professionalism" in health care, Lawrence provides information on how Kaiser compensates physicians. The leadership of each medical group determines base salary, which may be supplemented by limited incentive compensation related to regional financial performance, member satisfaction, and improvements in population health. Kaiser offers no incentives related to frequency of specialty referrals. When the medical group that serves Southern California proposed to extend incentives to nurses, nurse practitioners, and physician assistants, it drew the ire of the California Nurses Association (CNA). CNA leaders objected to the contamination of nursing by the sorts of conflicts of interest now common for physicians. Others might find this extension a welcome move toward greater egalitarianism among professionals in the health care field.[12] Perhaps suggesting a counter-trend, some Kaiser physicians have discontinued incentive payments for shortening hospital stays and prescribing less costly drugs.[13]

Clearly, members of the Kaiser organization are ambivalent about financial incentives. There is a sense that weak incentives, especially incentives tied to "quality," have generally positive effects, as prods to cost-awareness and the adoption of a true customer-service orientation. At the same time, there is fear that external incentives will erode internalized commitments to competence and compassion, and that patient trust in practitioners will suffer.

We need a reasonably clear specification of the meaning of "quality" to make meaningful comparative judgments among health plans. Yet agreement has proved elusive. Lawrence lists three critical elements of quality. The first is the relationship between patient and clinician. The second is the impact of care on populations and the application of knowledge concerning prevention, health education, and early intervention. We can measure effectiveness in this area by looking at mortality and morbidity rates by gender, age, and ethnicity. Cost is the third element and it is related to the second element: "Whether we are misusing those resources has a great deal to do with whether we will be able to meet the needs of various populations." Quality is related to accountability. Lawrence calls for a combination of government regulation and monitoring by what he calls "leading-edge employers," no doubt the kinds of corporations sophisticated enough to appreciate Kaiser's approach to health care.[14]

Lawrence concludes his comments on accountability by remarking that he would like to see the National Committee for Quality Assurance (NCQA) and similar organizations "expand their reviews to include the ethics of decision making related to benefits and care decisions—who makes the decisions, and by what process and ethical standards." Although some of Lawrence's statements would place him with rationalists who disdain moral language, this last comment is bound to endear him to ethicists and to those who believe that fact and value are intertwined. If "technical" or "scientific" judgments are also value judgments, then we must acknowledge this and openly discuss the values at stake. Explicitly incorporating ethical concerns into standards forces organizations to confront these issues, even if only in a cursory or superficial way.

Kaiser's Practices: Walking the Talk?

As I have said, Lawrence is an articulate spokesman for Kaiser.[15] This is a valuable quality in a leader. But the important question is whether Kaiser practices bear out his promises. The answer is yes—to a certain extent.

FINANCIAL INCENTIVES: THE CASE OF KIDNEY DIALYSIS

On the issue of financial incentives, there is evidence that Kaiser's integration of care and its mode of paying physicians, as aspects of Kaiser's distinctive corporate character, do make a difference.

In December 1995, the *New York Times* published a three-article series on kidney dialysis. The second article in the series focused on the practices of National Medical Care, at the time the largest provider in the competitive dialysis business in the United States. According to the *Times,* National Medical ensured the loyalty of kidney specialists by offering them profit sharing and extravagant perquisites. The supervisor of one clinic, a Dr. Roland, owned a Rolls Royce. National Medical reportedly paid for insurance on this vehicle and covered some of Roland's personal credit card bills as well. His partners were not pleased when they learned of this arrangement. "Worse," they discovered that National Medical "was also secretly splitting the clinic's profits with Dr. Roland: he was pocketing more than $250,000 a year, and in some years far more, for a few hours of work a week."[16]

Why was National Medical being so generous? Dialysis can be a very lucrative business. Payment is steady, since the federal government covers 80 percent of the total price tag for dialysis as a special item under the Medicare program. According to the *Times,* National Medical used old dialysis machines and reused disposable equipment to keep down costs. Dialysis providers in the United States have also been criticized for shifting duties from doctors and nurses to poorly trained, lower paid employees. Through profit sharing and more creative arrangements such as the one worked out with Roland, companies such as National Medical acquire access to the flow of patients controlled by kidney specialists and an "edge" on contracts to provide dialysis services to hospitals.

The *Times* reports that Roland's disgruntled partners eventually decided to do business with a new company started by defectors from National Medical. The new company, West Coast Medical Specialties, offered state-of-the-art dialysis machines, refused to reuse equipment, and offered better pay and benefits for nurses, along with profit sharing for physicians comparable to National Medical's. West Coast quickly attracted several hospital contracts, including three lured away from National Medical.

Displeased, National Medical severed its ties with Roland, and offered his old partners Roland's share of the spoils. The fickle partners promptly shifted allegiance back to National Medical. West Coast was reportedly informed that the partners, and their new patron, National Medical, would allow West Coast to keep the contracts it had already won, but only on condition that it not pursue any more contracts in the region. West Coast was awarded another contract, and was (reportedly) given an ultimatum: return the contract, or be driven out of business. West Coast refused to yield, and National Medical sued, accusing the company of stealing "trade secrets."

With the litigation in progress, West Coast's sources of funding dried up. The *Times* reports that National Medical used its size and financial muscle to dictate terms to area hospitals, which ensured it would get future contracts. Although we must treat the allegations summarized in this account cautiously, the article on National Medical Care at least points to some of the abuses that might arise in connection with fee-for-service payment.

According to the third article in the *Times* series, the annual mortality rate for dialysis patients in the United States is twice that of Japan and some European countries. But the picture is far from uniform. Government statistics reveal that Kaiser patients are hospitalized for less than a third as many days annually as the average dialysis patient, and are nearly twice as likely to work or attend school full-time. Further, even though Kaiser treats a larger-than-average number of difficult-to-treat diabetics, its annual mortality rate is sixteen percent, almost a third below the national average for all dialysis patients. Kaiser dialysis clinics do not reuse blood lines, and Kaiser lets patients choose between cleaned and reused dialyzers and new devices. (First use of new devices has been associated with adverse reactions.) Kaiser replaces its dialysis machines approximately every five years.

As an integrated health care system, Kaiser is motivated to keep patients out of the hospital; it knows it will end up paying the hospital bills. (In theory, an HMO could erect barriers to hospitalization, speeding its sickest and costliest dialysis patients to the grave. Its mortality statistics would suffer, but, in the past, HMOs have not been pressured routinely to disclose these rates.) Kaiser's *salaried* kidney specialists have no financial incentive to scrimp on care. Dr. Hock Yeoh, the medical director for Kaiser's Los Angeles unit, told the reporter for the *Times*, "Here, you're not driven by how much money you can get from the patient. You just do what is best for them."[17] One would hardly expect him, as a Kaiser employee, to say otherwise. Still, a specialist looking to get rich would never join Kaiser, where the average salary of around $150,000 is far less than one might earn elsewhere. Kaiser's integrated approach is also reflected in its staffing patterns. The dialysis unit in Los Angeles is staffed by at least two of its six kidney specialists, as well as registered nurses, dietitians, and social workers.

RESOURCE ALLOCATION DECISIONS: HOCAS AND LOCAS

Kaiser, like other managed care organizations, has made deliberate resource allocation decisions. Lawrence alludes to these decisions in a general way in his interview with Iglehart. Dr. David M. Eddy, a regular columnist for *JAMA*, who also happens to be a consultant to Kaiser Permanente Southern California

Region (KPSC), provides special insight into the decision-making process at Kaiser.

In one of his columns, Eddy describes how KPSC developed a practice guideline for the intravenous use of iodinated contrast agents for radiographic procedures such as computed tomography (CT) scans. Eddy states that nearly ten million of these procedures are performed in the United States each year. For decades, using agents with a relatively high osmolality—"high osmolar contrast agents" or HOCAs—was standard. According to Eddy, HOCAs have "excellent diagnostic properties," but can cause discomfort and adverse reactions. In the 1980s, researchers developed a new set of agents that lowered the risk of discomfort and adverse reactions. Known as "low osmolar contrast agents" or LOCAs, these agents cost ten to twenty times as much as HOCAs.

The KPSC guideline recommends the use of HOCAs, unless a patient has risk factors indicating a higher than average chance of an adverse reaction. The guideline was developed using a methodical approach consisting of four basic steps: "(1) analyze the evidence about the occurrence of reactions with HOCAs vs. LOCAs; (2) estimate the actual rates of different types of reactions in low-risk patients who receive the agents intravenously; (3) estimate the costs of the agents; and (4) determine if the differences in reaction rates are worth the difference in cost."[18] As Eddy first tells the story, a painstaking review of the literature was the basis for conservative estimates, which yielded obvious conclusions. Then Eddy gives the reader what he calls the "inside story."

In 1989, the American College of Radiologists (ACR) endorsed a large Japanese study establishing the benefits of LOCAs. The ACR also took the position that it remains reasonable to use HOCAs with low-risk patients. Initially, KPSC's associate medical director/physician manager of operations told the radiology chiefs to use LOCAs if they were medically indicated. He asked only for an estimate of expected use for budgetary purposes. Thereafter, the radiology chiefs directed that intravenous pyelograms and CT scans be switched to LOCAs exclusively. (Compliance with this directive was uneven across centers, radiologists and procedures.) Then the financial climate changed dramatically. Corporate customers wanted to be shown that they were getting value for money. Also, the amount actually spent on contrast agents greatly exceeded estimates.

A work group appointed by the radiology chiefs recommended using HOCAs for low-risk patients. Still, the group as a whole was reluctant to reverse the directive. According to Eddy, the major problems were concern for patients who, at a minimum, would experience increased discomfort, the radiologists' immediate responsibility for treating adverse reactions, a sense of exhaustion at the prospect of revisiting a popular decision, and a vague fear that any savings realized would not be reallocated to increase value. A desire to break the deadlock in a principled way set the stage for adopting the method described above.

When Eddy and his colleagues came to the cost-benefit analysis phase, Eddy says that they felt the issues were "too complex to solve in their heads." They sought some "beacon" to guide their deliberations. The "obvious beacon" was "the preferences of the people who would actually receive the agents, suffer the risks, and pay the costs—the members of our Health Plan."[19] The group favored a member questionnaire or poll.

Before conducting a large-scale member survey, they decided to use member focus groups to test the feasibility and accuracy of this approach. They presented focus groups with descriptions of the risks associated with HOCAs, then asked about their (members of the focus groups') willingness to pay to lower the risks. Eddy writes that, unfortunately, the strategy of putting cost-benefit questions directly to members did not work.[20] Thwarted in their attempt to find a beacon, Eddy's group began to look for a "sign": "We needed some sign from above that our budget had truly hit the point at which additional increases could not be tolerated and priorities had to be set."

They got their sign when a major customer asked KPSC to lower its rates; they stopped considering using LOCAs for all. They determined that using HOCAs in low-risk patients would "free up" approximately $3.5 million each year, and that spending a comparable amount on screening for breast and cervical cancer, or a cholesterol treatment program, would produce much greater health benefits. (Considering the funds saved as available for other uses seems somewhat at odds with the nature of the sign; surely adopting the guideline was intended to reduce spending.[21])

The final step was to consider "non-scientific and non-financial" issues. Eddy writes that these boiled down to three questions: (1) would they be sued; (2) would they lose a suit; and (3) would the costs of litigation and bad publicity wipe out any gains from adopting the guideline. The group believed that they *should* win any lawsuit. They had done everything right. The prospect of bad publicity (due to misunderstanding) continued to trouble them, but they felt such costs were outweighed by the principle at stake: "If we thought the guideline truly served the interests of our members, we believed we should stand up for it. To fail to make what we think are medically correct choices because of a fear of lawsuits would be to abrogate our overriding responsibility to our members."[22]

Outlining the factors that make this case a relatively easy one, Eddy concludes: "Finally, the value judgments, although they appeared so difficult when they were presented in qualitative terms, were really quite obvious once they were described with numbers. Who could fail to choose to prevent 35 to 100 cancer deaths over 40 severe but nonfatal reactions?"[23] This way of putting the matter entirely ignores distributional questions. What if the winners, or losers, all belonged to a particular racial group or gender? Further, questions concerning when to yield to payer pressures to control costs and how to address member concerns have entirely faded from view.

On the latter point, without identifying the organization involved, ethicists Laurie Zoloth-Dorfman and Susan Rubin describe how they were approached by nurses distressed over their employer's policy of using HOCAs for low-risk patients. The nurses asked whether patients should be informed that a more expensive option existed that greatly reduced the likelihood of side effects. They also wanted to deliberate about the fairness of a practice of giving a LOCA to the small number of low-risk patients who asked for it by name.[24]

Eddy does not mention how the KPSC guideline deals with patients who specifically request LOCAs. We are not told whether KPSC physicians routinely disclose the (non-) availability of LOCAs. The nurses who sought advice from Zoloth-Dorfman and Rubin had another concern: the policy at their institution did not take account of their actual patients' experiences with the less expensive contrast agent. Although Eddy reports a thorough literature review, and an attempt to solicit member preferences, he does not mention any systematic research into the effects of post-LOCA use of HOCAs. Obviously, the work group deliberations gave some weight to the radiologists' experience. But as far as we know, researchers made no provision for monitoring the consequences of the new guideline following its implementation.

Researchers and clinicians need to evaluate guidelines periodically, because guidelines can suffer from a number of deficiencies: they may be founded on research findings that are subsequently refined or discredited, neglect qualitative variables, gloss over uncertainties and contingencies, fail to make provision for "outliers" (or extraordinary cases), or rule out consideration of patient-specific value systems.[25] And pragmatic ethics counsels careful attention to the implementation process. If guidelines represent best practices, patients are harmed (or denied a benefit) if implementation is less than thorough. If guidelines deny a marginal benefit in the interest of cost-containment, incomplete or careless implementation is a positive injustice.

KAISER AND LAST CHANCE THERAPIES

Like Health Net, Kaiser has had difficulty controlling the use of bone marrow transplants. In the case of *Comer v. Kaiser Foundation Health Plan*,[26] a mother sued Kaiser in state court in connection with her son's death. Kaiser had refused to fund a bone marrow transplant it deemed "experimental." The U.S. Supreme Court declined to hear an appeal, and so let stand a Ninth Circuit Court of Appeals decision holding that the federal Employee Retirement Income Security Act preempts state tort remedies related to benefits provided by a self-insured employer. In other words, the court would not render a ruling on the propriety of Kaiser's actions. On the other hand, as described in greater detail in Chapter 5, Kaiser Permanente of Northern California now gives members seeking coverage for new therapies the option of consulting with an independent agency.

IMPROVING CARE AND CUTTING COSTS:
COOPERATIVE CARE CLINICS

Other "resource allocation" problems facing Kaiser and its practitioners and members are of a different nature. Caseload is not emphasized in the recent literature on ethics and managed care. But as medical sociologist Eliot Freidson points out, caseload is an extremely important factor affecting the quality of professionals' work: "Whether they work in private organizations devoted to maximizing profits or growth by minimizing production costs, or publicly supported organizations required to maximize production with minimal resources in order to keep taxes and political pressure low, an overwhelming caseload combined with a poverty of resources by which to handle it will at least discourage if not destroy both the inclination and the capacity to do good work."[27]

Many of the proposals for ameliorating some of the potential ill-effects of managed care assume that practitioners will be able to devote substantial time to explaining the new structures to patients.[28] If caseload or productivity requirements limit patient encounters to ten minutes, we cannot expect that conversation will fill the void left by technology. The solo practitioner can encounter the same difficulties under certain market conditions, e.g., when reimbursement rates are low. This is not only a "managed care problem." However, the managed care environment may exacerbate the problem by encouraging a victim mentality among physicians.

This may be particularly true of physicians in tightly managed, closed-panel HMOs: "The fee-for-service practitioner is often harassed, overbooked, and 'constantly on call,' but believes that these problems arise from the confidence of a loyal and growing body of patients and the esteem of referring physicians. Moreover, his income increases in direct proportion to his workload. The HMO physician, in contrast, may trace his feelings of harassment to the exploitation of the administration and the contractual rigidities of an HMO practice."[29] Once the psychological shift has been made, patients are readily classed with plan administrators as agents of harassment and overwork. Because plan members have a contractual right to care, they may assume the role of "bureaucratic client" in making and pursuing demands for services.[30]

Under these conditions character becomes crucial. A physician or an organization that values high-quality patient care, including meaningful personal relationships with patients, and has made a commitment to caring for a group of patients so large that it threatens to overwhelm available resources, is confronted with a problem. For pragmatists, this is the place to begin imagining alternative paths of response, not the point of resignation. The physician alone, the solo practitioner, may have more "freedom." He answers to nobody but himself. But the physician-as-employee, and the organization, may have more alternatives.

A Kaiser clinic in the Denver suburbs faced a major problem, arising from pressures similar to those described in connection with the HOCA/LOCA guideline, but the focus here is on the effects of such competitive pressures at the *clinical* level, rather than the development of region-wide policies. A writer for the trade journal *Hospitals & Health Networks* begins the story of the problem this way:

Each time John Scott hurried from one patient to the next that July morning four years ago, he sank a little lower. No matter how hard he pushed himself . . . , he left exam room after exam room feeling that he somehow hadn't met his patients' needs. At the front desk, Scott stopped to study the list of 10 people lined up to see him that morning. All were over 80 years old and suffering variations on the themes of aging and chronic illness. A glance at his afternoon schedule promised more of the same. The feeling of not doing enough suddenly became too much. "Comforting, teaching, explaining treatment options, discussing the emotions of aging and end of life—all of this is being dumped by the wayside in the name of efficiency," he says. "The way the world is going, we're being asked to do more and more with less and less. We end up compromising our beliefs about what our role as physicians should be."[31]

Scott's harried day in July of 1991 contrasts with the (relatively) leisurely pace of practice characteristic of Kaiser when he joined the plan in 1977. Back then, Kaiser was the only managed care plan in Denver, and Scott saw fourteen to fifteen patients a day.

On "that July morning" Scott finally aired his frustrations, and found that other doctors and nurses and clinic and central office administrators shared his frustrations. Together, they developed a "simple" solution that nobody else had apparently considered, what they called "cooperative care clinics."[32]

A managed care analyst comments that HMOs share with the health care field in general an emphasis on "diagnosing and curing" rather than "managing and maintaining." He adds, "Chronic care is the biggest ticking time bomb facing HMO's."[33] We should not be surprised to learn that most HMOs participate in the culture of short-sightedness. They concentrate on squeezing hospitals and other providers. In contrast, the cooperative care clinic concept takes the long view, but the driving force behind it was the immediate problem of providing high quality care to a particular group of elderly patients.

A cooperative care clinic consists in monthly meetings of twenty to twenty-five patients, overseen by the patients' doctor and a nurse. The Kaiser program targets patients over sixty-three with one or more chronic conditions. At the meetings, the group members receive routine check-ups, and they hear from Kaiser's in-house experts on exercise, diet, living wills, managing medications, and other topics of their choosing. Family members and friends acting as caregivers are invited to join in.

Patients have time to browse through their charts and question the medical staff. They receive preventive care like flu shots. There is also time for people who need private exams or special attention. "But what makes the biggest difference," according to the writer, is that "patients help one another over the rough spots of aging and illness, such as coping with the death of a spouse or a revoked driver's license. The groups become a forum for discussing events big and small that can chip away at independence and dignity, potentially sending patients into a spiral of depression and worsening health." Sharon Strammel, a registered nurse who helps run the clinics says, "Above all, these groups elevate patients to equal partners in their care—and hallelujah for that. We are not the experts on living with a chronic illness; they are. They deal with this much more openly and gracefully than clinical people do. And we learn from them."[34]

Note that Kaiser *as an organization* is able to do what no solo practitioner could easily accomplish, in terms of dedicating staff time to the task of organizing and evaluating the cooperative care clinics, and marshaling an impressive array of experts. Kaiser also has computer systems in place capable of tracking immunizations and flu shots and identifying people at special risk.

As numbers matter so much to some—and I think most of us would agree that *outcomes* matter—it is significant that over a one year period cooperative care patients experienced significantly fewer emergency department visits and repeat hospital admissions than a control group receiving traditional care. Also, both patients and clinicians in the experimental group reported higher satisfaction as compared with the control group.[35] Early on, Scott began making presentations to other HMOs and supported efforts to evaluate the cooperative care clinics rigorously and to disseminate the findings. He says, "I'd hate to see this concept used as one more tool in the vicious war between health plans."[36]

Current patients appreciate the "luxury" of spending more time with their own doctors, who can give extended explanations and still economize on time. The same is true for other health care providers, such as pharmacists and therapists. One patient with a spouse suffering from chronic lung disease comments, "We know a lot more people in the Kaiser system than we once did. . . . When you get older and need health care more often, you also need that sense of belonging." Patients have also developed a deep bond with Strammel, the nurse involved with many of the clinics. No longer an anonymous voice on the phone when the doctor is not immediately available, she now receives many of the calls. The article in *Hospitals & Health Networks* concludes with two themes, the common grace patients mediate to one another, and money:

> Naysayers at Kaiser predicted that patients would refuse to talk openly about sensitive topics or voice their fears to each other. But patients like Anne Temple proved them wrong. Scott was leading a session on arthritis when a woman in Temple's group spoke up from the back of the room, her voice breaking: "You mean I'm going to live with this for the rest of my life? How am I ever going to do that?" Temple, a 76-year-old widow with two artificial knees, a reconstructed shoulder and gnarled fingers, thanks to rheumatoid arthritis, waved a hand in the air. "Honey, look at this. I've been living this way for years. During our break, I'll tell you exactly how I do it."
>
> "I couldn't do that," says Scott. "I've never had arthritis. Not even a rheumatology specialist could tell her what Anne could. The amount of support people get from one another, not from some overburdened medical system, is astounding. And it doesn't cost anything, either."[37]

REACHING OUT TO THE COMMUNITY

Kaiser has also contributed institutional and financial support to community injury prevention and health promotion initiatives. Headquartered in Oakland, California, Kaiser has supported the development of protocols for domestic violence cases in the San Francisco Bay area. Working with parents and the School of Public Health at the University of California, Berkeley, Kaiser has helped to create a "violence-free zone" around a local middle school. A Kaiser psychologist involved in the project reports that skeptics doubted community members could be engaged as active partners. But, the skeptics have been proved wrong, he says. Parents are now walking the neighborhood, and stores are posting signs and offering safe haven for students.[38] Researchers are tracking the number of violent incidents at the school, truancy, and grades, and the early results are promising.

Kaiser Permanente Northwest provides up to two years of health benefits for displaced homemakers and other older women returning to school and their dependents. Kaiser collaborated with five area community colleges to develop the "Transitions" program. Kaiser executives view the program as a way to encourage preventive care to head off major health problems. They also hope to build up the confidence and capability of women who find themselves living precariously on society's margins.[39]

SOURCES OF UNEASE

Still, all is not well with Kaiser. Quality may vary significantly across regions.[40] Rationalization and standardization of practice may enable Kaiser to deliver reliable, cost-effective care to the majority of patients, but rationalization and standardization have their limits. As *Wall Street Journal* reporter George Anders says, even the best HMOs have one great vulnerability: the unexpected case. A baby with a fever is rarely suffering from a meningococcemia, a bacterial infection that only strikes about eight hundred infants a year. A 35-year-old man who experiences chest pain is rarely dying of a heart attack.[41] The accumulation of such rare cases opens HMOs—such as Kaiser Foundation Health Plan of Georgia, in this instance—to criticism. Is it possible, as a matter of standard practice, to respond to the exceptional? And what of the dollars at stake?

Research suggests that emergency room care is two and half times as expensive as similar care in an office or clinic setting.[42] In the non-emergency case, the extra expenditures are clearly waste, or so it seems until one starts asking questions. How easy is it for patients and their families to determine whether they have a "true" medical emergency warranting a departure from the standard procedures?[43] How much should they worry over the possibility of getting stuck with the bill as they decide what to do?

Consider the feverish baby.[44] There were three critical points in Kaiser Georgia's handling of the case. First, there was the initial screen. Lamona Adams, the baby's mother, asked for and received a same day appointment with a pediatrician. The examination failed to disclose the infection. There were no allegations of malpractice in connection with the exam, and experts testified that it would be unusual for any physician to diagnose the problem based on the baby's symptoms at the time of the exam. But the unusual becomes yet more improbable in light of the time constraints: Kaiser had just reduced its routine pediatric exam to ten minutes, from fifteen.

Second, there was the follow-up procedure. When the baby's condition worsened, Adams followed Kaiser's instructions and called the after-hours nurse advice line. Here the system clearly failed. Despite some alarming symptoms (communicated to the operator, who passed a "summary sheet" to the nurse), the nurse did not direct Adams to call 911. Indeed, she directed Adams to a hospital forty-two miles from the Adamses' home. The hospital had agreed to give Kaiser a volume discount. Third, there was the system's internal check. The nurse called a pediatrician at home to confirm her handling of the case. Based on the information given (which is disputed), the physician confirmed the treatment plan. The Adamses got lost on the way to the hospital, the baby's heart stopped, and they followed signs to a hospital just off the freeway. The baby survived, but his feet and hands had to be amputated.

In response to this case, Kaiser added the question, "Is there anything that makes you think that you should go to an emergency room right away," to its script for repeat callers to the nurse hotline. But Kaiser administrators refused to acknowledge any basic flaws in their manner of handling possible emergencies. A Kaiser spokesman denied that the issues had anything to do with managed care. In a sense he is correct. Miscommunication is possible outside of a managed care system. But in managed care "the system" makes miscommunication more likely by putting more links in the chain.

Anyone who has played the "telephone" game knows that messages become increasing garbled as they move away from the source. Further, the system makes communication less likely. Lamona Adams reported feeling rushed in the pediatrician's office, and a system of rules constrained her ability to seek reassurance by talking directly to a physician or by proceeding directly to the closest emergency room.

As if that weren't enough, a much publicized California Supreme Court case, *Engalla v. Permanente Medical Group*,[45] casts doubt on Kaiser's commitment to justice. In completing Kaiser's membership application form, the applicant agrees to submit monetary claims for injury or death to arbitration. Wilfredo Engalla signed such a form when he enrolled in a Kaiser plan. From 1986 to 1991, Engalla repeatedly visited a Kaiser clinic complaining of respiratory problems. The running diagnosis was either a common cold or allergies. When Engalla was finally diagnosed with inoperable lung cancer, he and his family retained a lawyer and initiated the arbitration process.

Whatever the merits of the underlying malpractice claim, Kaiser's handling of the arbitration does not bear up well under scrutiny. The California Supreme Court's review of the facts is a litany of horrors. Kaiser's defense counsel performed administrative functions, a clear conflict of interest not disclosed to members or potential members. The arbitration agreement specified that the party-appointed arbitrators select a third, neutral arbitrator. In fact, Kaiser's lawyer made the selection after consulting with Kaiser's in-house legal department. Kaiser's publications stated that a case would reach an arbitration hearing within several months' time. A statistical analysis of all Kaiser medical malpractice arbitrations found that delays occurred in 99 percent of cases. In only 1 percent of all Kaiser cases was a "neutral" arbitrator appointed within the timeframe Kaiser itself specified. The average time lapse between initiation and hearing was 863 days.

When Engalla's lawyer tried to schedule a deposition for his client, Kaiser's lawyer set a date more than five months away, well after Engalla was expected to (and did) die. Delays also arose in scheduling the depositions of doctors and nurses. When Engalla's lawyer asked Kaiser to agree that it would not capitalize on the delays—under California law, Engalla's death would alter the claims against Kaiser and significantly reduce the potential award—Kaiser's lawyer refused.[46] In sum, an appalling record.

There are also signs of increasing discontent among practitioners in some Kaiser regions. In the mid-1990s, someone leaked a critical memo from a group of Kaiser physicians in Northern California to the *San Francisco Chronicle*. The memo, which Kaiser later released to other members of the media, charged that "drastic cuts" were harming the "caregiver-patient relationship." The memo alleged that Kaiser had doubled the number of administrative personnel, while cutting "front line personnel" such as nurses. Trying to put the best face on things, a Kaiser spokesman described the memo as part of Kaiser's "democratic system." The memo was distributed internally in connection with an election battle over the position of executive director for the region.[47]

For more than a year, the California Nurses Association (CNA) waged a relentless public relations and legal battle against Kaiser in relation to a new collective bargaining contract. As part of that labor dispute, an administrative law judge ordered Kaiser to turn over information touching on the quality of patient care in the Northern California region.[48]

At least one regional plan has become embroiled in the scandal over gag rules and another tried to prevent the publication of a critical report. A directive from the Ohio Kaiser Permanente HMO to physicians prohibited them from discussing proposed treatments with patients prior to authorization, or even describing the authorization procedure to patients.[49] Kaiser Foundation Health Plan of Texas tried to prevent the release of a critical report prepared by investigators with the Texas Department of Insurance, arguing that it was protecting confidential patient and physician information, even though there were no patient or physician identifiers in the report.[50]

Some fundamental shifts in organizational structure accompany these tremors and missteps. The relationships between the plan and the professionals who provide the care are loosening, while the HMO is forming ties with organizations that do not share its history. These steps are responses to changed market conditions that introduce considerable uncertainty. In adopting a more loosely coupled structure, Kaiser may be evolving toward greater flexibility. It also risks betraying its basic commitment to comprehensive, coordinated care in favor of the business ideology and its equation of incentivizing with efficiency.

ASSESSING KAISER'S CHARACTER

Yet Kaiser is remarkable for the way it blends business and professionalism with considerable sensitivity to the democratic principle of developing the capacities of plan member-patients. We can evaluate Kaiser's "character" using the tools of character assessment.

Integrity and Responsiveness

Recall that, in simplified terms, integrity suggests integration and moral coherence, and that one test of integrity is the degree of fidelity to self-defined principles. Responsiveness requires openness and flexibility. Lawrence and Eddy stress integration and moral coherence in the accounts they give of their organization. The very fact of publication is significant. It is through the making of such records that Kaiser becomes "hostage to its history" as a public-spirited, innovative enterprise and opens itself to external critique. Through its integrated approach to health care and its system of rewards, and the kinds of administrators and physicians and nurses these structures attract, Kaiser both institutionalizes its commitments and helps ensure the preservation of its distinctive character through the changes a changing environment will bring.

Lawrence expounds on institutional identity, with responses that display consistency. His broad themes are responsiveness to members and to local community needs and commitment to comprehensive services integrated across the spectrum of care. Lawrence's discussion of quality suggests three concerns and related commitments: (1) a concern for individuals and a commitment to enhancing interpersonal relationships; (2) a concern for populations and a commitment to making general improvements in health; and finally, (3) a concern about costs and a commitment to eliminating waste, as a means of extending health services to a larger share of the population.

These concerns exist in some tension, but integrity does not consist in narrowing concern or pursuing a single goal single-mindedly. The question is whether Kaiser attempts to honor each concern at multiple levels of the organization, through its organizational structure, reward system, research and educational activities, and significant policies. The answer seems to be a qualified yes.

Regional variations challenge the integrity, and reputation, of the organization as a whole. The very same decentralization that promotes responsiveness to local community concerns permits the Ohio Kaiser Permanente HMO to issue a directive silencing its physicians and permits the Kaiser Foundation Health Plan of Texas to resist publication of a report critical of its operations.[51] These are clearly turbulent times at Kaiser, and it is not clear which forces will prevail. At least some Kaiser physicians fear that under competitive pressures the organization is in peril of losing its integrity.

As for responsiveness, Eddy describes Kaiser's attempt to involve members in policy making, which he concedes to have been a failure. It remains to be seen whether Kaiser is sufficiently committed to refine its strategy for member involvement in guideline development, or to experiment with other strategies. The difficulties the member-off-the-street may have in understanding resource allocation issues suggest that Kaiser might do well to cultivate groups of member-experts, groups defined by a shared interest in health care and a willingness to devote time to further study. As to involving members generally, I am inclined to think that Eddy and his colleagues asked the wrong kinds of questions. Despite, or perhaps because of, their extreme rationalism, they looked for signs, portents, and unambiguous numbers, and failed at the work of nuanced interpretation and meaningful conversation outside the medical-scientific circle.

Eddy and his colleagues offered participants in member focus groups calculations that had no immediate significance for them. Participants lacked a sufficient experiential "handle" on the problem.[52] Next time, Kaiser might consult with member-experts in developing more meaningful modes of involvement for the membership-at-large.

Plan managers should also recognize that involving members is certainly not philanthropy, and may be exploitation. Through involving plan members, however tangentially, plan managers may hope to shift responsibility without surrendering control. Further, member focus groups and surveys are an easy and relatively inexpensive avenue to the informational inputs needed for calculating cost-benefit.[53]

More generally, rationalism may inhibit organizational responsiveness to the full range of member concerns. Ultimately, this relates to a tension between two perspectives, what we might call *statistical rationalism* (a form of calculative rationality) and *encounter personalism*. Journalist George Anders charges that the managed-care industry as a whole "is dominated by people who see many statistics and few patients," who "want to be judged by how they treat healthy populations overall." He argues that the crucial test of a health plan is "how it performs when anxious families are fighting medical disaster."[54] This follows from his belief that the primary reason people seek health insurance is to be secure in times of medical crisis.

Focusing on populations and statistics rather than on persons and encounters devalues the experience of physicians and other clinicians, as well as slighting the concerns of people in crisis. Many share Eddy's belief in the number.[55] I would suggest that we need to consider experience gained in practice *and* statistics, persons *and* populations, and preventive *and* acute care, as well as care for those with chronic illnesses. Kaiser does not always strike the proper balance, but leaders like Lawrence and clinicians like Scott and Strammel are at least aware of the personal side of the equation.

Qualities of Character Nurtured in Persons:
Faithfulness, Openness, and Truthfulness

In addition, it is important to ask what qualities of character Kaiser nourishes in its leaders, and what qualities the organization and its leaders nourish in physicians, other clinicians, and member-patients. Consider Kaiser's leader, David Lawrence. Lawrence's own history suggests a strong commitment to social service. He articulates a vision in which the values of management and care exist in tension. The tension may not always be fruitful. Lawrence may consider abandoning some principles, such as pure community rating. But Kaiser has not abandoned the underlying moral commitment; rather the health plan has instituted various measures to promote wider access to its services among the disadvantaged. In Robert Nozick's terms, the principle not followed leaves "moral traces." The message is that Kaiser will compromise with the forces of the market, but not surrender. Lawrence is also politically astute. He realizes that Kaiser needs the support of intelligent regulation to maintain its distinctive character.

As for the clinicians, escalating productivity requirements, increasing constraints on resources, and de-skilling all diminish the internal goods of health care and make it difficult for clinicians to develop and display the virtue of faithfulness to patients. Clearly, Kaiser physicians and nurses are frustrated by the demands they face. Yet, when they choose to voice their frustrations, others within the organization, including administrators, may listen and respond.

Medical staff and administrators at the Denver clinic were able to mount a collective, effective response to one of the problems they confronted. They acted in a way that built on their collegial relationships, cutting across physician/ nurse and other professional and disciplinary boundaries, which ultimately enhanced relationships with patients. Further, the cooperative care clinics have developed the capacities of plan members to aid one another. They come to see what they have in common, and they help each other make sense of the losses of aging and the terrors of illness.

For the most part, Kaiser displays a praiseworthy commitment to openness. The silencing of physicians in Ohio and attempts to suppress information in Texas and California form lamentable episodes in Kaiser's biography. That biography also reveals many accomplishments in this area. For example, the HOCA/LOCA guideline could hardly remain a secret, but Kaiser displayed a commitment to openness in allowing publication of an "insider's" account of its deliberations. Kaiser's refusal to treat the concept of cooperative clinics as a trade secret is commendable. Further, there is some indication that Kaiser makes an effort to communicate these qualities to members and patients. According to Zoloth-Dorfman and Rubin, Kaiser circulates guidelines and policies to members for their review.

Kaiser has taken its distinctive character to its customers through advertising. Current print advertisements stress that Kaiser plans are not-for-profit and that its physicians are paid by salary, rather than capitation.[56] This is self-serving. But as noted in Chapter 3, much depends on the nature of the self served.

Democracy, Justice, and Community

On the compatibility of Kaiser's practices with the democratic vision, initially one must note that Kaiser *members* do not vote. Henry Kaiser believed that participation in the ownership and control of an enterprise is not a consumer perquisite (or responsibility); " 'you don't ask your corner grocer to share his ownership with people who buy at the store.' "[57] On the other hand, physicians elect Kaiser's professional leadership. Kaiser is also democratic in its adherence to the principle that physicians (collectively) should control their own work. One could only wish that the founders had extended this principle to practitioners other than physicians. The history of conflict between Kaiser and its nurses is not surprising, given the relative disempowerment of this group of professionals within health care, and the disappointment of hopes of something better from Kaiser and from managed care.

Several decades ago Kaiser expanded member representation on boards to meet federal requirements. I have reviewed some instances of member involvement in resource allocation decisions. A move toward more robust involvement in limited areas may be all we ask. Kaiser has performed well relative to other not-for-profit HMOs, and we might reasonably prefer management of health care plans in our interests, but also (for the most part) in our absence.[58] Concerns are lessened where democratic values are nurtured in other areas of the organization and in the relationships between clinicians and patients.

Concerning distributive justice, Kaiser has acted to subsidize the premiums of those who would otherwise be unable to afford its services. As demonstrated in the areas of kidney dialysis and caring for the chronically ill elderly, Kaiser favors restorative over maintenance strategies. On the other side of the ledger, Eddy's account gives us no sign of awareness of the distributional concerns raised by cost-benefit analysis.

In the area of commutative justice, Kaiser's record is mixed. Kaiser plans sometimes favor contractual language that gives members very little idea of what to expect. Kaiser plans in certain regions have been accused of treating members cavalierly, to put it mildly. Members do have a fair amount of freedom within the system. Patients in cooperative care clinics appear very satisfied, although we may assume that administrators did not arrange interviews with disgruntled persons. Still, some Kaiser patients are not getting treatments they want, such as bone marrow transplants. These treatments are clearly *desired*. Justice will prompt an inquiry into their *desirability*, given resource constraints. Certainly justice never requires arrogance or brutality; decision-makers can be humble about the limits of their own knowledge, and they can communicate their decisions with respect and compassion.

Is Kaiser just in its dealings with physicians and the other clinicians who actually care for patients? Some Kaiser physicians are discontented, but relative to physicians in other managed care organizations, Kaiser physicians have a great deal of control over their conditions of work. On the other hand, many of Kaiser's nurses have been profoundly unhappy with their working conditions.

Justice carries with it the notion of enforcement, whereas community is a voluntary ideal. The conditions for community can be put in place, but community itself is an "unforced flower." There may be those for whom even the finest achievements of communal health care are unappealing, who shudder at the prospect of attending a cooperative care clinic. Given the complexity of our world, the moderateness of claims made may be one test of their trustworthiness. Herman Weiner, a long-time advocate for the Kaiser style of practice, stated that the Kaiser model would not suit everyone. Early on, Kaiser insisted that groups joining the plan offer members another option.[59] Indeed, in keeping with a positive account of pluralism, we may hope for the flourishing of many different models for providing care. We will have criteria to assist us in evaluating these options, but these criteria will likely allow for a broad range of organizational structures.

FIVE

The Market, Professionalism, and Cooperative Egalitarianism in Health Care

> The central problem facing advanced technological societies [is] how to re-
> construct the either-or of economic growth versus social and cultural soli-
> darity into a both-and of technical progress in the service of a sustainable
> common good; how to develop leadership groups which will serve rather
> than undermine solidarity and collective self-development.
> —William M. Sullivan, *Work and Integrity*

In Chapter 2, I noted the strong influence of two ideologies, medicine and business, on the reception of managed care. In this chapter, I work toward a critical
reconstruction of the ideologies of business and medicine, reconsidering the
appropriate role of the market and professionalism in health care, and urging
a recovery of the cooperative ideal that informed the early development of
managed care.[1]

Features of health care render this "industry" resistant to many of the usual
forms of market discipline. Further, it is an illusion of the business ideology
that the market can stand alone.

I argue for a shift from economics to political economy and from business as
institutionalized avarice to business as a productive system. I revisit the concept of efficiency, attending to the relationship between means and ends and
the kinship between business and bureaucracy. Bureaucracy is a regular feature
of contemporary organization across sectors. This is not necessarily a cause for
alarm. The great peril is *substituting* market or bureaucratic methods of control
for collegial ones. Especially where social trust is weak, bureaucratic controls
may be perceived as manipulative and invite manipulation in turn. Bureaucracy
is most likely to go awry in large organizations.

Many pragmatists display considerable ambivalence concerning business and the market. In contrast, the professional ideal advanced by the ideology of medicine is dear to our hearts. Unfortunately, that ideal has often served as a cover for unwarranted group privilege. Fortunately, it is possible to reconstruct the professional ideal so that it is more compatible with a democratic social vision.

Difference is possible without hierarchy, and the professional ideal *is* democratic in the sense that it calls for people to control their own work. At the same time, the professional ideology has its characteristic pathologies. We can and should use market and bureaucratic methods to regulate cost and performance. We must also ensure that the specific methods chosen do not seriously undermine what is desirable in professionalism. I close the treatment of professionalism with brief meditations on the place of moral language in health care and the silence of mainstream medical ethics concerning power.

Although it is often forgotten, a third ideology, cooperative egalitarianism, played an important role in the genesis of managed care. As an outgrowth of the democratic vision, cooperative egalitarianism looks for the widest possible dissemination of power and the end of domination; it employs the rhetoric of community to those ends.

In this chapter, I aim to consider how the ideology of cooperative egalitarianism might serve to correct and complete the ideologies of business and medicine. The ideology is utopian in the positive sense of calling us to work toward something better than what we have. It can also offer guidance to those addressing some of the most pressing problems of the moment, including the development of fair and humane ways of handling requests for unproven "last chance" therapies and the fashioning of appropriate responses to the spread of large-scale organizations in health care.

THE IDEOLOGY OF BUSINESS REVISITED

The Profit Motive, Efficiency, and Economy

Those who are under the sway of the ideology of business celebrate the market. Like alchemists, they believe that activating the profit motive will convert a sluggish and inefficient health care sector into a lean and ferociously efficient industry, generating much gold for stockholders. I want to examine the concepts of "profit motive" and "efficiency" in greater depth.

THE PROFIT MOTIVE

Malik Hasan believes in the existence of a profit motive and the beneficent effects of its operation. The rhetoric of market proponents suggests a natural force such as gravity, but the forms of acquisitive behavior on display surely vary with the social environment. The business ideology tends to obscure the context in which acquisitiveness takes shape in multiple ways. The web of legal, political, and social structures that undergird actual markets becomes nearly invisible.

Participants in the market define and pursue their interests as defined by this range of structures, even as they seek to manipulate the structures to further advance those interests.[2] (Commentators have noted the co-incidence of the rise of large, for-profit corporations delivering health care, government programs such as Medicare, and tax policies favoring acquisitions, e.g., rapid depreciation allowances and full deductibility of interest on debt.[3]) They ignore the social shaping of individuals and behavior, along with the social resources on which the individual draws in his or her activity. As a result, they declare a careful assessment of the full range of social consequences following from each form of economic activity unnecessary.

The business ideology is forever losing sight of the fact that business depends on people's willingness not to exploit the trust others place in them. The business ideology does not counsel managers to work against the interests of shareholders whenever it suits their private interests. Why should shareholders and managers be told they have no reason to refrain from exploiting the public trust manifested in policies giving corporations benefits such as limited liability?

Or consider the complexity masked by the notion of profit-maximization. Choices that maximize long-term profit are not the same as those that maximize short-term profit.[4] The interests of long-term investors and speculators diverge. Actions that benefit the holders of common stock may not benefit the holders of preferred stock or bonds. Managers necessarily make difficult judgments that balance the interests of various groups.

Business is an activity that builds on a positive interdependence. This is nowhere clearer than in nations where social networks have broken down. We should acknowledge this, and straightforwardly grapple with the interests of all of the corporation's constituencies.[5]

EFFICIENCY AND ECONOMY

In Chapter 2, I alluded to the emptiness of efficiency as a slogan in the medicine-business polemic. Speaking from within the pragmatic tradition, in the field of economics, and signaling a more comprehensive vision by reappropriating the term "political economy," Charles Anderson argues that we can only assess efficiency if we specify the goal of the activity from the start. Then the end itself becomes open to evaluation. According to Anderson, efficiency is "fittedness to purpose—that technique and organization are as appropriate as possible to the end in view."[6]

Classical economic theory dwells on allocative efficiency, the adjustment of supply to demand, based on signals embodied in price, with equilibrium as the goal. Pragmatist political economy is at least as interested in dynamic efficiency—innovation or improvement of processes in the service of appropriate ends. In health care, the appropriate end must be something like caring for the sick, easing suffering, curing when possible, and educating in prevention.[7] If a form of organization compromises care for the sick and so on, then even if it saves money, it cannot be judged more efficient than forms better adapted to these ends. Efficiency also implies reliability, that is, some degree of standardization and quality control.

The moral significance of efficiency, defined in this manner, is bound up with the values and virtues productive activity can exemplify. In the pragmatic version of political economy, production is opposed to an abstract commercialism. This strand of pragmatism is particularly visible in economist Thorstein Veblen's analysis of the moral psychology of business. As Anderson writes, Veblen saw that "the 'pecuniary' and 'predatory' skills, which he associated with the more avaricious kinds of business leadership, with business perceived only as financial calculation, were parasitical on a productive system which was itself the product of 'idle curiosity,' or scientific inquiry and invention, a 'parental instinct' which connotes management as good stewardship, and a 'pride in workmanship' which was the foundation of rational, consistent performance, or efficiency." The distinction between business as institutionalized avarice and business as a productive system affects how the role of profit is understood: "The public function of the firm is to make a useful product. Profitability is a test of its performance, but not the definition of its purpose."[8]

This way of thinking makes sense, if one views social life in terms of practices. "Practice" is a commitment term. It indicates staying power, time for developing standards of good practice, technical and moral excellence, and so on. If one argues for the practical and normative significance of practices, one must also argue that there should be some resistance to the transfer of energies from one field to another. Obviously, there can be too much resistance to change. Productive activity has the satisfaction of human needs as an end in view. For a variety of reasons, a practice may become divorced from this end. Profitability represents an important, if not all-sufficient, test of performance and basic social usefulness, but it is *not* the end of productive activity. Linking efficiency to practices also draws attention to the satisfaction found by producers, or service providers, in doing good work.

"Economy" is a related concept. It refers to performing a function at the lowest possible cost consistent with purpose: what we think we are about in conducting cost-effectiveness analyses or seeking to reduce waste of all sorts. Economy requires us to assess alternative techniques within practices, within bounds set by efficiency. The moral significance of economy is linked to concepts like stewardship and sustainability.

Once again, we are led to the conclusion that expenditure of resources can only be judged waste in relation to a careful analysis of means *and* ends. The term medical-loss ratio, detached from the sphere where it made sense in relation to the ends of a practice (insurance), tends to suggest that all medical care is waste, but a low medical-loss ratio by itself tells us nothing about efficiency or economy in providing health care.

The business ideology suggests that for-profit corporations will have advantages in the area of motivation and therefore efficiency. For-profit health care corporations may be more efficient than their not-for-profit counterparts in maximizing reimbursements, but there is no good evidence of greater productive efficiency, or even the provision of services at lesser cost.[9] Indeed, two recent studies provide evidence that not-for-profit health care organizations perform better than for-profit health care organizations on measures of quality and cost.[10]

A Limited Defense of Markets

Delve into the pragmatic tradition and you will find considerable ambivalence concerning business and the market economy generally. Dewey saw wide assent to the proposition that productive activity must be stimulated by external goods (such as money) as an indicator of social distress, since he believed that human beings were by nature active creatures. Perhaps Dewey overcompensated a bit in a bid to do away with the view that work is a punishment, and that human beings are naturally slothful. Even assuming that all normal productive activity offers some intrinsic reward, the prospect of financial reward may sometimes serve as prod and reinforcement when work seems tedious.

Still, this is a modest role for gain at odds with economic orthodoxy. Jeffrey Pfeffer, a professor at Stanford Business School, is challenging orthodoxy when he writes, "people do work for money—but they work even more for meaning in their lives."[11] Pfeffer believes the classical economic view, that people can only be induced to work through a combination of rewards and sanctions, is a residue of Newtonian physics. This view does not fit with the empirical evidence establishing that large extrinsic rewards erode intrinsic motivation and may actually decrease performance in tasks that require creativity.

The current mania for manipulating payment structures reveals more about the power of institutional isomorphism than about the power of pay to improve performance. Pfeffer reports that when he talks to corporate executives about implementing payment systems that work, he hears, "'But that's different from what most other companies are saying and doing.'"[12]

In good pragmatic fashion, Reinhold Niebuhr combined skepticism concerning *homo economicus* with skepticism concerning attempts to dispense with economic man altogether. He wrote that the assurance of a "'pre-established harmony of nature' which transmuted all competitive strivings into an ultimate harmony, was obviously a more dubious doctrine than the basic assurance that men must be engaged primarily through their self-interest, to participate in the vast web of mutual services which has always characterized man's economic life and which increasing specialization of labor has made ever more intricate."[13] Niebuhr did not credit the unswerving pursuit of individual material advantage as a *comprehensive* explanation of human conduct. Hence, he saw no reason to expect the automatic harmonization of economic and social interests.

Niebuhr did credit certain claims made for markets: first, that the alternatives involve increasing the concentration of power in the hands of politicians and government administrators and second, that markets display some self-regulating tendencies and serve to foster initiative. (Adam Smith and Pope John Paul II agree that markets may nurture the virtue of industriousness.) Other benefits of markets include flexibility and responsiveness to consumers' desires. Commerce has also been credited with bringing people of diverse backgrounds together and hence fostering tolerance and combating prejudice.[14]

Markets and Health Care

Not all markets display these tendencies and realize these benefits to the same degree. The market for health care services provides a notorious example of an imperfect market, combining barriers to entry (licensing), differentiated products and services that are difficult for consumers, patients, and experts on quality to assess,[15] induced demand, and insensitivity to price owing to third-party payments. It also seems misleading to refer to "the market" for health care services, given regional variations. Further, there are forces working in any market that call for wider social direction and control. Competition can become predation. Corporate influence can corrupt the political sphere.

Adam Smith relied on government rather than the market to provide a range of public goods, and economists of various ideological stripes recognize the problems created by externalities. For example, health plans do not experience the productivity losses associated with illness and the costs of illness borne by informal caregivers. And given the current tax structure, individuals have an incentive to purchase "too much" insurance, shrinking public revenues available for other uses, and adding to the problem of overutilization of services. This is termed a "moral hazard" problem by economists because the individual has an incentive to take advantage of the system that shields him or her from the full costs of services by taking as much as possible, violating the actuarial assumptions on which the system is based, and ultimately undermining it. Another externality is associated with the underutilization of services such as vaccinations and other preventive measures. It is in each individual's interest *qua* individual to neglect these services, so long as others are diligent. This litany has led some to argue that market-oriented regulatory strategies aimed solely at making health plans more responsive to the demands of individual consumers are myopic.[16]

We must become more discriminating in judging markets, and more discerning in analyzing the relations between markets and other features of the social topography. Not all markets are the same. Markets for health care services have distinctive features. And some ways of understanding markets and their social effects are more adequate than others.

In a perceptive piece on corporate governance, James Boyd White argues that moderate critics of corporations have been misguided in focusing on the distinction between short-term and long-term profit. We do not advance very far by convincing corporate leaders that their task is to maximize the long-term profitability of the enterprise. According to White, the "real evil" is the economic model of wealth, "which takes in only exchanges." The model assumes that the social background is *stable*, whereas in reality, it must be perpetually remade. An ideology that allows the business corporation only one goal, to maximize profits, defines the corporation as "a kind of shark that lives off the community, rather than as an important agency in the construction, maintenance, and transformation of our shared lives."[17]

Business and Bureaucracy

An obvious but familiar fallacy links bureaucracy to "the government," rather than organizations as such, including insurance companies and managed care organizations. Adherents of the business ideology may score rhetorical points by portraying themselves as defenders of freedom over against the bureaucrats, but contemporary capitalism is neck deep in bureaucracy. In a sense, bureaucracy is merely an extension of the business ideology, reflecting the same instrumental view of other people. Although bureaucracy may mitigate some of the ill effects of cowboy capitalism, it may also reinforce (or amplify) the manipulative current in contemporary social relationships, sabotage efforts to maintain the fragile internal goods of practices, and support the channeling of the acquisitive drive in a purely pecuniary direction.

THE GOOD AND THE BAD OF BUREAUCRACY

Given its general disfavor, the first thing worth stressing about bureaucracy is that it has its benefits. Jeffrey Stout suggested investigating the potential for "bureaucratic enforcement of rights" to mitigate the bad effects of the marketplace on social practices and participants. The benefits of bureaucracy become clearer when one attempts to enumerate the features of bureaucracy in its ideal-typical form, rather than focusing immediately on its concrete failures. These features include, (1) fidelity to assigned duties; (2) accountability to the organization and its sponsors; (3) consultation as a corollary of the diffusion of authority; and (4) mitigation of arbitrariness through rule-governed decision.[18] While these are process values, they serve substantive interests. These features are associated with specific organizational principles, such as a fixed division of labor with clear lines of authority and responsibility, general rules to govern performance, and selecting personnel on the basis of technical qualifications.

Criticisms of bureaucracy typically fall into two categories, the technocratic and the moral. Technocratic criticisms are a sophisticated form of the common complaint about "red tape." Although Max Weber believed that one of the features of bureaucracy (or rational-legal authority) making it attractive to private industry was its ability to facilitate rapid response to change, decades of experience with bureaucracy suggest that this form of organization may rather hamper innovation.[19]

Appointment to positions based on technical competence and the establishment of clear lines of authority would seem to support prompt, effective decision making. In practice, however, systems may protect the jobs of incompetent officials or managers, and clear lines of authority may result in the slow movement of a proposal through multiple layers within and across divisions. Rules may be rigid and inflexible, not allowing for sufficient discretion.[20]

Further, the history of bureaucracy does not show organizations becoming ever purer and more rational. Feudal elements such as the exchange of fealty for protection have shown a remarkable resilience, flourishing amidst corporate charts, long-range strategic plans, and volumes of company policies and procedures. The rational bureaucratic-traditional hybrid is a creature sui generis.[21]

We cannot separate these criticisms altogether from distinctively moral concerns, but the latter stress the dark side of bureaucratic impersonality. Critics have used the word "domination" to describe the experience of bureaucracy by supplicants and lower-level functionaries. Initially, it may appear that domination is the necessary price to be paid for the benefits of bureaucracy, for it seems to stem from the very aspects that serve to mitigate arbitrariness, the ethos of system and governance by rules. While assuring evenhandedness and limiting corruption, these aspects of bureaucracy also seem to produce "a people-processing culture in which persons are treated as administrative objects and their special needs and circumstances are ignored."[22]

In concept, though, we should view discretion within limits as a necessary feature of bureaucratic administration, rather than as a threat to be minimized. Even where impersonality is prized, discretion restores some humanity to bureaucracy. When discretion is abused, it is this person, and not "the system" alone, who commits the wrong. Accountability is lodged with an individual as well as an organization. Sadly, our experience with bureaucracy reveals that it is exceedingly difficult to maintain discretion and limit at the same time.

POST-BUREAUCRATIC ORGANIZATION?

It is significant, then, that many close observers of the world of organizations have announced the arrival on the scene of the "post-bureaucratic" organization. Not surprisingly, there is some disagreement over the nature of the emerging phenomenon. Disputes have arisen over whether changes detected in organizations are merely reformist bureaucracy or a true break with the bureaucratic type. In any event, in many organizations, structures are becoming more fluid and rules are becoming more flexible, pushing authority and discretion down to lower levels.

Mitchell Rabkin, for many years chief administrator of Boston's Beth Israel Hospital, describes a "participative management" model that battles organizational opacity, as it affects those within the organization. An organization that operates according to the participative management model will keep staff informed of how the organization is doing and how their particular spheres of work are related to the success of the organization as a whole. It will create structures for staff to communicate ideas and concerns, and structures through which those ideas and concerns can be acted upon.[23] Post-bureaucratic organization may hold significant promise for health care. For the time being, however, we must address traditional bureaucracy, since it is far from moribund.

Bureaucracy and Health Care

THE PHYSICIAN AS DOUBLE AGENT

For many physicians and medical ethicists, the question of the fit between business-cum-bureaucracy and health care reduces to the following question, what are we to do about the physician's new role as a functionary in the health care system and an agent of social (usually financial) interests? The contrast is with the role of physician as patient advocate or agent for the present patient. I wish to quarrel with this way of framing the issue, while acknowledging that some physicians now see themselves as agents of social policy, a very undesirable development. (The worst constitute themselves as judges of the social worth of others—the physician still alone with his or her conscience, but with a change in the intended beneficiary from the present patient to an abstraction.[24])

The physician's role may be affected with a social interest in two ways. First, physicians function as social gatekeepers in a number of contexts, determining access to social resources and making judgments about fitness for social responsibilities. They served in such roles long before the term "gatekeeper" came into vogue. While these roles are problematic, there may be good reasons for them. I do not wish to argue the merits of involving physicians as experts in commitment proceedings here. The point is that physicians have long been functionaries in systems.

Second, in their ordinary activity, caring for patients, physicians have understood their role as one of agency for their particular patients, but only within socially established limits and subject to certain social considerations. The agents of society are dangerous, but so are physicians who serve only their patients' interests. The arena of medical research provides an example. Research has always had a certain moral dignity, even though it has led to some of the most egregious abuses of individual rights and social trust. Are we to applaud the physician who subverts a randomized clinical trial by "sneaking" her sickest patients into the treatment group?[25] Not every recognition of the claims of society, or other patients, is illegitimate. One may yield to such claims without "giving in" or abandoning the patient.

BUREAUCRATIC VERSUS COLLEGIAL CONTROLS

To rephrase the question, how do we assess, morally, the various means open to us for translating the legitimate claims of plan members as a group, present patients as a group, future patients as a group, the various communities to which we belong, and so on, into ordinary medical practice, while preserving meaningful personal relationships? The work of Eliot Freidson, one of the founders of the field of medical sociology, is an invaluable source of information about the effects of business concerns and bureaucratic structures on medical practice. The arrival of Medicare, Medicaid, and claims processing for private insurers was associated with a new emphasis on management and controlling physician performance. This regime forms the context for Freidson's investigations.

Freidson distinguishes bureaucratic from collegial methods of control. Bureaucratic controls rely on secondhand reports and tend to focus on what is measurable and quantifiable. Reviewing claims, and the many forms of utilization review, are bureaucratic controls. Collegial controls rely as much as possible on direct observation of performance and attend to qualitative as well as quantitative factors.[26] Since cost, a matter seemingly in the realm of the quantifiable, has been the primary concern in health care administration for decades, the stress has been on bureaucratic controls.

Beyond the obvious point that the administrative structure required is itself costly in economic terms, there are other sorts of costs associated with bureaucratic controls. For example, those who head and staff the program "develop an ideological as well as a personal vested interest in expanding it well past its true usefulness" and "its very logic of operation will reward conformity to statistical standards even when what is being dealt with actually falls outside the norm."[27] Insofar as bureaucratic controls are perceived as manipulative, and foster manipulation as a mode of resistance, they invite particular scrutiny within an ethical framework that focuses on the quality of social relations.[28]

Bureaucratic controls are most questionable when financial incentives directed to individual physicians represent the primary means of ensuring compliance with the rules. Acknowledging the pedagogical role of organizations, we might inquire into the "lesson" of this practice. It seems to be something like this: "People are greedy, out to get as much as they can for themselves. We are realists, we recognize this, and bright as you are, we think you do too. So get as much for yourself as you can, and help us in the bargain. (We're greedy too, we wouldn't put the proposition to you unless we thought we'd get something out of it.)"

But why should converts to the gospel of greed care much for the interests of the proselytizers? Doubting the truth of this particular gospel, we may believe that many will "stay honest." They will either work within the system while doing their best to ignore it, or leave it altogether. But what reason have the converts to refrain from manipulating the system, or subverting it, in order to maximize their own earnings potential?

As for the others, the virtuous remnant, they may find it impossible to escape altogether the pressures to conform, the pressures to play the system's game or "game the system."[29] And they will, no doubt, be demoralized. According to Freidson, "the profound weakness of neoclassical economic assumptions" is that "financial incentives tend to subvert policy goals by stimulating the efforts of those most inclined to put gain before any other end and discouraging the others."[30]

SUBVERSION OF BUREAUCRATIC CONTROLS: DRG CREEP

Freidson uses diagnosis-related groups (DRGs) to illustrate the process of manipulation and subversion of bureaucratic controls. "DRG creep" describes a host of questionable practices, from selecting patients with diagnoses that have favorable reimbursement rates for the facility or health plan, to selecting diagnoses with favorable reimbursement rates for the patients one has.

DRG creep "suggests how vulnerable the system is to those who create its records," since "service is not exactly and irrevocably specifiable independently of the discretionary judgment of the 'worker.'"[31] Manipulation may extend well beyond patient selection and creative record-keeping. Providers may alter a patient's course of treatment, or disregard her wishes, in order to ensure that her care is reimbursable.[32]

Administrators would not have adopted such a system without faith that responses to financial incentives under the system would be counter-balanced by professional and moral considerations.[33] The policy presupposes a kind of character at odds with the lesson it teaches. The lesson might be different were the policy embedded in a larger network of practices nourishing trust. But the relationship between practitioners and administrators has long been adversarial.

Freidson himself identifies the variable of trust as significant, when he remarks that "[a]n enormous variety of empirical studies carried out over the past half-century has shown that, *when they feel no loyalty to it,* people do not passively obey, but instead actively seek ways of 'getting around the system' wherever they can."[34] In general, we might expect greater respect for limits where these limits are perceived as legitimate. It is not merely a matter of perception; limits *are* more or less legitimate, according to the processes that create them, their compatibility with an organization's particular values and principles, and the consistency with which organizational members adhere to them.

The DRG example underscores the connection between financial incentives and manipulation.[35] Other examples suggest that the lack of subtlety in many strategies to measure performance, combined with ordinary desires to do well or to avoid criticism, may be sufficient to produce similar dysfunctions.[36] Massive funding of social programs without accountability is a recipe for disaster. At the same time, the judgments called for are difficult, not obvious or "technical." Most organizations that attempt to evaluate outcomes neglect qualitative factors. Managers should make an effort to link the limited tools of quality assurance monitoring and outcomes evaluation to the organization's mission, goals, principles, and values. They should also credit the intelligence of their staff and clientele.

A BALANCED VIEW OF BUREAUCRACY

Realizing the benefits of bureaucracy within managed care organizations requires well-designed systems, adequate resources, well-trained and motivated staff working in an organizational culture that reinforces conscientious performance, and effective methods to correct inadequate performance.[37] Bureaucracy is less a dragon to be slain than a complex of organizational features that can be beneficial or destructive depending on details of implementation and the spirit which animates the process. This dual nature comes through in the story of Christine deMeurers and Health Net.

As the narrative unfolds, we encounter both too much and too little bureaucracy, or perhaps Health Net had many of the vices of bureaucracy without its virtues. Too much bureaucracy, when corporate decision makers display so little sensitivity to the average person's experience that they seem shocked when their rulings are received as death sentences and vigorously contested. The vices of bureaucracy, when recalcitrant physicians are brought into line by calls from headquarters. Too little bureaucracy, when physicians seem poorly integrated into the organization's philosophy of care. An absence of the virtues of bureaucracy, when the decisions rendered seem totally arbitrary from the viewpoint of plan members.

Problems of Organizational Scale and Complexity

Large size may exacerbate the problems associated with business and bureaucracy. Hence, it is disturbing to find ourselves in a period of unprecedented consolidation in health care. Defenders of large organizations argue that they offer significant benefits in terms of efficiency and economy. For example, large corporations can absorb greater research and development costs than smaller organizations. Innovativeness might be a property of size; there is some evidence of this in certain industries.[38]

Defenders of large managed care organizations argue that they require great concentrations of capital, not so much for building physical plant as in the past, but for developing and implementing sophisticated information management systems. Managed care organizations may generate significant administrative and cost savings by consolidating purchasing. Some argue that only a managed care organization with a monopoly or near monopoly in a particular geographic area has an economic incentive to take responsibility for community health.[39] However, not all the "efficiencies" large corporations achieve are productive. Large health care organizations may use their resources to secure favorable treatment from those charged with protecting the public weal, undermining accountability and contributing nothing to the realization of the proper ends of health care. Further, much of the consolidation has to do with financial manipulation rather than innovation, gains from exploiting provisions of the tax code or speculation rather than improvements in service delivery.[40]

Growth can also be associated with organizational dysfunctions such as bureaucracy run amok in outdated rules and improperly invoked hierarchies.[41] Health economist James Robinson has drawn attention to three negative features of large organizations: incentive attenuation, influence costs, and organizational insularity.

Incentive attenuation occurs when rewards and responsibility for performance become disconnected from daily activities. The pragmatist will relate this dysfunction to the loss of sense and the general problem of organizational opacity exacerbated by scale. Connections to other people are also attenuated, and responsibilities blur. The result may be a situation in which no one takes responsibility, as suggested by studies in which the presence of a large group of observers diminishes the willingness of any one to help a person in need.[42]

Influence costs arise when there is "surplus value," i.e., resources are loose in the organization and "the potential rewards for haggling, coalition-building, and back-scratching exceed rewards for effort, innovation, and entrepreneurship."[43] The pragmatist will set the economist's concern within a larger frame, asking how the rewards of nonproductive activity come to exceed the rewards of productive activity. Growth may foster neglect of internal goods.

Finally, organizational insularity refers to a fortress mentality that nourishes corporate culture, but blocks information and ideas from outside. In other words, growth may upset the balance between integrity and responsiveness. In each case, the pragmatist will push for a description that highlights the continuity between economic and moral concerns, suggesting that corrective action should be guided by an enlarged vision.

Greater size is usually associated with increased organizational complexity, and organizational complexity creates its own set of difficulties. Considered purely in terms of the project of organization, complexity is almost always an evil because it leads to internalization of costs and risks that could be externalized in a firm-to-firm relationship. HMOs are exceedingly complex organizations.[44]

Health care managers are becoming increasingly aware that organizations can achieve many of the benefits of consolidation through collaboration and "virtual" organization, pooling resources among a group of corporations to fund research and software development, creating purchasing cooperatives, and so on. Although these kinds of alliances may become conspiracies posing perils comparable to the corporate colossi (and require monitoring), their very nature as more "loosely coupled" systems lessens our concern about enormous concentrations of wealth and power in the hands of a very few.

THE IDEOLOGY OF MEDICINE REVISITED

Philanthropy Debunked: Hippocrates or Hypocrisy?

The ideology of medicine offers us professional commitment to competent performance and dedication to patient welfare, if only physicians are free (or freed) from the intrusion of market forces and bureaucratic controls. Pragmatists suspicious of markets may embrace this ideology. Yet there are good pragmatic reasons for skepticism in this area as well. Pure philanthropy is neither possible nor desirable, and the pretense is corrupting. The ideology of medicine shares the "pathologies" Freidson ascribes to professional ideologies generally:

> [T]he collegium becomes more concerned with its own welfare than that of its customers; it expands the scope of its monopoly well past its capacity to serve public needs; it actually resists efforts at rationalization that would reduce the cost of its work and the range of its jurisdiction and control, and practices featherbedding with impunity; it becomes preoccupied with refining its knowledge and skill for their own sake, irrespective of public need; stratification develops internally, dividing its members. Cost, distribution, and quality are virtually uncontrolled by the regulatory processes that the collegium claims it exercises. Quality varies widely—from extraordinary virtuosity to perfunctory routine and even negligent incompetence.[45]

In *Doctoring Together*, Freidson describes how professional etiquette, as an expression of occupational solidarity among physicians, takes priority over efforts to realize the ideals of dedication to service and technical proficiency.[46] No wonder radical critics of medicine such as Ivan Illich cite his work. The same physicians who react defensively to scrutiny by administrators and patients may also resist "intrusions" by colleagues in the form of peer review. Most of us dislike having our work subjected to criticism, and defensiveness is first nature. Yet the "sham of perfectionism," the inability to "tolerate error or acknowledge mistakes because this lessens one's image among peers as a technically proficient caregiver," is harmful to clinicians and sometimes lethal to patients.[47]

A CRITICAL RECONSTRUCTION OF PROFESSIONALISM

R. H. Tawney's critical defense of professionalism is a useful point of departure on the road to reconstruction. Writing in the 1920s, Tawney had little sympathy for claims to exclusivity of expertise or virtue which were mere ornaments for the monopolistic drive. On the other hand, Tawney valued the association of profession with high standards, even if these standards were not always attained. He wrote, "[t]here is all the difference between maintaining a standard which is occasionally abandoned, and affirming as the central truth of existence that there is no standard to maintain."[48] (Of course, any standard so remote from practice that is it is only occasionally *attained* has the bad odor of hypocrisy.) Tawney considered the professional attitude an antidote to the "acquisitive society," and proposed extending professionalism to all areas of productive life.[49]

Tawney's work holds out the hope of difference without hierarchy. Because all fields of human endeavor will eventually be professionalized, there will be no moral hierarchy of occupations. At the same time, different standards will be appropriate to different kinds of work. Each practice will have its own distinctive complex of internal goods and rules. The goods of health care and automobile repair will differ, although there may well be areas of overlap.[50] The ethical code for physicians will not be identical to the code for auto mechanics. In each endeavor, faithfulness will have a distinctive shape. Other spheres of human activity will have their own goods, codes, and models of excellence.[51] Health care administration would itself constitute a practice.[52]

Tawney sensed the dangers accompanying the annihilation of difference. Health care, and the fields of human endeavor comprehended by the term "business," lose their distinctive shapes as practices when treated as meaningless means to the sole or primary end of generating income and profit.

Tawney feared the industrialization of the professions, and he used medicine as an example. Precisely because he saw no unexpungeable divisions, no ontological necessities, Tawney wrote, "It is conceivable, at least, that some branches of medicine might have developed on the lines of industrial capitalism, with hospitals as factories, doctors hired at competitive wages as their 'hands,' large dividends paid to shareholders by catering for the rich, and the poor, who do not offer a profitable market, supplied with an inferior service or with no service at all."[53]

As a mode of organizing work, professionalism can be highly compatible with the pragmatist's vision of democracy. It is based on the democratic notion that "people are capable of controlling themselves by cooperative, collective means and that, in the case of complex work, those who perform it are in the best position to make sure that it gets done well." It is founded on the assumption that when people can control their own work, and that work is challenging, "they will be committed to it rather than alienated from it."[54]

The important next step is to move away from a privatized understanding of professionalism and the goods pursued through professional relationships. Where health care is framed as a purely private act of philanthropy, or commerce, we lose sight of the public dimension, the social networks in which health care is embedded and on which it depends, and the social values this work can embody and advance.[55]

What we need is a chastened medical profession that can accept some measure of external scrutiny, relinquish the sham of perfectionism, recognize competence and dedication to patient well-being in other practitioners, receive lay participation as a contribution rather than an affront, and accept some sacrifice of financial reward in order to preserve internal goods such as pride in the quality of one's work, the respect of colleagues, and the (deserved) trust and gratitude of patients.

Fee-for-service payment, like capitation, tends to sharpen the physician's awareness of his or her economic interest in performing a service, and in favoring certain recommendations over others. Independent contractor status may lessen a sense of subservience to corporate interests, but foster insensitivity to legitimate demands for accountability. As Freidson notes, engineers, priests, and scientists have traditionally been employees with modest salaries, without losing their intellectual or moral excellence. Ironically, many managed care organizations go to great lengths to avoid employing physicians, in order to limit the organization's malpractice exposure.

The potential for medicine to survive as a practice is linked to the creation and maintenance of virtuous organizations. It is a mistake to think that either professionals or professions can survive without adequate institutional supports. Should we enthusiastically greet physician efforts to organize their own managed care enterprises? The story of the Connecticut State Medical Society's M.D. Health Plan in Chapter 2 suggests that physicians who have not resolutely accepted some sacrifice of external goods as the price for preserving professionalism are all too ready to sell out when the price is right.[56]

HEALTH CARE PROFESSIONALS AND UNIONIZATION

Caution may be appropriate in relation to recent efforts to organize physicians. Indeed, the ambiguous moral status of professionalism is laid bare in the current debate over unionization and organized medicine's intensive lobbying campaign to win a special exemption from federal antitrust laws to permit independent physicians to jointly negotiate fees and working conditions with health plans. According to public statements by AMA representatives, they are pursuing unionization and an antitrust exemption to empower physicians to serve as more effective patient advocates.[57]

Federal officials who oppose antitrust exemption point out that antitrust guidelines already permit physicians to join together to discuss raising standards of care and to form networks to improve care. Economists suggest that the AMA's current strategy has more to do with shoring up income and status, and preserving autonomy at the expense of accountability, than disinterestedly pursuing patient welfare.[58] They also point out that profit margins for most managed care organizations are small, and the likely effect of widespread collective bargaining by physicians will be higher premiums for patients.

While financial issues are intertwined with patient care issues, that relationship is complex. Although care is likely to suffer where physicians are impoverished and overworked, it is unclear whether making doctors rich is the best way to promote high quality care. At the very least, the AMA's form of action, lobbying for a blanket exemption, fosters skepticism, and even cynicism, concerning the alleged justification. Even if AMA representatives believe their own rhetoric, the idea that unaccountable power will not be abused is terribly naïve. Physicians must avoid collapsing patient interests into their own.[59]

FEARS CONCERNING PROFESSIONAL AUTHORITY

This leads to the more general question of physician authority. For some bioethicists, the ideal is a strong doctor-patient relationship as the locus of control in health care.[60] Physicians as a professional group, drilled in the creed of patient autonomy and patient rights and freed of financial conflicts of interest, are considered trustworthy guardians of the principles and values that should guide the healing enterprise. Not so with others. Going back at least as far as the seminal work of Robert Veatch, some have questioned the alignment of professional values and patient or public values.

These individuals have expressed two concerns about the traditional role of the physician as patient agent, as well as the newer, and more controversial role of the physician as bedside rationer or policy advisor. First, physicians, by reason of their socialization and professional role, may overvalue health relative to other goods. Second, and related to that, physicians may give too high a priority to beneficence, pursuing every procedure or treatment that may potentially benefit a patient. These two concerns add up to a fear that physicians will resist the constraints on medical practice required by patient autonomy or justice, and that their own view of what justice requires will be skewed by a bias toward health, the good to which they have dedicated their professional lives.[61]

Because these concerns are not baseless, it is worthwhile to consider possible correctives. One option is to take some authority from physicians and vest it in others. To a limited extent, the view I have endorsed entails some circumscribing and diminishing of professional authority. While emphasizing intraprofessional discipline, I have recognized the beneficent role of bureaucrats (plan managers and government regulators) in ensuring that practice is accountable, consistent with plan philosophy and with public values. I have advocated transferring power to those the health professions are intended to serve, i.e., consumers. I will develop this theme further in the next section.

Another partial solution is reshaping the professional ideology. Bioethicists have enjoyed modest success in altering physicians' socialization, thereby creating a place for patient autonomy in the professional ethic. That experiment suggests there may also be room for justice and a more balanced view of the goods of human life.

Such halfway measures are important, since certain considerations seem to weigh against another option, the complete overthrow of professional authority in health care. I will touch on three. First, many have argued that professional authority is integral to the healing process. Illness has been described as an "ontological" and not merely a physical assault. Even in the United States, in a culture that emphasizes self-determination to an unusual degree, studies reveal that many patients would experience taking responsibility for the details of their day-to-day treatment as a burden.[62] The physician's professional authority is rooted in the relationship between one in distress, seeking hope and help, and an "other" who offers hope and help according to the approved cultural pattern. Therapeutic power is vested in the person and the social role, as well as in the specific techniques brought to bear on the disease.[63] As Howard Brody warns, "defanging" the powerful physician may give us a person who can neither harm nor help.[64]

Second, a system in which patients must acquire sufficient knowledge to displace professional authority would seem irrational. By definition, a patient is an expert on her illness. Laypeople can become informed concerning disease processes and clinical tools. However, these are not substitutes for medical training and clinical experience.

Third, concerning professional authority to ration, patients in an insurance pool have an interest in restraining costs out of concern for their own medical well-being, assuring that resources are available when most necessary and that insurance is affordable, as well as their general economic interests and their concern for others who depend on the pool. Mark Hall argues that purchasing insurance creates a kind of incapacity, insensitivity to costs, that necessitates delegation of cost-benefit trade-off decisions.[65]

Certainly for major categorical decisions, such as coverage exclusions, the best response to the problem of individual insensitivity to costs is the development of limit-setting rules by bureaucratic, or if possible, cooperative means. Although there is little evidence to support fears that physicians differ systematically from the general population in their understanding of justice or in their readiness to sacrifice vulnerable groups to maximize utility, there is no reason to believe they are immune from general kinds of bias.

On the other hand, for routine, day-to-day clinical decision-making in the gray areas of medical practice, careful analysis seems to favor clinical discretion constrained by rules and subject to various forms of internal and external bureaucratic oversight over the alternatives.[66] Surveys suggest that most people would choose to allocate decision making authority in this fashion.[67]

It is important not to take this too far. Illnesses vary by kind and degree in their disabling effects. Focusing energy on the work of healing, work that may require an unusual degree of reliance on the judgment of others, must be distinguished from regressing to an infantile state of dependence. And, with reference to the empirical studies and public opinion surveys, people's preferences are shaped by what they have been taught to expect. Jay Katz has argued that while physicians point to the fact of regression and patient disinclination to make decisions in rejecting the model of shared decision making, they themselves engage in practices that foster regression, or at least do nothing to restore a sense of agency and power in the midst of illness.[68]

Moral Language in Health Care

Even when Freidson and other social scientists are clearly engaged in social criticism, they strive for measured neutrality. If they do not yield to a sense of outrage over the discrepancy between the announced ideals of the medical profession and actual physician conduct, they also tend to discount the significance of moral standards and values in general.[69] Freidson, unlike Tawney, cannot recognize ideals as potential elements of ideology, in the negative sense of a smokescreen for a power grab, and yet allow for their beneficial operation in guiding and judging practice. Certainly, we should not expect virtue or conscientiousness to prevail too long, or among too many, without encouragement. We should not test the limits of virtue too frequently; it is always best to have incentives and conscience working in the same direction.

This is not, however, equivalent to an argument for discounting the effects of an ideal altogether. It may be that Freidson is simply wiser than Tawney. But restrained cynicism, like anything else, may originate in ideology, or habitual patterns of thought. It protects one against disappointment. It also supports a certain flattening out or homogenizing of experience. What is being lost, or left out?

At the very least, many people still act as if values matter. Differences over values seem to be extremely significant in the intramural conflicts among the various groups of health care professionals. I do not wish to slight the importance of power in battles between nurses and physicians, physicians and administrators, and nurses and administrators. But in the nature of things, even battles over power are partly battles over what power shall be used for.[70]

Physicians want power, resources, and freedom, in part, to preserve life, which they sometimes conceive of as holding off death to the last possible moment, and in part, to advance medical knowledge through research. Nurses want power, resources, and freedom, in part, to demonstrate care, and to resist physician demands that counter a patient's interests, as they conceive those interests based on their more intimate association with patients and families. Administrators want power, resources, and freedom, in part, to conserve resources for future generations, and to resist demands by physicians and nurses which they regard as improvident or as insensitive to the interests of the organization as a whole.

Each professional group has legitimate claims. I do not believe it would be an advance if they were to sideline questions of value and focus on the "real issue," whatever that might be. One of the most attractive things about the health care field is that people within it still do, on occasion, speak frankly about moral concerns. In the business world generally, talk about morality must often be disguised in the language of cost-benefit analysis or efficiency and effectiveness.[71]

The answer is not to train people to care less about what they care deeply about. Rather, the solution to the dilemma, inevitably partial, is to create structures that cross professional boundaries. If nurses serve on planning committees, they will better understand the sources and the moral weight of administrators' concerns about costs and budgets and the efficient implementation of initially cumbersome new information management systems. If administrators spend one week a year or one hour a week "on the floor," they will better understand nurses' concerns about understaffing and the lack of effective processes for ensuring that patients' wishes are known and honored.

Retaining the focus on moral and ethical issues, I am sympathetic to Daniel Chambliss's indictment of traditional medical ethics as inattentive to power.[72] One can make this criticism in a blanket way, but Chambliss, looking at the moral world of nurses, has a quite specific concern.

Medical ethics has been concerned with resolving difficult moral questions or quandaries. The task of ethics basically ends with the identification of the preferred solution. That sort of approach used to work for physicians, who had the freedom to act based on their understanding of what was right. But what of the health care worker faced with a situation that is problematic, not because the preferred solution is unclear, but because the worker lacks the power to act? Short of a revolution in which the morally right are automatically gifted with power, the solution to this dilemma requires attending to organizational structures. The task is to interest persons who do have power in the issue of powerlessness, and to establish channels for the less powerful to communicate their concerns outside the "chain of command." Whistle-blower protection policies help, but action will often be attended by risk.[73]

Professionalism and Faithfulness

Finally, we ought not to divorce a discussion of professionalism from the passionate sense of calling expressed by some health care professionals. For these men and women, what they do is holy work, not because they themselves are god-like creatures, but because they minister to the sick. They have a profound awareness of their responsibility in the face of human vulnerability. They select words like "reverence" to describe their feelings toward those they serve. To capture this relationship, William May chose the word covenant over contract, suggesting that what is owed is faithfulness rather than strict enforcement of agreed-upon terms.[74]

These doctors and nurses display faithfulness to patients not only in heroic acts demanding great personal dedication and professional skill, but also in ordinary acts of caring that show respect and compassion for human beings vulnerable in body, mind, and spirit. What must survive the increasing visibility of market and bureaucratic forces in health care, and the recognition of the legitimacy of certain limits, is this sense of calling, and structures that support rather than undermine faithfulness.[75]

THE IDEOLOGY OF COOPERATIVE EGALITARIANISM RECOVERED

When Michael Shadid initiated a prepaid health plan in Elk City, Oklahoma, he was inspired by the cooperative, and more particularly, the farmers' grain cooperatives common in that region of the country. Shadid wanted to make comprehensive health care available to everyone at reasonable cost, and he wanted customers to have a stake in the enterprise. He cordoned off the area of clinical practice for professional control, but the rest was to be left to collective deliberation and judgment. Shadid subscribed to the ideology I have labeled "cooperative egalitarianism."

The practical force of cooperative egalitarianism will vary depending on where the emphasis is placed, as between cooperation and equality, although the joining of the two concepts expresses their close relationship. If we accent cooperation, the focus will be on nurturing participatory democracy, or what some term deliberative democracy. One asks what difference it makes to think of health care as a project in which all participate as moral equals, a project in which each person is both a contributor and a recipient. In this area, the ideology of cooperative egalitarianism offers action guides such as "those affected by a problem should participate in its definition and resolution" and "favor structures that build cooperation over structures that place persons in relationships where some command and others obey."

If we accent equality, we return to distributive justice. Rejecting the simplistic view of equality as equal shares, I focus on those without the social and material supports for moral equality. Many impairments to health form potential barriers to personal development and social contribution. We have a social obligation to address health impairments that are amenable to reversal or amelioration, meeting needs for health care as communal resources permit. Working out the implications of this kind of egalitarianism through processes that incorporate elements of participatory democracy is important in rationing. In this area, the ideology of cooperative egalitarianism offers action guides such as "consider the plight of the least advantaged"—those who are most vulnerable and, therefore, most dependent on others (on us) for support and respect.

Facing the Difficulties

The proponent of a more prominent role for cooperative egalitarianism in health care immediately faces certain difficulties. First, history suggests that cooperative egalitarianism is hard to sustain in organizations. Indeed, history suggests that cooperative egalitarianism is hard to sustain period. Many people have shown little interest in participating, and many movements aiming to open up organizations and make them more accountable seem to depend on strong leaders for their success. These phenomena pose a challenge to the ideology.

Second, cooperative egalitarianism, both as participation on terms of moral equality and as distribution to assure moral equality, appears incompatible with efficiency. Third, although we can defend professionalism as democratic, it is not easy to reconcile professional organization with the demands of cooperative egalitarianism, either as to relations among professionals or relations between providers and clients.

ROBERT MICHELS AND THE LIMITS OF COOPERATIVE EGALITARIANISM

The work of Robert Michels represents a good place to begin working through these difficulties. Michels is known for his account of the demise of democracy in organizations and the so-called "iron law of oligarchy."[76] Even organizations with strong commitments to participation on terms of equality readily drift toward structures incompatible with their founding principles. To achieve their objectives, leaders must attend to the task of building an effective organization; this creates the risk that standard criteria of organizational effectiveness will displace the original objectives. The oligarchic tendency Michels described is linked to abandoning direct, participatory democracy in favor of representative democracy in response to problems of scale.[77] However, even small organizations likely tend toward concentrations of power.

Despite the "iron law" rhetoric, Michels identifies two regulative principles that check the drift toward oligarchy and mitigate its effects. First, democratic participation in any area of life tends to stimulate and strengthen member capacities for criticism and control. Abilities developed in one arena can and do spill over into others. Second, oligarchy can be limited when power is available to check power. The involvement of elites is essential if critical movements are to be sustained over time.[78]

There is some tension between the first and second principles. After all, is not the gathering of power in the hands of elites the first step toward oligarchy? Even if elite power is not transformed into domination, because elites are multiple and serve to check each other, is not the very notion of an elite antithetical to democracy and to cooperative egalitarianism?

I understand democracy as the fullest possible development of individual capacities and powers, including their social dimensions. If a person has an interest in and talent for exercising social power, he or she can use these gifts for social purposes. The term "elite" may refer to the beneficiaries of class privilege, or to a special class of experts. It may also refer to those from whatever walk of life gifted with enthusiasm for social work, political intelligence, and leadership ability.

We need leaders. There is nothing scandalous in the fact that some are leaders in some areas, so long as power is as fully dispersed as possible, authority is structurally limited and open to contestation, and leadership in one area does not translate into dominance in other spheres of activity. Indeed, one mark of democratic as opposed to authoritarian leadership is that it is not threatened when others act as leaders. To the contrary, democratic leadership nurtures the leadership capacity in others.

Further, the model of democracy as universal participation in governance scarcely works in the political arena. Extending it to the management and practices of health care organizations is, at present, unrealistic. No one has fully articulated the means for accomplishing such a revolution. It is difficult to imagine middle-class Americans, let alone those worrying about having enough money to buy food and pay the monthly utility bill, becoming health care activists en masse, in response to the call of civic duty. Then, too, being committed to cooperative egalitarianism as participatory democracy may work against efficiency and the other productive virtues, creating organizational paralysis, or permitting a small but vocal group to bully others, because they are prepared to bring the organization to a halt. In his comparative analysis of HMOs, Lawrence Brown concluded that the cooperative model crippled two organizations, to the detriment of members as well as managers.[79] In short, some of us may want health care organizations to be "managed in our interests, but also in our absence."[80]

Yet, we should always be striving for something more fully participatory. Health care touches us more closely than many an issue debated in Washington or the state capitol, and understanding the ways in which organizations condition what goes on in the doctor's office and the surgical suite should be part of health education in school and beyond. No one should be satisfied with the communication of this sort of information through sound bites, infomercials, and billboards with beaming moms and babies and the promise that your managed care organization will provide "ALL THE HEALTH CARE YOU DESERVE."

Participation frequently suffers due to a lack of resources, and people may be "apathetic because they are powerless, not powerless because they are apathetic."[81] Improving existing conditions may certainly be feasible. We need to become more active and responsible in relation to our own health and health care; this sort of democracy, in the broad sense, is a realistic goal. Various forms of local involvement may also serve to "stimulate and strengthen in the individual the intellectual aptitudes for criticism and control," and may even furnish the basis for more properly political activity, without being merely instrumental to this purpose.[82]

The activity of elites will likely remain a significant factor in monitoring and checking the political activity of health care organizations and shaping their internal politics, policies, and decision making.[83] Still, organizations seeking to facilitate broader participation can provide the missing resources, or better, use their resources to develop the potentialities already present in communities.

Lack of information is another barrier to participation. Organizations have many reasons, some more legitimate than others, for restricting information flow, e.g., concerns about the confidentiality of patient information, protection of trade secrets, fear of litigation. If an organization struggles to diminish opacity by increasing openness, then, even if it makes no directed effort to facilitate participation, it has made participation more likely.[84]

EQUITY VERSUS EFFICIENCY

One of the great difficulties in the area of resource allocation is what philosophers refer to as the trade-off between equity and efficiency. Should we distribute health care resources based on need or based on efficiency? I recognize the problem, while constructing it in a slightly different fashion. If efficiency is understood as fittedness to purpose, the appropriate matching of technique and organization to end in view, then efficiency cannot be set up in opposition to equity.[85] Rather, the conflict or tension is with the principle of utility, which would make maximizing health (or wealth) the end in view.

There is also a conflict or tension internal to the principle of distribution according to need, since we cannot meet all needs, and needs are not always commensurable. Norman Daniels provides an excellent account of the perplexities that arise when we try to set priorities among services that provide different sorts of benefits to different sorts of people. These priority-setting dilemmas confront us under certain conditions, specifically when (1) a scarce resource is "lumpy" (not easily divisible), (2) the competing claims are legitimate, (3) general principles of distributive justice underdetermine the outcome, and (4) moral disagreement exists about how to establish priorities.

Three dilemmas concern trade-offs between maximizing good health outcomes and meeting the most intense or concentrated needs: the priorities problem ("How much priority should we give to treating the sickest or most disabled patients?"), the fair chances/best outcome problem ("Should we give all who might benefit some chance at a resource, or should we give the resource to those who get the best outcome?"), and the aggregation problem ("When do lesser benefits to many outweigh greater benefits to a few?").[86]

Daniels does not propose a solution to these dilemmas, and I am similarly bereft of answers. However, I would propose three guides.

First, if we are persuaded by any account of distributive justice in health care that centers on need, or aims to secure fair equality of opportunity, we will tend to give a higher priority to the sickest vis-à-vis the relatively healthy than would the utilitarian.[87] We will also tend to favor fair chances in circumstances (comparability of need) where the utilitarian would pursue best outcomes. We will do this knowing that we will have less-than-maximal aggregate benefit in terms of health. Even so, most of us boggle at the prospect of enormous expenditures for infinitesimal benefits. At some point, our commitments are constrained by a sense of proportion and limit, e.g., no kidney transplants for persons in persistent vegetative states.

The aggregation problem is a particularly tough one for the principle of distribution according to need (or fair equality of opportunity), because it may pit preventive against acute care. The promise of preventive care is a future in which needs for health care, and the toll taken by illness and disability, are substantially reduced. The weight of "lesser benefits to many" relative to "greater benefits to a few" should depend on whether the "lesser benefits" arise from true preventive care that averts significant disability, or rather from care addressed to the kinds of minor aches and ills that occasionally annoy but seldom impair.

Second, the "practice" concept may be relevant to how we view these dilemmas, even if it provides no answers. As I have said, the proper goal of health care must be something like caring for the sick, easing suffering, curing when possible, and educating in prevention. Distortions appear when those within or outside the practice begin acting as if the aim were to overcome death or to deliver us from all the tragedies of life. We have physicians ordering aggressive life-sustaining treatment for the dying and parents demanding ventilator support for babies born without brains. There are some needs that cannot be met with health care, but rather belong to the sphere of religion or philosophy. Religion may serve as an umbrella term for practices that address ultimate questions and offer rituals that allow individuals and communities to come to terms with tragedy and loss. As Robert Veatch says, the principle of justice asks who is worse off *and how can they be helped*.[88] Sometimes help will lie beyond the powers of medicine.

Third and finally, when we are in a gray area, in terms of either the demands of justice or the appropriate goals of medicine, we can allow for choice. Pragmatists both recognize and value pluralism. Some argue that we should offer consumers multiple lists of services, each with the same expected cost, eliminating the need to create a single definitive list of covered services. This may prove the best course, although we must consider the costs vis-à-vis a system that mandates a uniform benefits package: some increase in administrative complexity, some loss of comparability among plans, some decrease in the ease with which consumers can evaluate their options,[89] and some rise in the potential for risk selection, as some plans tailor their benefits schedule to appeal to the healthy. Of course in this as in other areas, we can search for a compromise that honors both sets of concerns. For example, we might standardize the benefits packages (plural) across organizations, and regulate plans to minimize the favorable selection of risk.

Moral Equality in Policy Making: Setting Standards

The highly visible process by which Oregon brought explicit rationing to its Medicaid program has often been the paradigm for attempts at community involvement in policy making. Rather than rehearse the virtues and serious imperfections of that process here, I will offer another paradigm.

The Ethics of Managed Care

In 1995, Denver's Rocky Mountain Center for Health Care Ethics sponsored a conference entitled "Ethical Managed Care: Avoiding an Oxymoron." Some of the participants—200 consumers, patients, providers, purchasers, employers, and representatives of managed care organizations—expressed a desire to continue their dialogue. The goal would be to create a code of ethics for managed care in Colorado.

The Center staff first gauged the degree of interest in the project, then made a commitment to lead it. They recruited a Steering Committee of twenty from the various stakeholder groups. The Steering Committee adopted a goal and four objectives. The former was stated as follows: "The goal of this process is to create a Code of Ethics for Managed Care in Colorado with the participation of consumers, patients, providers, purchasers, employers and payers."[90] The four objectives were to (1) identify and prioritize ethical issues and concerns associated with managed care; (2) engage in structured reflection and dialogue to consider these issues and concerns; (3) create ethical standards for addressing ethical issues and concerns; and (4) increase public and personal involvement and accountability in healthcare delivery.

Once they identified ethical issues and related these issues to four organizing themes, they created work groups. The themes were economics and resources (e.g., profit, incentives, uncompensated care, enrollment discrimination), relationships and responsibilities, information, and allocation of resources (e.g., medical appropriateness, mechanisms of decision making, new technologies). Rather than focus on the conflict between business and medicine, or elect business ethics or medical ethics as the standard for evaluation, the process centered on the tension between the Hippocratic tradition and population-based health care.

The work of the work groups involved more than 100 persons. The Steering Committee incorporated the work group recommendations into a draft Code. The preamble of that draft Code affirms a commitment to fairness, honesty, respect for persons, justice, caring, and compassion, and states that the standards articulated are intended to guide individual and organizational stakeholders.

The structure they adopted for the document relates standards to seven "key issues" and associated value statements. The seven key issues are: (1) improving the health of the public; (2) appropriate resource usage; (3) fairness, equality, and just treatment; (4) exchange of information, education, and shared decision making, (5) privacy and confidentiality, (6) stakeholder relationships, and (7) creating ethical environments.

"The Code of Ethics for Managed Care in Colorado: Working Document" is a thoughtful piece of work. Yet, it is scarcely revolutionary. One might even say that the content is common—and therein lies its charm. It is the product of an effort directed toward a shared (common) goal. Not incidentally, it is also the product of an effort people initiated because they were excited by the prospect of working with others who would bring different perspectives to the project. The Code's title is a reminder that this product is also a process. In the project's Phase II, the Steering Committee planned to submit the Code to criticism by broader groups of stakeholders, who would then disseminate and operationalize it.

One of the specific objectives for Phase II was to "continue testing and refining the Code by increasing the number of active participants and broadening the demographic and geographic boundaries."[91] Weaknesses already identified by a consumer group included an absence of accountability mechanisms, neglect of physician-patient relationships and funding for research and education, and a lack of specificity in the standards. Even so, midway in the process, some managed care organizations were beginning to implement the directives. The project directors reported that in conducting an internal assessment, members of one organization discovered two structures or practices needing change: financial disincentives to hospice referrals, and the release of patient-identifiable data to employers.

Skeptics may be wondering who funded this project, fearing the undue influence of managed care organizations. These fears would be partially justified. Managed care organizations funded Phase I; money and influence being closely related, the suspicion is not groundless. The Center obtained community funding for Phase II, which may reflect a concern to avoid even the potential for manipulation of the process, as well as the existence of the draft Code as a platform for fundraising. Skeptics may also distrust claims to diversity. How were the representatives of the various stakeholder groups selected? Staff members reported that they advertised in the newspaper, and also worked through known individuals. Anyone interested could participate.[92]

This summary does not prove that cooperative egalitarianism works. At first glance, though, this collaborative effort appears to justify a modest optimism concerning the prospects for cooperative egalitarianism in health care, where there is a will and a willingness to learn. The Colorado process also illustrates an important aspect of the pragmatist understanding of community, that participation (the process) may be considered an end in itself, as well as a means to other ends (the Code). In pursuing the defined goal, and their own private goals, participants may experience the conversation itself as immensely stimulating and valuable.

Moral Equality in Policy Making: Setting Limits

Most people who have studied the issues accept that we do not have sufficient resources to meet all legitimate needs for health care. Even in an ideal system that minimizes waste, demographic trends and technological advances, combined with our commitment to goods other than health care, quickly take us to the brink. In a truly ideal system, the United States would be more generous in funding programs to improve health and well-being in other countries, creating an even greater strain on communal resources.

Since we cannot meet all health needs, justice itself impels the setting of limits. In a decentralized system, managed care organizations are central actors in this drama, as we have seen in the deMeurers case. In considering what moral equality implies for limit-setting decisions, there is some symmetry in revisiting the difficulties surrounding the treatment of high dose chemotherapy with autologous bone marrow or stem cell transplant (HDC/ABMT) for advanced breast cancer, and other "last chance" therapies of unproven efficacy.

Norman Daniels and James Sabin have studied this issue by interviewing medical directors and managers at several managed care organizations. Their analysis is guided by this question, "Under what conditions should the public begin to view MCOs [managed care organizations] as a legitimate locus for making limit-setting decisions?" Initially, they rule out the option of submitting conflicts to some canonical decision rule. They note that while adherents of the major approaches to ethics and justice will recognize certain sets of patient-centered and population-centered concerns as valid, they will differ over weights and priorities.[93] Hence, the necessity of resorting to fair procedures, fairness being defined by four conditions: (1) Limit-setting decisions or policies and their rationales must be publicly accessible. (2) The rationale must make clear how the policy supports providing "value for money" in meeting the health needs of a population under reasonable resource constraints. (3) There must be a mechanism for challenge and dispute resolution. (4) There must be regulation to ensure conditions 1–3 are met.

The Group Health Cooperative of Puget Sound is an outstanding model of deliberative democracy. Governed by a lay board elected by members, it holds annual meetings that stand in an advisory relation to the board, and it sponsors town meetings on especially significant or controversial decisions.[94] Although Daniels and Sabin do not make member and patient participation in the processes that lead to the initial articulation of limits and rationales a condition of fairness, they hope to foster democratic deliberative processes in other ways. For example, the second condition is intended to protect against victory by brute force alone. Decision makers must support all decision with reasons. The third condition, the availability of an appeals mechanism, may open up the process of decision making: "[G]ood arguments that plausibly challenge the original decision are provided a visible and public route back into the policy formulation process. . . . Conversely, those affected adversely by the original decision are compelled to engage in the process of constrained reason-giving that informed the original decision."[95]

While Daniels and Sabin do not tether limit-setting decisions directly to a principle of distribution according to need or fair equality of opportunity, they require that a rationale have a certain shape. Even those who "lose out" (in the sense that they are disadvantaged relative to others) must recognize that the decision rests on the kinds of reasons that appropriately play a role in deliberation. Much will depend on the translation of theory into practice. In particular, the formal due process rights favored by bureaucracies may be poor proxies for democratic engagement, where the process is so daunting that few people take advantage of it.

Drawing on their empirical research, Daniels and Sabin describe three "exemplary practices" adopted by managed care organizations in addressing the problem of limit-setting in the area of HDC/ABMT. The three practices form a continuum from procedures most heavily weighting patient-centered concerns to procedures most heavily weighting population-centered concerns.

Aetna initially implemented the first procedure, which incorporates both internal and external reviews. If a patient requests coverage for an unproven but promising treatment not covered by existing company policy, a consulting oncologist within the organization will review the clinical situation. The consulting oncologist is only empowered to approve requests. If he or she does not approve a request, the consultant will forward the file to an independent agency providing review by an expert panel with no affiliation to the company or to any potential provider. According to Daniels and Sabin, this is not a technology assessment, but rather an expert clinical assessment of the value of using the technology for the particular patient.

Kaiser Permanente Northern California has since adopted the Aetna procedure. Managers there reported that when concerns about trustworthiness and potential conflict of interest were addressed in advance by the offer of independent consultation, "patients and families were much readier to enter into a reflective dialogue with their Kaiser physicians about what treatment approach really made sense for them."[96]

Oregon Blue Cross Blue Shield developed the second procedure. The health plan employs a full-time transplant coordinator, a clinically experienced nurse, who works with patients and families, transplant programs, employers, and the benefit system to create consensus on individualized treatment plans for patients. In speaking with the various affected parties, the coordinator uses both scientific evidence and moral argument, for example, asking those seeking coverage to use a universalization test to assess the justice of their claims. The highest priority is open communication and shared deliberation. Another priority is supporting clinically important research. If a promising but unproven treatment is available in a scientifically sound clinical trial, the plan will cover the costs of patient care. The transplant coordinator told Daniels and Sabin that, as of the time of their visit in June 1996, no patient had sued and a significant number had decided against the unproven treatment.

Minnesota's HealthPartners is the source of the third procedure. The HealthPartners benefit contract expressly excludes coverage for investigational treatments. The plan nevertheless covers unproven therapies, if they meet certain standards. In other words, HealthPartners follows the traditional model for technology assessment and eschews case-by-case decision making. This procedure accords the greatest weight to population-centered concerns.[97]

All three of these approaches offer more in the way of cooperation and equality, participation and equity, than the original Health Net procedure for evaluating Christine deMeurers's request for a bone marrow transplant. At the same time, the differences are subtle rather than huge. First, consider the Health Net procedure vis-à-vis the Aetna and HealthPartners procedures. Health Net initially convened a panel of experts to make its limit-setting decisions. Like the Aetna consultants, they were not organizational employees, but unlike the Aetna consultants, they were not truly independent because Health Net engaged them directly. Further, at least some belonged to organizations that depended on Health Net for a substantial portion of their business. Hence Health Net's original procedure did not solve the problem of trust and trustworthiness or the problem of conflict of interest.

The HealthPartners procedure may appear as an analogue to the Health Net procedure, but HealthPartners does not use "investigational" or "experimental" status as its sole criterion. Even if a therapy is investigational, it will be covered, if it meets certain standards. The HealthPartners procedure will itself fail to satisfy Daniels and Sabin's conditions, if the plan fails to offer appropriate rationales for decisions and denies members a forum for challenging denials and dispute resolution.

After the deMeurers case was resolved, Health Net adopted a procedure like Aetna's. Indeed, health plans, patient and consumer advocacy organizations, and legislators who agree on little else unite in supporting external reviews. Critics have challenged the wisdom of the approach on the grounds it goes too far in favoring individual patient-centered concerns over population-centered concerns, such as promoting research to establish efficacy.[98]

The procedure developed by Oregon Blue Cross Blue Shield, which would not preclude an external appeal mechanism as a fallback measure, seems the most consistent with the ideology of cooperative egalitarianism. Accenting cooperation, there is reason to favor a procedure that seeks agreement among all affected parties, and seeks to ground that agreement in scientific and moral evidence rather than coercive power. Accenting equity, there is reason to favor a procedure that promotes individualizing a treatment plan to match the needs and values of a particular patient, yet lays down certain general rules with the rationale of promoting good science. The crowning virtue of the procedure is its open-ended nature, for neither therapies nor science stand free of our interpretations, and they do not stand still.

Even as evidence from clinical trials of HDC/ABMT casts doubt on the value of the procedure for advanced breast cancer, therapy proponents recast negative findings ("no advantage over standard therapies") in positive terms ("at least equivalent survival compared with standard therapies"), and urged others to suspend judgment pending several more years of follow-up. Refinements to the transplant procedure itself suggest that in several years trials of the primitive technology may be of doubtful relevance.[99]

Moral Equality in Clinical Practice

The issues differ somewhat when we shift from the prospects for consumer or patient participation in policy-making to the prospects for cooperation and equality in the day-to-day working arrangements among providers and recipients of health care. "Cooperative egalitarianism" does not rule out a world in which persons occupy roles with distinctive, but mutable, properties. However, in practice, the world in which persons have occupied the roles of physician (mostly men) and nurse (mostly women) has ordered those roles in a rigid vertical hierarchy. Physicians have commanded and nurses have obeyed.

In practice, functional differentiation has been inegalitarian. In the last several decades, there has been some diffusion of power and some mixing of genders, though scarcely enough to satisfy critics. A systematic reconstruction of roles would greatly advance cooperation.[100]

The same concern extends to other workers. Physicians and nurses are often allied in their disdain for the "clerks" employed by managed care organizations. If clerical workers are poorly trained, the solution is to train them better. If clerical workers are poorly supervised or given inappropriate tasks, the solution is to manage them better. Defects in the employing organizations do not supply the grounds for treating clerical workers as non-persons, lacking the ability to learn or the capacity to experience moral distress when asked to perform tasks for which they are unqualified.

In their contempt for clerks, medical and nursing personnel express two questionable assumptions. First, they assume that poor performance by clerical workers reflects an innate deficiency, rather than system failure. Second, they assume that clerical workers do not make valuable contributions to the enterprise of patient care. Surely, the value of excellent clerical support is demonstrated by the chaos that emerges in its absence.[101]

For patients, participating as a patient in one's own treatment differs from participating as a policymaker in a debate concerning macro-level issues, even if the patient's perspective is what one brings to the policymaking table. Cooperative egalitarianism does not require ending all distinctions between professionals and those who come to them for help. It does require a different way of thinking about the relationship between patients and health care professionals.

Cooperative egalitarianism applies a greater emphasis to the role of professional as teacher (doctor) and gives the teaching relationship a more democratic cast. As an exemplary teacher, Paulo Freire, has said, "One does not teach what one does not know. But neither, in a democratic perspective, ought one to teach what one knows without, first, knowing what those one is about to teach know and on what level they know it; and second, without respecting this knowledge."[102]

Cooperative egalitarianism can be reconciled with a reformed professionalism that values lay knowledge. In 1984, Jay Katz envisioned a world in which meaningful communication replaces the silence between physician and patient. "Only after physicians have professed their esoteric professional knowledge and patients their esoteric personal knowledge, and both have confessed (another meaning of profess) to what they can do and what they expect, can a mutually satisfactory recommendation emerge."[103]

Cooperative egalitarianism is also a prod to pursue avenues to cooperation among persons seeking care, including innovations such as cooperative care clinics, mainstream approaches such as support groups, and more radical ventures such as health collectives, the most famous being the women's health collective that created *Our Bodies, Ourselves.* Consistent with democratic theory, a sense of confidence nurtured among persons facing common problems often translates into more effective social and political action.

Another example, "Partners in Policymaking" has been a successful school for personal as well as system advocacy. The program, an intensive leadership training course for parents of children with disabilities and adults with disabilities, originated with the Minnesota Governor's Council of Developmental Disabilities in 1987. The curriculum includes an introduction to self-advocacy and the history of the independent living movement, techniques for advocating for services, skills for providing testimony to or meeting with public leaders, appreciation of the "difference you can make," and a vision for the future.

A number of states now offer this course. It is free to participants, who are also paid for travel, personal assistance services, and respite care. They receive money for child care, meals and lodging where necessary, meaning barriers to participation are minimized. Core funding comes from the federal government; many of the discussion leaders are volunteers. Graduates report that the program helps them work out problems in their own lives, rather than becoming discouraged and giving up, and inspires them to help others by founding local support groups or advocating policy change. One participant says she finished the program feeling a "moral imperative" to become involved in reforming the system.[104]

COOPERATIVE EGALITARIANISM AND
THE "CORPORATIZATION" OF HEALTH CARE

Whatever their merits or demerits in terms of efficiency, certain kinds of organizations are clearly detrimental to the democratic cause and the social vision of cooperative egalitarianism:

> Individuals can find the security and protection that are prerequisites for freedom
> only in association with others—and then the organization these associations take

on, as a measure of securing their efficiency, limits the freedom of those who have entered into them. . . . The predicament is that individuality demands association to develop and sustain it and association requires arrangement and coordination of its elements, or organization—since otherwise it is formless and void of power. But we have now a kind of molluscan organization, soft individuals within and a hard constrictive shell without. Individuals voluntarily enter associations which have become practically nothing but organizations; and then conditions under which they act take control of what they do whether they want it or not.[105]

Regulation is a partial response to problems created by "molluscan" organizations. Critics of government intervention seldom note that corporations are creatures of the state. Further, the danger that large corporations will dominate the government and the political process is at least as great as the danger that the government will dominate its citizens through expansionary policies intended to control corporations.

Law may be less significant as a system of punishments than as a standard and a help to those who wish to do the right thing, by freeing them from unscrupulous competition.[106] For reasons I expressed in the section on bureaucracy, we may have some reservations about administrative rule. Dewey believed the problem of corporate impersonality, in particular, could only be effectively addressed by cultivating "face-to-face" associations:

The situation calls emphatic attention to the need for face-to-face associations, whose interactions with one another may offset if not control the dread impersonality of the sweep of present forces. . . . It involves even more than apprenticeship in the practical processes of self-government, important as that is, which Jefferson had in mind. It involves development of local agencies of communication and cooperation, creating stable loyal attachments, to militate against the centrifugal forces of present culture, while at the same time they are of a kind to respond flexibly to the demands of the larger unseen and indefinite public.[107]

By incorporating the notion of community into a developmental trajectory for the organization, we express the hope that the entities that simultaneously sustain and oppress us might themselves assume a more democratic character. Yet, alongside the rise of the corporation, we observe the transformation of the notion of community itself by a calculating rationality.

Sociologist Robert Merton coined the term "pseudo-Gemeinschaft" to describe the manipulation and exploitation of sentiment. The rich, positive associations of "community" are mere fodder to those "'for whom a tree is not a tree, but timber'" (Karl Mannheim). Christopher Lasch coined the term "Gemeinschaftschmerz" to label the pious twaddle that has always been the great temptation for the communitarian tradition.

The rhetoric and ideal of community are deeply woven into the fabric and history of health care. Community hospitals have opened with much public fanfare, and many have been a continuing source of local pride. Along with the school and the church, the hospital has been one of the pillars of small rural communities and embattled urban neighborhoods. Often, when these institutions shutter their doors, the community dies.

Roman Catholic medical ethics, in particular, has long displayed a particular affinity for the language of community. The religiously informed vision of community and service is linked to a sense that Roman Catholic health care institutions and providers have a distinctive mission or calling, but it tends to lead away from a narrow parochialism.[108] There is also the concept of "community-oriented primary care." In the dry, technical public health vocabulary, a community may be simply a "defined population." Nevertheless, the community-oriented primary care model incorporates principles that reflect a more robust conception of community. Under favorable conditions, it has developed along lines consistent with such a conception.[109]

In an article entitled "Paradigm Lost: The Persisting Search for Community in U.S. Health Policy," health policy analyst Mark Schlesinger describes two particularly significant shifts in the terms of engagement between communities and organizations that provide health care. In the first decades of the twentieth century, actual control of health care *by* lay people in the community declined as the rhetoric of service *to* the community spread. In the 1960s romantic revival of the concept of community, policy makers strove to carve out a place for community participation in health care. But, as federal funding and attention dwindled, community control gave way to control by interest groups or experts. Further, "market-based models of policy reform encouraged health care providers to respond to the interests of individual consumers rather than to the collective concerns of local communities."[110]

For-profit hospital chains continue to benefit from the services of volunteers, an incongruity that demonstrates the resilience of the old spirit of community and volunteerism.[111] Some for-profit corporations do what they can to foster this sort of confusion. Note the frequent use of the word "community" in the names of for-profit hospitals and managed care plans. Some hospital chains have even retained or invented religious sounding names. One hospital made its post-partum discharge policy sound like a community service and the ultimate in family values, in a flyer for patients entitled "Positive Thoughts Regarding the Eight-Hour Discharge."[112]

Of course, attitudes toward community are not uniformly positive. For some, community effort suggests ineptitude or amateurishness.[113] These uses and abuses of the language of community alert us to the need for a critical and discerning eye when we consider the ways in which cultivating community may answer the challenges posed by the increasing prominence of large organizations in health care.

SIX

Making Sense of Managed Care

Over the past 150 years, health care delivery has expanded from what was largely a social service provided by individual practitioners, often in the home, to include a complex system of services provided by teams of professionals, usually within institutions and using sophisticated technologies. As a result, problems develop . . .

—Preamble, A Shared Statement of Ethical Principles for Those Who Shape and Give Health Care (The Tavistock Group, 1999)

I have argued that the managed care debate is not being advanced very far by the trading of barbs between proponents of the ideologies of business and medicine. Health care professionals' fears concerning the effects of business practices on health care have some foundation. The business person's impatience with business-as-usual in health care is not without cause. One is asking a lot, then, in asking the proponents of both sides to put aside their barbs, fears and impatience, and to sublimate the passion aroused by mere mention of the term "managed care" in inquiry.

For health care professionals in particular, a world is under threat, patients are at risk, and a pall hangs over the future. But it is that future and the possibility of affecting it that counsel against simple intransigence. If managed care is neither all good, nor all bad, nor set for all time, then there is room to work, and the time to commence the effort is now.

The first step is to establish a framework for inquiry, and I have provided an outline of one approach that draws on the resources of the pragmatic tradition. In this chapter, I want to synthesize the perspectives presented in preceding chapters by bringing them to bear on five aspects of managed care practice and regulation. First, I will look at two of the most controversial practices associated with managed care, use of financial incentives and gatekeeping.

The method of inquiry I presented in Chapter 3 was intended as a help, not a dogma. But in general, the analysis of these topics will follow the path I initially indicated. I use stories to draw attention to some key dimensions of the problem. This prompts an analysis of options leading to the elimination of some alternatives in light of the risks they pose. I follow through with other options to elicit the promise they may hold. I will argue that some forms of incentive compensation and some forms of gatekeeping fall outside the range of acceptable options, and that some forms of incentive compensation and some forms of gatekeeping are realizing the ends and values given prominence within a pragmatic social ethic.

Managed care has also focused attention on the "master problem" of consent. Hence, this chapter includes a discussion of disclosure rules and consent processes. In particular, I subject the theory of *economic* informed consent, which seeks to wrap the doctrine of informed consent to medical treatment around rationing, to critical analysis. The theory is fashioned for a world of choice far from our own. Even if the situation were to be radically transformed, the theory would founder on the existential difficulties to which I alluded in Chapter 2. I conclude that, in the area of rationing, consent can bear some weight, but it cannot do all the work.

The next section of this chapter explores the role of the ethicist or ethics committee in a managed care organization. Some have touted formal ethics structures as a big part of the solution to the ethical problems of managed care. While these structures can enhance the process of moral deliberation within organizations, they are no panacea. Ethicists and ethics committee members are enmeshed in the same personal and organizational tensions and conflicts as other human beings, and they cannot function effectively as advisors to organizations without steadfast support from organizational leaders.

Given the likely insufficiency of internal structures in ensuring that organizations pursue the good, or at least refrain from wrongdoing, I review the forms of external regulation and oversight available to sanction abuses and advance ethical conduct. I consider the contributions and limitations of the media, the courts, and federal and state legislative and regulatory bodies briefly.

I end the chapter by considering the "outcomes" of managed care, in particular, evidence concerning the effects of managed care on the well-being of the least advantaged members of society. I conclude that while the evidence is equivocal, we must be vigilant in certain areas. Some experiments in caring for vulnerable groups have been extraordinarily successful, but under fairly stringent conditions. In addition, outcomes research cannot capture all we care about in health care.

AREAS OF CONCERN: FINANCIAL INCENTIVES

Managed care raises a wealth of issues, including the broad question of the relationship between medicine and the marketplace. I have addressed some of the global issues in previous chapters. It is also important to deliberate about particular practices or dimensions of managed care. Two appear to arouse the most concern: financial incentives and gatekeeping. The pragmatic method I have outlined is receptive to using storytelling as an aspect of inquiry. Here, then, is a story of financial incentives.

On a business trip, Patrick Shea was hospitalized for severe chest pains. When he returned home, he made several visits to his primary care physician or PCP, mentioning his extensive family history of heart disease and indicating that he was suffering from chest pains, shortness of breath, muscle tingling, and dizziness. Despite all this, Shea's primary care physician said a referral to a cardiologist was unnecessary. (Shea belonged to an HMO that covered specialist visits *only* if a primary care physician approved them.) When Shea's symptoms did not improve, Shea offered to pay out of pocket for a visit to a cardiologist. Shea's primary care physician then persuaded the forty-year-old man that he was too young to be experiencing heart problems and that his symptoms did not justify consulting a specialist. Shortly thereafter, Shea died of heart failure.

Shea had reason to trust his primary care physician's judgment. He had been lucky enough to find his longtime family doctor on his HMO's list of preferred providers. Although he did not know it, he also had reason to distrust his primary care physician's judgment. Under the HMO's payment arrangements, PCPs were rewarded financially if they refrained from making covered referrals to specialists; they were punished, docked a portion of their fees, for making too many.[1]

The Fundamentals of Financial Incentives

We will return to Patrick Shea and to the questions his story raises after some preliminary mapping of the terrain. Financial incentives are so central to managed care that we must expend some time and effort in understanding and evaluating *specific* incentive structures. The first thing to underscore is that financial incentives are pervasive. Where physicians are paid a fee for a service, there is an incentive to perform more of that service. Where there are treatment alternatives, and physicians are paid a higher fee for one alternative relative to the others, there is an incentive to recommend the most highly compensated treatment.

Under traditional indemnity (fee-for-service) insurance policies, the costs involved in performing surgery were typically reimbursed, while patient education and other cognitive services were not. Predictably, the tendency was to neglect the latter. Inpatient services brought more generous payments than outpatient services, if outpatient services were covered at all. Accordingly, patients were admitted to hospitals for procedures and tests that might have been performed on an outpatient basis. These fee-for-service incentives could be particularly perverse in system terms. A frequent result was higher cost and greater risk to patients of iatrogenic harm (harm caused by medical care) without any corresponding benefit.

THE THREE BASIC OPTIONS:
FEE-FOR-SERVICE, SALARY, AND CAPITATION

Managed care has multiplied the range of reward systems employed in health care. Typically, the focus has been on the physician. There are now three major ways of structuring physicians' basic income: fee-for-service, salary, and capitation. As noted, physicians have traditionally been paid on a fee-for-service or "piecework" basis. This mode of payment is sometimes considered exploitative of workers, as in the garment industry. Physicians have favored it because the immediate payers, mostly insurance companies, let physicians set their own rates and control the manner and pace of their work. In other words, physicians were able to maximize their income and their autonomy.

Although managed care and fee-for-service payment can coexist, the rules for fee-for-service have changed. Managed care organizations negotiate discounted fee schedules with selected physicians or physician groups, and they employ measures such as pre-authorization procedures for hospitalization to control utilization. This limits both income and autonomy.

Managed care organizations may also attempt to control utilization through adjusting fees. An HMO might pay an obstetrician $1,025 for delivering a baby with a one day hospital stay, and a much lower fee of $600 if the patient stays in the hospital for three days.[2] Finally, the company may utilize embellishments such as bonuses and withholds, features I will describe momentarily.

Payment by salary is fairly uncomplicated. Utilization is a concern for the physician only as it affects the economic viability of the enterprise that employs her. A physician may recognize that her continued employment depends on the wise use of resources by her and her colleagues, but her base income is not affected by the number of services she performs. In theory, then, there is no general incentive to overtreat or undertreat, although the considerations reviewed in the preceding sentence tend to support a *conservative* practice style. For this reason, many in academic circles favor this mode of payment. Of course, the salaried physician also has no incentive to increase her productivity, apart from the prospect of a salary increase in future years, internal pressures to perform, or a sense that her contribution is important to the enterprise. For this reason, many HMOs have erected other incentive schemes atop the basic structure of salary, introducing the complications "salary" seemed to escape.

Capitation in relation to physicians involves paying a fixed amount per month (or other time period) to the participating physician designated as the primary care physician or PCP for a plan member. The physician is responsible for providing all the services specified in the contract for the particular member over the period. (Specialists may also be capitated. At least one HMO with a policy of open access to specialists makes flat per member per month (PMPM) payments to networks of specialists, while paying primary care physicians on a fee-for-service basis. This arrangement is termed "reverse capitation.") The incentive is for primary care physicians to keep services to a minimum by keeping patients healthy, by reducing inappropriate tests and referrals, or by simply limiting care whenever possible, assuming the malpractice risk created by any particular omission is not too great. Organizations that use a capitated payment structure typically rely on patient satisfaction surveys and other quality assurance mechanisms to discourage the latter strategy.

SOURCES OF COMPLEXITY: TIERING, BONUSES AND WITHHOLDS, AND RISK-ADJUSTMENT

There are two primary sources of complexity. First, capitation more than any other payment mode stimulates the development of various techniques for segmenting and adjusting risk, including bonuses, withholds, and stop-loss protection. Second, there may be tiers of compensation, especially in the case of independent practice associations (IPAs) or network HMOs. In a network HMO, for example, members select, or are assigned to, an individual physician who belongs to a particular IPA or physician group. A managed care plan and physician group might be capitated, paid a certain amount per member per month, and yet physicians treating patients might be paid on a fee-for-service or salaried basis.

Any of the basic modes of payments may be combined with additional features intended to alter or enhance incentive effects. I referred to bonuses and withholds as embellishments, but these are far from ornamental. Bonuses are straightforward in conception, and highly variable in practice. The basic idea is to reward certain desirable practices with a payment over and above base income. A bonus is supposed to be a carrot, a reward promised for good behavior. Also, a bonus is usually small relative to total income. If base income is low, a bonus begins to resemble a stick, and a big one at that. The formula for determining bonuses may be very complex, including factors such as productivity and patient satisfaction as well as utilization.[3] The time frames for which bonuses are calculated may vary considerably.

Managed care organizations usually combine withholds with capitation or fee-for-service arrangements. A percentage of the per member per month payment to the physician, or the fee paid to the physician according to the managed care organization's fee schedule, is held back and placed in a special account or "risk pool." In capitated plans, managers use the funds in a risk pool to pay for referrals to specialists, laboratory tests, hospitalizations, or extraordinarily costly treatments, or separate pools may be established for each category. The nature of the items covered will depend on the extent of the risk assumed by physicians.

The exact nature and structure of the risk pool(s) is a matter for negotiation.

In fee-for-service plans, a risk pool may be used to fund payments to physicians that exceed the plan's forecasts of utilization. At the end of some period, usually a year, plans may distribute any remaining funds in a pool to physicians, or physicians who meet certain criteria. For example, physicians who have drawn heavily on a pool may be excluded from the distribution. If a pool has a "negative balance," that is, if funds prove inadequate to cover expenses incurred in the period, physicians may be required to make up the difference.

In capitated plans, risk pooling for extraordinarily expensive treatments is one of the options for addressing the problem of patients who are cost "outliers," to use an ugly but serviceable term. Plans may also purchase stop-loss insurance, or cap the amount of a physician's liability for care for a single patient in a particular period. Finally, plans may adjust capitation payments to physicians to compensate for risk. (The same is true of payer payments to plans.)

While risk-adjustment remains a very inexact science, progress is being made. It is, in any event, a misconception that highly accurate forecasts of expenditures for individuals are either possible or necessary for effective risk-adjustment. The goal, especially at the level of the plan or practice, is to adjust premiums and payments to compensate for *predictable* risk, not unpredictable risk, so that plans and physicians will gladly serve individuals with predictably higher needs. In other words, the primary aim of risk-adjusted payment is to reorient plans and physicians by scattering "money-losing" and "profitable" members-patients across all levels of need. For risk-adjustment to work to change behavior, it need not be an exact science.[4]

The use of bonuses and withholds is widespread and increasing.[5] On the other hand, certain factors have tended to blunt the force of these incentives. First, many payment arrangements are complicated, and we can expect a "learning curve" in physician understanding of and responsiveness to incentives. Second, many physicians and physician groups participate in multiple managed care plans, each with its own distinctive incentive structure. This may flatten out the learning curve. More importantly, the evolution of managed care toward non-exclusive relationships—IPA HMOs are growing much faster than arrangements in which an HMO and its providers deal exclusively with one another—means that responses to incentives will be highly variable, depending on the constellation of plans and incentives in a particular practice.

THE CONCEPT OF INCENTIVE INTENSITY

Stephen Latham employs the concept of "intensity" to describe the force incentives have in practice, or their effects on actual clinical encounters and on the decisions physicians make concerning the care of particular patients.[6] The simplest case is one in which the amount of money a physician receives is tied to a specific decision, such as when to discharge a patient from the hospital; intensity clearly increases with the amount. Incentive intensity *decreases* as the number of clinical decisions over which risk is spread increases, the significant variables being the length of the period and the size of the group for which the incentive payment is calculated.

Incentives that are lump-sum rather than graduated are more intense due to the "end-of-the-year effect," the tendency to err on the side of spending at the beginning of the fiscal year and on the side of not spending towards the end of the fiscal year, as the financial picture becomes clearer.[7] An incentive scheme that applies to a physician group will reduce the end-of-the-year effect, because it is easier to predict costs for a large patient population, so uncertainty decreases. Over a number of years, or over a number of physician practices, costs will even out.

What Latham refers to as the "tipping phenomenon" shifts our attention to the difference made by case mix, the proportion of a practice that consists of patients in managed care plans and how physicians perceive their practice. In some regions of the country, only a small percentage of a practice may be composed of patients in managed care plans. Even where most patients belong to managed care plans, the number in any one plan may be quite small. The patient group subject to particular managed care incentives may be perceived in two ways: as a separate "line of business," in which case incentives may be very intense, or as part of the total practice, in which case intensity is diminished. While limited data suggest that the second perspective is more common, there is anecdotal evidence that when 40 percent of income is derived from plans with financial incentive schemes tied to utilization, physicians begin to take those incentives much more seriously.[8]

The Influence of Incentives

At present, we have a paucity of data concerning the effects of particular financial incentive schemes on practice, on physicians' behavior and patient care. The data do show that some types of incentives affect utilization, but do not appear to affect crude measures of outcomes.[9] Also, most of the research (limited as it is) dates from early in the experience with managed care, and the findings may not be generalizable to the present or future. If there is a learning curve and a tipping point, we would expect to find greater changes in behavior among today's more knowledgeable, more thoroughly "incentivized" physicians. Beyond this, it is difficult to extricate the effects of financial incentives from the influence of other factors.

An incentive that is not intense in one situation may be very intense in another. As one expert says of capitation, the mode of payment "is never an isolated factor in determining the patterns of care," because its effects "depend on many other factors in the organization of care, such as the form of the delivery system, the risk relation, the cultural norms, and the specific methods used to try to mold physicians' behavior."[10] For example, non-financial incentives such as peer pressure may be extremely significant. In one setting, a strong sense of professionalism may counteract financial incentives to limit care, while in another, a culture of fear or greed may give added weight to an "identical" incentive scheme. It follows that the problems researchers have had in isolating incentive effects are not easy to solve. We cannot separate behavior neatly from character; nor can we separate individual character neatly from organizational character.

The most recent evidence concerning financial incentives and quality is weak but worrying. A 1996 survey of primary care physicians practicing in California found that more than one-third reported receiving bonuses as part of their compensation packages.[11] A subgroup reported earning more than $40,000 annually in the form of bonuses. Similar proportions of office-based and HMO-based physicians in the bonus group reported incentives indexed to productivity and using referrals and hospital services. Incentives linked to prescription drugs, quality of care, and patient satisfaction were more common among physicians in HMOs. Over half of the physicians in the bonus group felt pressured to limit the number of referrals, and 17 percent believed this pressure compromised the quality of care. A substantial majority (75 percent) felt pressure to see more patients, and 24 percent believed this pressure compromised the quality of care.

Just over one quarter reported pressure to limit what they told patients about treatment options. As compared with physicians in office practices, HMO physicians felt less pressure to limit referrals or discussion of treatment options in ways they felt compromised care, but greater pressure to see more patients. Incentives based on productivity were associated with lower physician satisfaction ratings, while incentives based on quality or patient satisfaction were associated with higher physician satisfaction ratings.

This study had a number of limits. Self-report is associated with strategic bias, i.e., the incentive respondents have to strategically shape their responses, when they believe those responses will influence policymaking that may affect them. The study did not measure the actual effects of incentive arrangements on patient care and outcomes. Still, the researchers are likely correct in concluding that "high-quality care is unlikely to flourish in an environment that leaves physicians demoralized and leads many to believe that the standards of care have been compromised."[12]

Incentives are pervasive. The cause for moral concern cannot be that now we have financial incentives where formerly there were none. What is new in health care is that managed care organizations are consciously manipulating incentives to effect certain goals. Although these goals are usually articulated as cost containment *and* quality improvement, one problem in this area is the tendency to reserve the second consideration for ceremonial occasions. Efficiency and economy are important. One need not apologize for considering the economic effects of various policies and practices, but efficiency in the pragmatic sense demands that cost and quality be held together. In addition, *manipulation* in the service of a goal, however worthy the goal, is highly problematic.

Making Sense of Managed Care

The Ethics of Incentives: Four General Considerations and a Principle

Drawing on material in the preceding chapters, I would put forward four general considerations and a principle as guides in deliberating about particular payment arrangements, before proceeding to an analysis of the options.

BEWARE CRUDE INCENTIVE STRUCTURES
First, as the discussion to this point suggests, we need to beware of incentive structures that are crude tools ill-adapted to ends. An incentive is crude if it is unintelligent, put into effect without a clear idea of its effects, or short-sighted. By "short-sighted," I mean imposing significant burdens on others, or disregarding the long-term harms. For example, an HMO may discourage referrals to specialists through financial incentives, by making specialist referrals a covered service under a capitation arrangement or creating a referral risk pool, or through cumbersome referral procedures. The HMO gets an immediate windfall because specialist care is expensive. At the same time, specialist care may resolve certain medical problems more efficiently.[13]

The HMO managers may be indifferent if the costs of inefficiency are borne by the primary care physician (who has to provide more care over a longer period of time) or the patient. One would hope for more inclusive sympathies. Still, even in strictly financial terms, there may be long-term gains to the HMO from practicing more efficiently, not simply more cheaply, e.g., reduced hospitalizations for conditions that recur if inadequately treated. Also, the consequences for the primary care physician and the patient may eventually come back to the HMO. The primary care physician who accepts too much treatment responsibility to avoid a costly referral may make a mistake leading to a malpractice suit against practitioner and HMO. The patient may disenroll from the HMO, rather than suffering patiently or switching primary care physicians. The patient's employer may scrutinize a report on medical absences for employees enrolled in the HMO and conclude that it should take its business elsewhere.

BEWARE OVERLY REFINED INCENTIVE STRUCTURES
Second, we need to beware of incentive schemes that are too refined. MacIntyre observes that we are losing the ability to distinguish between manipulative and non-manipulative social relations. MacInytre is concerned about the manager's *attitude* toward others, a consideration independent of whether the behavior rewarded (or sanctioned) is right or wrong, desirable or undesirable. I have stressed the unfortunate consequences of a thoroughgoing behaviorism for character. The designer of an incentive scheme that is precisely calibrated in every particular treats others as mere instruments of her purposes. Consider a concrete example offered by Latham.

A plan offers obstetricians a fixed end-of-year bonus if their average inpatient length-of-stay (LOS) for deliveries stays below a certain target figure. How is the target set?

> An unrealistically low target . . . would be out of the question for every conscientious physician and would amount to no incentive at all. . . . On the other hand, the requirement must not be too simple to obtain or the incentive will fail to squeeze out all the savings . . . In short, an incentive planner should set the average LOS that triggers the bonus at the most difficult possible level which a conscientious physician would be willing to attempt to obtain. If a planner sets the perfect target level, the entire bonus amount would effectively be at stake in each individual clinical decision.[14]

Latham's planner, if only as a matter of realism, allows for a standard of "conscientiousness" that limits physician responsiveness. Were she to ask how far physicians could be pushed to compromise their standards through financial incentives, and not through any direct effort to persuade them to change their standards for given reasons, any sense of what it means to treat others as ends and not as means only would be lost.

The project of designing a precisely calibrated incentive structure may also be self-defeating. Behavior may fail to conform to expectations, because people do not understand the structures confronting them. Active physician subversion is another possibility. MacIntyre's jeremiad against faith in management, the organizational system theorist's reservations concerning ambitious "programming," and Pfeffer's cautions concerning the effects of emphasizing extrinsic rewards counsel some degree of humility on the part of managers.

BEWARE DIRECT TIES BETWEEN RATIONING AND REWARD
Third, concern is in order when plan executives substitute financial incentives for careful, deliberative approaches to rationing. Where financial incentives are designed and implemented solely to reduce the practitioner's referrals for or use of services, payment functions as a non-specific rationing technique. Defenders of incentives to limit the use of services or to undertreat argue that these incentives merely compensate for the excesses that resulted from fee-for-service incentives to overtreat. Somehow "appropriate utilization" of services is supposed to emerge from the mix.

However, there is a flaw in this logic. "In essence, an HMO takes the same physicians who it thinks abuse fee-for-service incentives and trusts them not to underserve their capitated patients, while giving them direct incentives to do just that."[15] The plan administrators provide little or no guidance concerning justified and unjustified decisions to withhold services. The diffuseness of incentives employed in this manner may prove a barrier to monitoring effects on practice.[16]

In addition, some critics argue that incentives to ration services are more dangerous than incentives to provide services, because they work invisibly. The patient whose doctor recommends surgery knows that there is a decision point and has an opportunity to seek a second opinion. The patient who never learns that surgery is an option has no such opportunity. Skepticism about the patient's ability to serve as an effective monitor of potential abuses under the first scenario (and hence skepticism about the benignity of incentives to over-treat) does not mitigate the concerns raised by the second scenario.[17]

Where reducing services produces a direct financial benefit to the individual practitioner, there is a heightened risk that the question of who benefits, or whose benefit matters more, will enter into the practitioner's decision making. This sort of incessant questioning can only erode the quality of the practitioner's work.

BEWARE SUBVERSION OF OTHER INCENTIVES

A fourth and final question to ask of any particular financial incentive is whether it supports and reinforces other types of incentives that influence practitioners, or rather tends to undermine them. I would join the commentators selecting salary as the best method for paying practitioners because that payment structure is relatively neutral and creates space for professional incentives to operate.

As I noted in Chapter 5, not all professional incentives are good by nature or in their effects (e.g., occupational solidarity), but many are (e.g., commitment to the work and to quality). Minor departures from straight salary, such as modest bonuses, might be linked to patient satisfaction or service on inter-disciplinary committees, both remedying some of the deficiencies of professional incentives.

KEEP FAITH WITH PATIENTS

Patients expose themselves to physicians and to other health care professionals in the expectation that their vulnerability will not be exploited. Patients trust those who poke and prod and ask them intimate questions, soliciting information that may be shared with no one else. They also trust those unseen networks of communication and administration that compose the infrastructure for clinical interactions. The obligation to keep faith is especially strong for clinicians, but it extends well beyond them. Offering and providing care are both an invitation to trust and an assurance of trustworthiness, a ratification of patients' expectation of safety from exploitation. Keeping faith is a more inclusive obligation than keeping promises, because the relationships that arise in health care are covenantal rather than purely contractual.[18]

Covenantal relationships, such as relationships with patients, have a para-doxical quality; they can be both freedom-restricting and freedom-enhancing. On the one hand, the consequences for the patient necessarily become a consideration in any choice that is made. The professional–patient relationship forecloses consideration of certain options, and decision making for the professional becomes more complicated because he or she must also involve or give an account to the patient affected by the decision.

On the other hand, keeping faith is freeing, because many options that would tempt professionals with the prospect of financial reward or prestige are readily rejected. These goods, which so often seem to control us, lose their power in relation to the greater goods at stake in fulfilling obligations to patients.

While the principle of keeping faith is demanding, its demands are not unlimited. Keeping faith is not equivalent to meeting every expectation, or satisfying every spontaneous desire. These limits create the potential for conflict with patients. Unfortunately, fidelity to the principle of keeping faith is no guarantee against the *perception* of betrayal of trust.

Bad Incentives

Although many considerations weigh in favor of salary, few persons outside the sociological and medical ethics communities, and medicine's academic elite, favor this method of payment.[19] If we will have a variety of payment arrangements for the foreseeable future, the necessary next step is to identify and rule out those that are clearly bad.

In 1995, the AMA's Council on Ethical and Judicial Affairs released a report entitled "Ethical Issues in Managed Care."[20] The report avoids setting forth any hard and fast rules concerning financial incentives; rather it counsels decision-makers to pay attention to such factors as the percentage of provider income placed at risk, the frequency with which incentive payments are calculated, and the size of the professional group whose performance becomes the basis for judgment. The idea is to blunt the force of incentives; the drafters assume that weak incentives will operate only at the margins or in the "gray areas" of medical uncertainty. However, even incentives that appear weak may be significant in a particular context. Incentives are all the more dangerous where susceptibility to incentives is denied.[21] The drafters of the AMA report paid little attention to the logic of particular incentives. For the most part, they treated incentives as non-specific rationing techniques.

The current rules for managed care plans that participate in Medicare and Medicaid, imitated by several states, prohibit payments to physicians or physician groups as an incentive to limit medically necessary services to a specific individual. The rules also require plans to limit potential financial losses for physicians at "substantial" financial risk for any referrals they make. Physicians are at substantial risk if their group is asked to give up more than 25 percent of its potential payments to cover the costs of referrals. In other words, risk is calculated without regard to the income effects of services that group members provide.[22]

The adequacy of these rules is open to question. The flat prohibition is aimed at a practice that has not been popular among managed care organizations—implementing incentive schemes that target single-patient transactions.[23] The loss containment provision focuses on protecting physicians from financial risk, rather than protecting patients from the potential harms of intense financial incentives. This provision is therefore incomplete, although it addresses one dimension of the incentive problem: physicians and physician groups desperate at the prospect of losing income may be readier to take risks with patient care.

ASSESSING THE ALTERNATIVES

Research on incentives is too meager to aid much in line drawing, and we cannot suppose that a percentage point or two will make a great difference. At the same time, it seems sensible to conclude that the dangers posed by incentives increase with intensity, and hence to focus on the factors that make incentives more or less intense, such as the size of the panel subject to incentives and the frequency with which incentives are calculated. Further, if one fears the effects of general financial insecurity as well as incentives that bear on particular clinical decisions, one will want to limit the percentage of physician income and group revenue at risk, allowing for some adjustment in the case of a group, to account for factors like size.

While the specific numbers selected are bound to be somewhat arbitrary, the range is not. Twenty-five percent seems too high, five percent too low for a *legal* ceiling. Policy makers have the task of specifying the outside limit within a range of reasonableness, and regulators, such as state insurance commissioners, have the task of assessing the intensity of each particular incentive scheme that comes in for review. Administrators and physicians must go beyond mere compliance with the law and locate the danger points in their own organizations or practices. Financial incentives linked to quality and patient satisfaction appear consistent with the goals of health care; they are also associated with higher physician satisfaction. Accordingly, the case for totally avoiding these types of incentives is weak. On the other hand, financial incentives linked to productivity and referrals need strong justification given their association with physician dissatisfaction and perceived deficiencies in care.

One might still ask why we should accept a "somewhat arbitrary" limit, based on a common sense belief that, in general, the magnitude of the effects on behavior will vary with the proportion of income at stake, among other factors. Part of the caution has to do with the non-specific nature of popular incentive schemes. In most cases, rewards depend on reducing the level of overall utilization. How a practitioner achieves these reductions depends in part on the practitioner's character, the patient's sophistication and persistence, and the extent of the managed care organization's quality assurance monitoring.

In a good number of cases, the practitioner will not succumb to the temptation to skimp on patient care to enhance her own income. In a number of cases where the practitioner attempts to cut corners, a vigilant patient or a peer review program will keep the practitioner in line. We may expect real problems in a relatively small number of cases. Yet the risks involved in learning more about the nature of the risks may be, and, I believe, are, unacceptably high, especially given the effects of incentives on trust.

Consider again the story of Patrick Shea. Clear and direct financial incentives to limit referrals may have played a significant role in his doctor's decision not to refer Shea to a cardiologist. If so, we have a betrayal of trust, a violation of the principle of keeping faith with patients.

Alternatively, this may have been a simple case of poor judgment, or even a case of appropriate judgment within a gray area of medicine. The uncertainty introduced by the financial incentives extends to the phase of the relationship in which Shea offered to pay the expense of the cardiologist visit himself, and his doctor persuaded him that no visit was necessary. There are several ways to view this episode. Did Shea suspect that his doctor's reluctance to refer could be traced to financial considerations? Did the doctor dissuade Shea from paying for the cardiologist visit out-of-pocket because he "really" believed the visit was unnecessary, or because he needed to believe that his judgment was not affected by financial considerations? Or did he simply want his patient to believe that his judgment was not affected by financial considerations? Given the nature of the particular financial incentives in this case, none of the participants in this tragedy can have peace of mind.

Permissible Incentives: Criteria for Evaluation

The discussion of bad incentives leaves open the question of how to evaluate incentives that are not morally or at least prudentially out-of-bounds.

FROM INDIVIDUAL TO SYSTEM
In determining what kinds of incentives to prohibit, administrators usually focus on effects on the choices of individual physicians. The objective is to make physicians aware of cost without creating risks of gain or loss so great that their concerns about income overwhelm all other considerations. But as an astute observer has pointed out, a form of payment such as capitation may affect quality of care in two ways: by influencing individual decisions, and "by encouraging *systemic* integration and innovation in the design and delivery of services."[24]

Administrative attention to the systemic dimension becomes the basis for developing general criteria of desirability. When one asks whether a particular payment structure promotes integration and innovation, one is no longer using an incentive scheme as a non-specific rationing technique. Rather, one is using incentives intelligently to effect certain results. At the same time, one is not regarding others as manipulable objects, but encouraging creativity.

For example, a capitation contract must specify the services that the plan, physician or group is expected to provide in exchange for the fixed monthly payment. Certain services may be explicitly carved out and reimbursed separately on a fee-for-service basis. In determining whether to include or "carve out" a service, the plan's creator asks whether the health care provider that will become the risk bearer has the capacity to redesign the pattern of care to improve quality, while simultaneously reducing costs. If the provider lacks that capacity, the service should be excluded. If too many services must be excluded, the provider should not be offered a capitation contract.

Risk-adjustment of capitation rates also requires attention. Where capitation rates do not reflect the higher costs of caring for needier patients, plans and providers have incentives to engage in strategic behavior to avoid the sick, as well as those more likely to become ill. Poorly designed capitation can be disastrous for people with disabilities or chronic illness; "[p]roperly designed capitation can broaden time horizons, clarify areas of interdependence, and encourage cooperation, all of which can improve the quality of care."[25] The latter are all highly desirable from a pragmatic point-of-view. Of course, these kinds of incentive effects are not confined to capitation as a payment method for patient care. Payments to clinicians for efforts on behalf of the managed care organization or system that may reduce practice time, such as service on a quality improvement or ethics committee, would produce similar benefits.[26]

ANOTHER STORY: CARE FOR THOSE WITH ASTHMA

The ideal is to aggregate payment for the total care of a defined population, reducing the stake fragmented providers have in preserving inefficient, uneconomical patterns of care. As I recounted in Chapter 4, Kaiser Permanente's investment in kidney dialysis made economic sense under a comprehensive capitation arrangement because reductions in costly hospital care ultimately offset the expense.

Asthma treatment can serve as another illustration of the benefits of capitation at the plan level. Asthma is a serious, chronic illness, affecting five of every hundred children and resulting in more than ten million lost school days, one in six of all pediatric emergency visits, and 200,000 child hospitalizations annually. Child deaths from asthma have doubled since 1980. Proper treatment at an early stage is crucial, since the inflammation that is characteristic of asthma can thicken and stiffen the membrane in the bronchial airways, which damage becomes irreversible over time.

In asthma outreach programs, educators teach patients and families in their homes about preventing acute episodes. As compared with the traditional approach of waiting for patients to show up at a doctor's office or hospital, these programs are more efficient in preventing and easing suffering. Further, when all the costs associated with the two approaches are aggregated and compared, outreach programs appear superior in terms of economy.[27]

Unfortunately, current reimbursement structures may pose a barrier to this type of program. In a fragmented payment system, providers may be fully reimbursed for office visits and hospitalizations, while receiving little or nothing for educational home visits. Where payment is aggregated, the costs associated with a beneficial innovation like home outreach or intensive case management can be paid for with cost-savings from reduced office visits and hospitalizations.

Harvard Pilgrim Health Care Plan, a not-for-profit HMO in New England, has made asthma treatment a priority. Initially, Harvard Pilgrim used its databases, established to track costs, to identify members with asthma. Next, Harvard Pilgrim began a program of intensive education for physicians, creating a clinical pathway from national guidelines and emphasizing the importance of giving patients and families the technology to manage the disease themselves. (This involved educating patients and families on the proper use of the technology. This was extremely important since many asthmatics leave the office with inhalers they don't know how to use.)

To address the broader social context, social service workers, allergists, and other professionals joined the treatment team, and outreach nurses took responsibility for maintaining regular phone contact with participants. Program benefits have included a decline in hospitalizations and fewer emergency room visits, along with patient improvement on multiple measures of ability to function.[28] Capitation may prove beneficial at the individual and system levels.

AREAS OF CONCERN: GATEKEEPING

As illustrated by the story of Patrick Shea, financial incentives to restrict care are often intertwined with gatekeeping by primary care physicians. An inquiry into "gatekeeping" quickly leads one to conclude that gatekeeping is not a single practice, but a range of practices.

Gatekeepers as Coordinators of Care

For many managed care organizations, "gatekeeping" simply means giving an individual physician or advanced practice nurse control over the full range of health services, including specialist referrals and hospitalization. The stories of Patrick Shea and Christy deMeurers highlight the role of the primary care physician in blocking referrals. It is important to note that in deMeurers's case, some of the gatekeepers were themselves specialists.

Proponents and critics of managed care have long recognized the potential for a different form of gatekeeper program, one in which the managed care organization assumes responsibility for the *competence* of health care professionals acting as providers of primary care and coordinators of other services that might benefit individual patients.[29] This would involve more than credentialing. MCOs might educate providers on the role of case management, and they might carefully monitor the adequacy of the referral network of specialists and supportive care agencies, both in terms of quantity and quality.

The next step for organizations is to put information management systems and clinical guidelines in the service of case management. One managed care organization is using its massive medical-billing and pharmacy database to evaluate physician adherence to well-established guidelines for medical practice. This information is then provided to physicians.[30] Other managed care organizations are bringing primary care physicians and various specialists together to develop guidelines and to improve patient care.

HealthSystem Minnesota and the Institute for Clinical Studies Integration have developed and implemented more than twenty clinical guidelines, covering common illnesses and procedures. These include breast cancer detection, childhood asthma, hypertension diagnosis, lower back pain, and stable coronary artery disease.

The breast cancer detection guideline is one of the success stories. Prior to development of the guideline, a positive diagnosis could take up to three weeks. With a team of primary care physicians, radiologists, surgeons, and others working together, the time from mammography to ultrasound to needle biopsy was reduced to three hours.[31] This significant improvement in service would not have been possible if an organizational commitment to cooperation and the reward system had not been working together. One significant change was to have radiologists use stereotactic methods for most biopsies. The surgeons might not have supported this innovation had they not been working within a capitated system.

Under some circumstances, then, designating a particular health care provider as gatekeeper, like the use of certain forms of capitated payment, *may* serve the cause of integration and innovation, continuity of care, and coordination across the whole spectrum of care. But one must also note the potential pitfalls. A managed care organization may invest in a network of competent, caring primary care physicians, and yet compromise patient care, and place these physicians in a terrible bind, by entering into cut-rate deals with deficient providers of specialty care and ancillary services.[32] A rigid commitment to primary care gatekeeping may compromise the care of persons with serious disabilities. Not less important, it may rob them of dignity by forcing them into the role of bureaucratic supplicant, forever pleading for access to the specialist.

Indeed, one may use a qualitatively different term, such as "caretaker" or "care counselor" to indicate the qualitatively different practice of taking care or providing guidance, whether or not one is delivering services. Two psychiatrists, James E. Sabin and Carlos Neu, observe the difference between gatekeeping and caretaking in the case of a defensible exclusion of certain services from coverage: "If a patient's suffering or dysfunction will not receive insurance coverage because it does not arise from a mental disorder, an ethical or just managed care program would ask the clinician to advise the patient on alternative directions to take (that is, identifying other gates through which the patient can pass) not simply to send the patient away (i.e., closing the gate)."[33]

As a care counselor, a primary care physician can assist patients who are not sure they want an intervention recommended by a specialist in assessing the risks and benefits in light of the patients' own values and goals. A patient may find it difficult to conduct this kind of assessment directly with a specialist, given the specialist's investment in the tools of his or her subdiscipline and the patient's fear of offending. A 1997 survey of patients with chronic health problems in managed care found an overwhelming majority valued having a single identified primary care physician and found it helpful for that primary care physician to participate in decisions about specialty care.[34]

Gatekeepers as M.D.s-in-the-Middle

In 1988, Dr. Henry Scovern described his experience as a primary care physician in a for-profit, staff-model HMO in the pages of the *New England Journal of Medicine*. Scovern found that high turnover among enrollees and physicians in his HMO meant few patients had established relationships with their primary care physicians. First contact was often made when a patient showed up at the emergency room of a nonparticipating hospital. Scovern frequently had difficulty contacting and gaining the cooperation of physicians who were strangers, and he was put in the difficult position of negotiating treatment without personal knowledge of the patient or an opportunity to perform an examination.

To the patients, Scovern was also a stranger. He wrote that "patients were understandably uncomfortable when the preauthorization of emergency care was withheld on the basis of a telephone conversation with an unfamiliar physician." Even when patients were admitted to participating hospitals according to the rules, headaches would arise when it fell to the primary care physician to cajole the specialist or subspecialist in charge of the patient's hospital care to engage in discharge planning. Scovern found himself in the position of "nagging (at best) or appearing to be telling a subspecialist his business (at worst)."[35]

Scovern's conclusions concerning gatekeeping as he experienced it are fairly damning of the practice: "The intense involvement of the primary care provider in authorizing referrals, making rounds among hospitalized patients on nonprimary services, and monitoring and promptly transferring patients from nonparticipating to participating hospitals was promoted as 'total involvement' with patient care. It is obvious, however, that these efforts primarily served the interest of the HMO in tracking, predicting, and controlling expenditures. In addition, the large administrative component in these endeavors was a waste of physicians' time."[36]

These problems were exacerbated by an absence of job security. Given the standards for evaluation, Scovern speculated that manipulation would become commonplace. Where the gatekeeper role amounts to "M.D.-in-the-middle," it is simply untenable, demoralizing and ultimately corrupting for physicians, and harmful to patients. Surveys of patients and physicians confirm the lessons derived from Scovern's experience. The 1997 survey that elicited positive responses to care coordination found that perceptions of referral barriers were a strong predictor of low trust, low confidence, and low satisfaction ratings.[37]

Gatekeepers as Rationing Agents

The term gatekeeping often identifies not merely selecting a single clinician to manage care in the interests of better coordination, or cost-cutting, but also charging that clinician with imposing limits on care using cost-effectiveness or cost-benefit analysis. Clinicians become medical *and* economic agents for their current patient and for the population of patients the plan serves. This form of gatekeeping is highly controversial. Some, including the AMA, object to any consideration of cost in clinical decision making; if there is rationing to be done, it must be done at another level.

Many ethicists concur, arguing that while rationing may be morally acceptable under some circumstances, it must be totally excluded from the clinician's job description. Someone else, a non-clinician health professional, a manager, or a board of patients or members will do the rationing. This will free up the clinician to be a militant, loyal servant of the individual patient's interest. The position has intuitive appeal. Divided loyalty is morally problematic, and dual agency requires complex judgments.

Primary care physician and ethicist Howard Brody refers to this view—the physician serves the patient and the administrator serves the whole society by constraining costs—as the "division of labor" model. He considers it both wrongheaded and unworkable. When the attempt is made to protect clinicians from making any of the trade-offs associated with other forms of human activity, cost containment necessarily becomes a crude and often brutal business, a matter of remote control. Brody points out that some trade-offs are built into medicine. No physician limits herself to one patient at a time. Hence, each physician must ration her time among a group of patients using her best clinical judgment. According to Brody, this is the kind of limited, knowledge-based, contextual rationing that *properly belongs* to the physician as gatekeeper.[38]

Mark Hall's comprehensive rebuttal to the advocates of the strict division of labor model buttresses Brody's argument from his experience as a clinician. Hall begins by considering rationing by rule alone. He argues that such an approach is neither feasible nor desirable. It is not feasible because the research infrastructure to generate sound clinical rules—properly termed protocols rather than guidelines—does not exist. Even if it did exist, such protocols cannot completely substitute for clinical judgments: "Physicians make these judgments either through a type of gestalt pattern-recognition process that they are not able fully to articulate . . . or by constructing in their minds a narrative, cause-and-effect explanation of what is happening to each patient and the physiology of the proposed intervention."[39] Clinical protocols would eliminate this aspect of professional practice.[40]

Hall argues that rationing by rule alone is undesirable because rules are removed from the scene (their advantage from the perspective of the proponents of the division of labor model) and necessarily reductionist, and because relying on rules to do all the moral work may erode a sense of personal responsibility. One is either contemplating an additional layer of bureaucratic review on every clinical decision or accepting that the rationing councils will operate by means of a general rule, with all the limitations that attend such an approach.[41] Apart from the practical problems, the impetus for this kind of proposal is the view that trade-offs are external rather than internal to medicine, a view against which Brody argues strenuously.

The alternative is to make clinicians responsible for prudently trimming marginally beneficial services, while taking account of the particular patient's values, preferences, and special needs. Clinicians are not continually generating cost-benefit analyses, and no one should confuse judgments of treatments as not "cost-worthy" with judgments of the patient as not "worthy of the treatment." Additional work must be done to move the concept of "marginally beneficial" out of the theoretical realm and into conversations with patients. One paradigm would be along these lines: "I could prescribe x now, but the situation may resolve itself in a month or two. If you still have y symptom two months from now, we can reassess the situation. Shall we wait and see?"

We should rely on rules to do two things: to define which treatments are entirely excluded and when last chance therapies cannot be endorsed or paid for, and to set the broad parameters for routine management of care. Professional and legal norms and publicity and other forms of internal and external oversight should be supported to discourage abuses of power. True, clinicians *may* make value trade-offs atypically. Rules and other constraints are necessary. True, in the area of values, clinicians have no special expertise, apart from claims to knowledge arising from a certain body of experience. On the other hand, there is little evidence to support claims of a special handicap.[42]

In practice, clinicians make trade-offs. We accept that the clinician must reconcile her obligation to any one patient with her obligation to each of her other patients. The new question is whether we can accept physician economizing on marginal benefits as legitimate practice aligned with our interests, and whether the healer's charismatic power can work when the patient knows that some economizing is going on.

I am inclined to believe that the answer to the question is yes, although I admit to some unease. Clearly, physician rationing is least tolerable where the financial consequences to physicians are direct, or where it takes the form of M.D.-in-the-middle. Hall's response to our queasiness about rationing is to extend the notion of informed consent to the enrollment decision.[43] I discuss the difficulties that attend that project in the next section.

DISCLOSURE RULES AND CONSENT PROCESSES

Consumer consent to the terms of a health plan, including any procedure employed to ration health services, has generated nearly as much discussion as financial incentives and gatekeeping. Ethicists and moral philosophers supportive of the free market join their more skeptical colleagues in advocating for more complete disclosure. Information sharing may have intrinsic value. It is also a necessary aspect of the kind of consent that confers legitimacy on professional interventions and social projects.

Disclosure Rules

JUSTIFICATIONS FOR DISCLOSURE

E. Haavi Morreim argues that disclosure has three primary justifications. First, certain information is a kind of property to which the plan member or patient has a right. Second, the plan member or patient is likely the weaker party in the transaction with plan or professional, and, therefore, needs protection. By increasing the patient's knowledge, disclosure makes the relationship between the parties more nearly equal. Third and finally, disclosure enhances autonomy, understood as the capacity to make one's own decisions in light of one's own values and goals, and then to take responsibility for those decisions.[44] This last consideration will have special force in a form of pragmatism informed by the principle of subsidiarity, if it is not taken to imply an atomistic understanding of the individual.

THE SCOPE OF DISCLOSURE

Disclosure rules, whether adopted voluntarily or imposed, must identify the kinds of information to be communicated and assign responsibility for communication. The AMA proposes a division of labor between managed care organizations and physicians. The managed care organization must be responsible for ensuring disclosure of benefit restrictions and any incentives the organization offers providers to limit care. The AMA is more complacent about fee-for-service incentives to overtreat.[45]

The President's Advisory Commission and the American Association of Health Plans (AAHP) largely concur.[46] Physicians must be responsible for disclosing treatment alternatives, financial incentives affecting their own practice, and any contractual agreements restricting referrals. On the last point, patients may be unaware that IPAs or physician groups sometimes have an internal understanding that all referrals will be made within the association or group.

Information concerning financial incentives is especially sensitive. Current regulations for Medicare managed care plans only require summary disclosure, and then only when individuals request it. Yet, I have heard few persuasive arguments against stronger disclosure requirements. Certainly, if an incentive is of sufficient magnitude, and the connection between the incentive and services delivered is clear, disclosure will undermine patient trust and the healing alliance between patient and professional. This is not an argument against disclosure, but an argument against employing the incentive.[47]

THE SPECIFICITY OF DISCLOSURE

The specificity of disclosure is a related issue. Disclosure rules that seek to capture all possible nuances will likely prove unworkable, another reason for addressing financial incentives and other features of managed care with substantive regulation as well as disclosure requirements. Morreim published an article in a trade journal with a model disclosure statement for health plans. Written for the most part in vague "happy talk," it nevertheless states clearly: "No matter what payment or incentive system a group uses, Healthplan limits the total economic risk to our doctors. No doctor can lose, or gain, more than 15% of his or her salary or capitation fee."[48] This statement provides the kind of bottom-line information consumers need, and need to pay attention to, versus definitions of all the forms of compensation the plan has in its arsenal. A consumer who understands how incentives operate would also want to know the maximum amount at risk in caring for any single patient.

A further question is whether a physician should disclose every potentially beneficial test or treatment option. Some standard of materiality, of what a reasonably prudent patient would wish to know, is probably in order, for two reasons. First, maximal disclosure is not necessarily in the interests of patients. Disclosure may raise needless anxieties or hinder judgments of significance. This is a common complaint about the current practice of informed consent, which favors revealing every risk, however remote, in a litany of potential calamities.

Second, since people may respond differently to information, judging how any particular person will be affected by any particular piece of information is difficult. Telling a patient about treatments the plan won't cover may be cruel; some may wish they had never been told. But others will appreciate the honesty, even if they choose not to act, or vow to go down fighting the coverage limitations, or set about raising the funds to pay for treatment.

The most difficult case may be presented by all the relatively trivial "marginal benefits" that may be selected against by guidelines, formularies, or clinician judgment. Some disclosure is obviously in order, but is a general statement that the plan saves money where it can sufficient? One resolution would be for the plan and physician to present the member (or patient) with a kind of global disclosure, with opportunities for more specific disclosures in each episode of care.[49]

The plan's global disclosure would include instructions on how to obtain more information. Interactive computer programs that allow people to access information selectively are promising, and some leading health services researchers have called for more study of community-based models for disseminating information.[50] Efforts are already underway to supplement standardized disclosure with more personal communication using computer bulletin boards.

As critics of the current practice of informed consent continually point out, the "how" of disclosure is as important as the "what," or the information conveyed. When physicians impart information, they must consider the viewpoint of the plan member or patient, trying to make the information meaningful by relating it to the other's experience, and at the same time, responding adequately to questions and concerns. In place of an extended discussion of the difference between sensitivity and a cowardly reticence concerning an unpalatable reality, consider this example excerpted from one of Sabin's cases.

A psychiatrist (Jones) proposed monthly sessions for a depressive patient who had demanded long-term therapy with frequent visits; the patient expressed his belief that the HMO "was only interested in saving money." Jones explained that while the public generally thinks of psychotherapy as weekly or even more frequent sessions, and while much of the professional community locally agreed with that view, outcomes research does not answer the question and his own experience suggested that they could achieve their objectives in the plan he was proposing. He acknowledged that the HMO did try to save money where possible, making funds available for other aspects of care.[51]

Jones is not a communications virtuoso. On the other hand, he does take his patient seriously as a partner, someone who should be offered the reasoning behind a procedure. Note, too, that the final statement is only truthful within an organization that retains its earnings and channels those funds into improved patient care.

MARKETING AS (DIS)INFORMATION

For other observers, a concern with disclosure suggests the importance of undertaking more ethical scrutiny of marketing. Advertising may be mere puffery (ALL THE HEALTH CARE YOU DESERVE), or it may be misleading or outright false.[52] Loosely monitored sales personnel interested in rapidly increasing enrollment may employ questionable tactics.[53] Sadly, patients are often surprised to discover that the plan's "comprehensive" health benefits do not extend to their participating in clinical trials for promising new, potentially life-saving therapies, or that their "free choice of provider" does not extend to their long-time physician or neighborhood health center. When expectations are created that cannot be met, patients, providers, and relationships all suffer.[54]

Consent Processes

Morreim notes that one justification for increasing disclosure is to enhance autonomy as the capacity to make decisions in light of one's values and preferences *and* to take responsibility for those decisions. The traditional doctrine of informed consent can also be viewed from two angles. From one angle, the doctrine of informed consent empowers the individual. She can either give or withhold her consent to treatment or to participation in research. Many managed care critics see extending the doctrine of informed consent as a way to correct certain power imbalances. From another angle, the informed consent doctrine confers legitimacy on what would otherwise be questionable or wrongful acts or projects. Having consented, the individual loses the legal or moral power to protest the consequences.

CONSENT AS JUSTIFICATION FOR RATIONING

This second aspect of informed consent has emerged as especially significant in the debate over the moral justification for rationing. Mark Hall is one of the most sophisticated proponents of the view that informed consent can operate to confer legitimacy on economic arrangements, just as it can operate to confer legitimacy on medical interventions. Hall develops what he calls a "theory of economic informed consent."

In a nutshell, Hall argues that if people consent to a plan for rationing up front, when they enroll in a health plan, we (and they) have no grounds for objecting to the consequences on moral grounds. Hall's theory bears a family resemblance to Waymack's argument that an ethic of autonomy holding consumers to purchasing decisions should replace an ethic of beneficence that seeks to do what is best for the particular patient in his or her present circumstances. However, Hall distinguishes between the standards that govern arm's length commercial transactions and the more demanding fiduciary standard that should govern transactions concerning health care. Not minimal fairness alone, but full disclosure, fair substantive terms, and a reasonable range of choice are required; both beneficence and autonomy are operative.[55]

The greatest practical challenge to Hall's theory is its dependence on conditions that are not satisfied under the current system. As long as there is little or no solid information (and much disinformation) available about plans, little or no regulation to ensure fair substantive terms, and little or no choice among plans for most people, the prerequisites for informed consent for rationing will be lacking. The more basic challenge to Hall's theory has to do with existential constraints on choice, a concern that emerged in the discussion of choice in Chapter 2.

Hall sets up his argument with a reasonable call to recognize bias. He notes that the clinical orientation of mainstream bioethics "causes many bioethicists to ask what forms of resource allocation are proper only from the perspective of a presently sick patient seeking treatment and discourages them from examining the perspective of healthy potential patients contemplating how to structure an insurance arrangement."[56] He makes a second reasonable point, which I would frame this way. Persons in an insurance pool have an interest in restraining costs, both out of concern for their own medical well-being, since prudent stewardship assures that resources are available when they are most necessary, and out of regard for their economic interests. The difficulty arises when Hall argues that all the moral weight can be borne by consent at the time of enrollment. In effect, he affirms the perspective of the healthy potential patient as wholly adequate in defining what is acceptable in the way of restraining costs.

Hall acknowledges that this is a departure from traditional informed consent in the medical context. In the case of medical informed consent, one's situation at the time of consent to a procedure is virtually identical to one's situation at the time when the procedure is performed. Indeed, if one's situation changed, the consent would likely be nullified. If I have consented to surgery for a brain tumor and then discover that I have been misdiagnosed, it would be very odd to insist that I go through with the surgery.

This example also makes the point that medical consent is a matter of revocable permission rather than obligation.[57] Hall identifies the new element in economic informed consent vis-à-vis traditional informed consent as "precommitment." He writes: "[T]he validity of precommitment turns on the strength of a variety of factors. The first is the possible degree of deprivation that advance irrevocable consent can cause. We are also more inclined to honor precommitment commands if they are designed to protect against anticipated periods of irrationality or extreme temptation and if they govern events that are not too distant in the future."[58] Unfortunately, the validity of precommitment to the rationing of health care seems questionable along every one of these dimensions.

Advance irrevocable consent to rationing may be associated with serious deprivation, depending on the quantity and quality of the rationing in the particular case. It is difficult to know what to make of anticipation, where the eventualities to be considered may be very remote from one's experience and may come on suddenly or never. Hall raises but does not resolve the fundamental issue. He acknowledges that "[t]he terminally ill patient's last-gasp desire to receive any and all possible treatment may be so overwhelming that a healthy individual could not truly appreciate it through mere psychological projection."[59]

Even if the concept of informed consent will not accomplish all the work Hall would like it to, it is important as a partial help. Where the standards of disclosure, substantive fairness, and voluntariness are satisfied, the individual's decision to enroll in a plan that has adopted certain arrangements for the rationing of services ought to increase our level of moral comfort with the rationing of services to that individual in accordance with those arrangements. But the existential constraints we face as individuals push us beyond the doctrine of informed consent and individual autonomy, or rather, remind us of the importance of intersubjectivity, even here.

If the healthy learn from those confronting illness, they will make better decisions as individuals. Further, a community in which this kind of conversation occurs will do better at ensuring justice through standards of substantive fairness. It will also do better at promoting the internalization of a sense of justice by its members. In his conclusion, Hall notes: "Too often, we think of our health insurance as giving us individual entitlements to make limitless demands on anonymous resources. A communitarian vision helps us see that insurance creates a collective interest in a shared resource that entails both individual rights to demand support and individual obligations of restraint."[60]

ETHICISTS AND ETHICS COMMITTEES: THE CURE FOR WHAT AILS MANAGED CARE ORGANIZATIONS?

Problems and Possibilities

Laurie Zoloth-Dorfman and Susan Rubin have emphasized the role of ethicists in debates about health care's future. The term "ethicist" in this context indicates a member of a somewhat ill-defined body of persons with credentials from a broad range of disciplines, persons who devote themselves to solving problems of an ethical nature in the health care context. Some professionals, especially physicians and nurses and other clinicians, pursue this endeavor alongside their remunerative work. For others, who work as consultants or are employed by an academic institution or health care organization, "ethics" is a career.

Zoloth-Dorfman and Rubin recognize that ethicists do not stand outside the health care system. Regardless of their place on the spectrum, ethicists are participants, not spectators. However, Zoloth-Dorfman and Rubin also want to claim a certain objectivity for ethicists. They argue that "the social stance of the clinical ethicist *as outsider*" is becoming increasingly important, as the conflicts of interest at the clinical level become ever more direct.[61] The point is that ethicists, who have focused on clinical decision making for particular patients, need to take a greater interest in the management decisions that shape policies and ultimately affect the direction of health care.

Ethicists seem especially well suited to this task because they straddle the boundary between "inside" and "outside." Yet this posture makes them as vulnerable as any boundary-spanner; Zoloth-Dorfman and Rubin do not mention the ethicists' own conflicts of interest. Ethicists, like others, wish to please their employers and colleagues. For years, they have been criticized for adopting the agenda of medical professionals, physicians in particular; their interests have been shaped by the institutional world they inhabit. Without denying the many contributions of the ethicist, the role is no panacea. It represents a limited institutionalization of ethical concern, as does the development of ethics committees.

Proposals for extending the ethics committee concept to HMOs and other managed care organizations stress both departures from and continuities with traditional hospital-based structures.[62] Although commentators emphasize that ethics committees should not be given, or attempt to take on, resource allocation, utilization review or cost containment functions, committees will operate within an environment constrained and sometimes defined by these functions.

Hence, some organizations charge their ethics committees with arriving at a sharpened understanding of terms such as "futile," "marginal, and "experimental."

Such conceptual work cannot be too sharply separated from the concrete practices of the organization overseen by other committees. This suggests that cross-representation and cross-fertilization between committees is desirable. Some would argue that interpenetration would compromise the ethics committee and its task. There are dangers associated with this approach, for example, that the ethics committee's deliberations will become a sort of Good Housekeeping seal of approval on policies established outside of its purview. Maintaining a lively awareness of such dangers is the best defense against them. The alternative is to ensure purity by building in irrelevance. Furthermore, it is to accept a highly questionable model of the ethics committee's function, one in which the committee becomes the conscience for the morally suspect "body" of the organization.

Pragmatism weighs in against this kind of dualism and the hierarchy it implies. In addition to developing or refining the conceptual frame for resource allocation decisions, topics of great urgency in the managed care context include the following: proprietary practices, that is, the growing tendency to view innovations that improve patient care as trade secrets to be kept from competitors rather than as knowledge to be communicated freely for the benefit of all; ethical aspects of care in non-hospital settings, including the home; and protecting privacy and confidentiality in light of the increased collection and wider diffusion of data.[63]

We should not sneer at proposals to extend structures such as ethics committees and the position of ethicist to managed care organizations. Neither should we disdain proposals to extend the scope of responsibility of ethicists and ethics committees to management and policy. On the other hand, one must remain alert to the limits of these structures. A managed care organization in which the decision makers in the first or last instance (the executive officers of the corporation) are not already sensitive to ethical considerations will not support an ethics committee committed to integrating ethical considerations into decision making at all levels as part of its mission. The ethicist or ethics committee can only be effective within an organization that has some ethical commitments.

THE HARVARD PILGRIM ETHICS PROGRAM

Harvard Pilgrim has been a leader in institutionalizing ethical concern through a formal ethics program; it remains to be seen how that program will weather the organization's near demise in the Spring of 2000. In a letter opening its 1997 Annual Report, the Chairman of the Board and President and Chief Executive Officer noted that accolades for superior performance do not necessarily win over a public concerned about the relationship between cost and quality, financial incentives, medical decision making, and confidentiality.[64] In essence, the letter presented the business and technocratic case for ethics. It also established the background against which Harvard Pilgrim's development of a program to address ethical issues became a point of pride.

The letter referred to the "gap between [public] perception and reality," but one might also describe the gap as one of accountability. Some areas of public concern, especially those extending beyond technical proficiency, had not been on the HMOs' agenda; and the contributions of some HMOs toward improving the quality of health care had not been communicated effectively. The leaders of Harvard Pilgrim recognized the problem, even if they failed to perceive some of its dimensions.

In a question and answer format, Lisa Raiola, the founding director of the formal ethics program, detailed the approach to ethics adopted by Harvard Pilgrim.[65] Raiola described the Harvard Pilgrim program as an opportunity to create a "common language" and an explicit "ethical compass" for the organization. The ultimate goal is to preserve and enhance trusting clinician-patient relationships by strengthening the health plan's ability to act as an ethical leader in its clinical and business activities. Raiola identified the first step toward that goal as understanding the paradigms implicit in the practices that comprise the organization. This is necessary to augment the skills of participants in recognizing and articulating ethical tensions, and to supply participants with a methodology they can use in negotiating those tensions. Equally important is promoting dialogue among members of the organization and external stakeholders. For this project, "commitment to openness is key."

The program's core is the Ethics Advisory Group. Members of the group include managers, staff, clinicians, representatives of area employers, and plan members. The group meets monthly, and at each monthly meeting a manager requests consultation on a specific case. The meetings are open, in the sense that anyone can attend, and cases are published in a newsletter. The group tries to conclude each meeting with a recommendation, but will not create policy or issue mandates. Owing to a belief that all advice should reflect the diversity of the group's composition, they do not try to force consensus. The group's "customers" find value in articulating divergent opinions, and in confirming that sometimes there are no simple solutions.

Creation of a code of ethics was not a top priority. Raiola was concerned that a code would give the program a punitive cast. She wrote that codes can be "flat" or lifeless, especially if they are perceived as the work of "a detached group of experts who think they know what's best for everyone else." At their best, codes convey what ethics means to particular organizations in capsule form, and provide a framework for evaluating the institutionalization of ethics within organizations. To function in this way, though, a code must be the result of an open process of exchange rather than a point of departure.

Raiola saw recognition of the program's practical value as its greatest achievement: "Our CEO, as well as senior executives, operational committees, community physicians and even Board members, have turned to the Ethics Advisory Group for help in sorting out challenging decisions with serious ethical implications. Not only have they sought out the program, they've allowed us to publish their cases in the spirit of organizational learning . . . [L]eadership recognizes that the ethics process enhances the way we do business." Raiola's description of the program suggests that the "common language" fostered by the program represents a melding of high ideals and practical wisdom (or common sense in a non-pejorative sense) and business logic and terminology. This is borne out in a presentation concerning the operation of the program by a senior executive.

At a 1998 conference devoted to constructing an ethical framework for managed care, corporate medical director and senior vice president Joseph L. Dorsey described how members of the Ethics Advisory Group identified five "ethical guideposts" to assist senior management in decision making about drug coverage: (1) whenever possible, avoid patient harm; (2) within the bounds of responsible stewardship, be "the ethical leader in the market"; (3) ensure that product design and reimbursement methodologies support financially neutral clinical decision making to the extent possible; (4) advocate for industry change or reform when the external environment promotes "deselecting of bad risk" (i.e., avoidance of persons who are likely to have above-average needs for health care); and (5) begin to address *long-term* issues, such as the inadequacy of resource allocation processes, and more specifically, introduce issues such as the incorporation of stakeholder values and the design of global budgeting methodologies in discussions at the senior management level.[66]

The Harvard Pilgrim project is both admirable and sensible. It is also unstable. Harvard Pilgrim's decision to limit drug coverage for seniors drew criticism from consumer advocates and state regulators, along with lots of negative press. If the ethics program is justified primarily by its capacity to close the gap between image (bad) and reality (good), what becomes of a process that may have contributed to an ethically sound judgment, all things considered, but failed to solve the HMO's public relations problem? Unless the leaders recognize the process of deliberation as an end as well as a means, they are unlikely to maintain it through difficult times.

EXTERNAL REGULATION AND OVERSIGHT

If internal structures for oversight and correction, such as ethicists and ethics committees, are no guarantee against ethical lapses by managed care organizations, we must ask whether and how external structures might fill in the gaps.

Media Scrutiny

Publicity can shame corporate leaders into more ethical conduct. Media attention often provides the impetus for the lawmaking that may be necessary to free the morally disposed from unscrupulous competition. News reports awakened public outrage over "gag rules" (restrictions on communication in physician contracts) and "drive-through deliveries" (early postpartum discharge). Yet a vigorous public press may be met with a wall of silence. Journalist Dave Lindorff found that physicians affiliated with for-profit corporations were often unwilling to criticize their business partners.

Unfortunately, the press may compress material to fit within its own space-time matrix, the available space on the page or time on the air, or to fit with a perception of "what the public wants" by way of drama or simple truths. Note the catchphrases for the abuses already exposed. The complexities and ambiguities described here are often neglected by the media.[67]

Threat of Litigation

The courts are another external mechanism for disciplining individual practitioners and managed care organizations.[68] Defenders of financial incentives to limit services cite malpractice liability as a deterrent to deficient, as opposed to conservative, physician practice. We know that the threat of liability has some influence on the behavior of some physicians. We also know that malpractice liability is not a predictable outcome of bad practice. Hence, one would not wish to rely on it exclusively. Such reliance would be especially foolhardy in light of proposals to sharply limit the amount or availability of relief.

A number of malpractice suits have named the managed care plan itself as a defendant. The view of corporate moral responsibility I presented in Chapter 3 supports this practice. It is edifying to observe how some managed care organizations have tried to shield themselves from liability for conduct they promote. Either they have availed themselves of the protection of a flawed federal law or they have gone through contractual contortions to deny, on paper, the influence they exert in practice.[69] Managed care officials have undertaken similar efforts to dodge liability for wrongs committed directly by the organization, such as bad faith denial of benefits.

Government Regulation and Oversight

Nearly every ethicist who has examined managed care ethics has called for increased regulation of managed care organizations. The analysis of the market and bureaucracy I presented in Chapter 5 suggests that we should not fear regulation generally, so much as bureaucratic rigidity.

The perspective of the social experiment weighs in favor of a certain freedom. It is difficult, and indeed counterproductive, to attempt to regulate creativity or virtue too directly. Congress can scarcely mandate that every HMO have x units of innovation or integrity. Regulators do have the power to support or undermine, hinder or advance, creativity and virtue.

Regulation also supplies the regularity necessary for intelligent innovation. Hence, the pragmatist will be somewhat skeptical of industry arguments against regulation framed as altruistic concern about innovation.[70] In addition, proponents of laissez-faire seem overly sanguine about the possibility of reversing course if the bad consequences predicted along a certain path do materialize. In psychological terms, actions become habits resistant to change, just as, in sociological terms, practices become entrenched in institutions. The problem at the societal level is greater, since social reform usually requires concerted effort across diverse groups, which is very difficult to achieve.

The pragmatist's general instructions to regulators might begin: Renounce obfuscating language, use sticks (prohibitions and penalties) to establish a floor, and offer any available carrots to the creative and the virtuous. Beware of impulses to dominate or micromanage, and favor modes of regulation that build consumer voice.[71]

Federal and state governments regulate managed care by setting standards for participation in the Medicare and Medicaid programs and benefit programs for government employees, as well as through general laws.[72] Unfortunately, governments often seem to lack integrity in this area, adopting a rule of "do as I say, not as I do." The Medicare program has fought judicial intervention to reform an appeals process that fails to meet standards proposed by the administration for private insurance.[73] This posture has fueled doubts about government as a positive force in health care. Program administrators have also been complacent in the face of disruptions engendered by market forces.[74]

RECENT LEGISLATION

Physicians' organizations have lobbied vigorously for state legislation that would require managed care organization to contract with any physician willing to accept their payment rates and basic terms. Such bills are often termed "Patient Protection Acts," a rather disingenuous label, since this type of legislation seems intended to protect physicians.[75] Few seem concerned to distinguish between physician selection criteria that have to do with quality and those that have to do with a history of low utilization, for example. Other provisions give plan members the ability to go out of network at will, undermining a plan's ability to control cost and quality.

Many legislators have not been terribly enthusiastic about these acts, favoring proposals that give patients direct access to certain specialists, mandate minimum stays for certain procedures, adopt a prudent layperson standard for access to emergency services, make provision for transitional care (where a relationship between a chronically ill, disabled, or pregnant plan member and her provider is disrupted because of the member's involuntary disenrollment or the provider's termination without cause), establish standards for handling grievances and appeals, arrange for independent review of disputed cases, and set requirements relating to network adequacy and financial solvency.[76]

At the national level, partisan positions on a "Patients' Bill of Rights" initially developed in a polarized way that was particularly unhelpful. Republicans tended to link any reform by external means to an increase in the number of uninsured. With the exception of a few defectors, they did not reflect on whether the health insurance maintained for existing beneficiaries and perhaps extended to others would be of a kind worth having. Being insured is small comfort, if you cannot trust your doctor or rely on the availability of a core set of services in time of need. Democrats, for the most part, ignored the problems associated with increased regulation in favor of broad statements of principle which often degenerated into slogans playing on fears and stereotypes— slogans such as, "physicians should control medical decision making, not accountants."[77]

Many legislators have neglected the qualities of relationship so essential and yet so elusive in health care today. For example, expansions of public programs are often associated with new bureaucratic controls and the relentless ratcheting down of payment rates to providers.[78] Politicians may not consider the damage that can be done between the time of implementation and the time of response to cries of pain from providers and patients, percolating up through the state and federal bureaucracies. Often, committed providers who struggle to meet the needs of patients without cutting corners, while complying with a tangle of rules and regulations, are the first casualties of mandates and payment policies that neither legislators nor health administrators have carefully thought through.[79]

Government regulation is necessary to establish minimum standards and to give aid and comfort to the morally disposed. Still, regulation has its limits. By its very nature, regulation tends to generate procedure rather than goodness. A law prohibiting gag clauses should prevent a plan from "deselecting" a physician for the stated reason that she discussed the plan's coverage limits with a patient. But it will not give the physician the kind of freedom associated with participating in a plan that truly values openness.

Finally, the political sphere is also the playground of large corporations and other interest groups. Reviewing some of the recent legislative and administrative battles over managed care scarcely inspires confidence. In any event, we should not rely upon legislative and regulatory processes as the ultimate guarantors of ethics, or quality, in health care.

OUTCOMES AND THE PLIGHT OF THE LEAST ADVANTAGED

Concerns about ethics and concerns about quality are not entirely separate. If managed care has greatly improved the quality of patient care, why all the fuss? Much depends on how one defines quality, and how the goods one means to capture with the term are distributed. If justice commands special attention to the plight of a society's least advantaged members, then we cannot purchase improvements in the quality of health care for the well and well-off at the price of neglecting the poor and the sick.

Making Sense of Managed Care

Outcomes in Managed Care versus Fee-for-Service

It is difficult to argue that generic "fee-for-service" practice produces health outcomes superior to generic "managed care" practice. A number of research studies, some involving vulnerable populations, seem to demonstrate that managed care results in similar or improved health outcomes.[80] For example, a study of patients with rheumatoid arthritis found similar utilization and outcomes for persons with that diagnosis in fee-for-service and prepaid group practice settings.

Women with breast cancer enrolled in HMOs in San Francisco-Oakland and Seattle-Puget Sound showed long-term survival outcomes that were at least as good as those of women receiving care in the fee-for-service system; they were also more likely to receive recommended therapy in the early stages.[81] Further, HMOs that seek accreditation are assessed according to an extensive set of performance measures, introducing a form of accountability lacking in traditional fee-for-service medicine.[82]

On the other hand, we cannot ignore the troubling findings of the Medical Outcomes Study (MOS). The MOS was a four-year observational study of 2,235 patients aged 18 to 97 with hypertension, non-insulin-dependent diabetes mellitus, recent acute myocardial infarction, congestive heart failure, and depressive disorder. Researchers collected data in 1986, with follow-up in 1990. They analyzed the data for patients over 65 covered by Medicare and low-income patients (200 percent of poverty) separately. The study compared practice styles and outcomes for patients treated in staff-model or IPA-model HMOs and patients treated in large multispecialty groups, small, single-specialty groups, or solo practices compensated on a fee-for-service basis.

The investigators found that physical and mental health outcomes did not differ for the average patient; however, outcomes did differ for sub-groups of the population differing in age and poverty status. Outcomes favored fee-for-service over HMOs for the poverty and elderly groups; outcomes favored HMOs over fee-for-service for the non-poverty and non-elderly groups.

Elderly and poor patients were more than twice as likely to decline in health in an HMO versus a fee-for-service plan; 68 percent declined in physical health in an HMO versus 27 percent in fee-for-service. There was one exception. In one of the three study sites, mental health outcomes were better for elderly patients in HMOs relative to elderly patients treated on a fee-for-service basis.[83]

Likewise, the RAND Health Insurance Experiment found that while the average patient did very well in an HMO, people who were both poor and sick were likely to suffer in a system requiring co-payments or using other incentives to decrease patients' inappropriate use of health care services.[84]

Given the demand of pragmatic justice that people be enabled to meet their own needs, the findings of a Health Care Financing Administration (HCFA) sponsored study command special attention. Researchers found that HMOs handled their home-care patients faster, cheaper, and less effectively than providers compensated on a fee-for-service basis under traditional Medicare. The HMOs spent an average of $877 per case and approved an average of 12.7 post-hospitalization home-care visits, compared to $1,305 per case and 18.8 visits for traditional Medicare. The patients with traditional Medicare had significantly more favorable outcomes. They were more likely to be able to feed themselves, toilet on their own, manage their medications, and shop for themselves. The lead researcher concluded, "HMOs tend to approach some aspects of home health care with more of a 'maintenance' philosophy rather than a rehabilitative or restorative philosophy."[85] Another study found that Medicare beneficiaries enrolled in HMOs who suffered strokes were more likely to be sent to nursing homes, and less likely to be discharged to rehabilitation hospitals or units, than beneficiaries with similar diagnoses in fee-for-service settings.[86] Doctors and nurses believe that managed care has negatively affected the quality of care.[87]

Medicaid Managed Care Programs

A review of Medicaid managed care programs by Deborah Freund and Robert Hurley yielded mixed results. Freund and Hurley observed programs across a spectrum, from fee-for-service primary care case management to HMOs. States reported cost savings from managed care in the range of 5–15 percent. Emergency room use declined, while effects on inpatient hospitalization and use of primary care were uneven across programs and states. Access improved according to objective measures (e.g., 24-hour availability, travel, and wait times), but patients generally perceived reduced access, likely owing to restricted access to specialists.

Freund and Hurley also found that dissatisfaction tended to correlate with having a *new* physician in the gatekeeper role, rather than gatekeeping per se. Finally, evidence on quality was extremely limited, leading the authors to conclude, "Irrespective of which position one adopts, the scarcity of good, sound evidence about the impact on quality of programs now serving almost 10 million beneficiaries is reason for significant concern."[88]

Another troubling aspect of Medicaid managed care is the perpetuation of below market reimbursement rates for Medicaid patients enrolled in managed care, leading to the segregation of this patient class.[89] It may be true that "the increasingly competitive environment has made the Medicaid beneficiary more attractive to providers and plans, especially those who have historically not been responsive to this population."[90] It may also be true that Medicaid beneficiaries have become most attractive to plans and providers who expect to compensate for low payment rates by engaging in cherry-picking or underservice, believing that a medically unsophisticated population will be less likely to detect or act upon any deficiencies.

Finally, managed care is likely to worsen the situation of the uninsured. Somewhat ironically, many of the newly desirable Medicaid beneficiaries will quickly join this group of unfortunates; nearly half of those who are enrolled in plans under Medicaid lose their coverage within a year.[91] When managed care organizations, convinced that there is money to be made in care for the insured poor, skim off the healthiest either legally or illegally,[92] public hospitals and community health centers are left to care for the sickest insured at a loss and to provide uncompensated care to the uninsured.[93] There may be a silver lining to this situation, a gathering of will to address a newly visible problem. But in the meantime, the suffering occasioned by the disruption of settled patterns for coping is increasing.

MEETING THE NEEDS OF PEOPLE WITH DISABILITIES:
THE COMMUNITY MEDICAL ALLIANCE

For persons with disabilities, managed care represents the best and the worst of times. Persons with disabilities "have much to gain from a truly and responsively integrated delivery system." At the same time, they "bring atypical and complex service needs to managed care and may (thus) introduce an element of unwelcome clinical and financial risk."[94]

The promise of managed care for people with disabilities, given proper motivation and adequate financing, is illustrated by an experiment termed the Community Medical Alliance (CMA).[95] CMA, a Boston-based not-for-profit HMO, was founded precisely to serve those with "atypical and complex service needs." The group initially included people with quadriplegia, then HIV or AIDS. CMA was the brainchild of Dr. Robert Master. Drawing on 20 years as a doctor in a community health center and three years as the director of the Massachusetts Medicaid program, Master set out to test whether flexible financing and preventive care could improve health outcomes for people with quadriplegia. Master saw this project as a return to the roots of managed care as the development of novel strategies to prevent health problems.

CMA proved successful on a number of levels. The program was structured to cultivate strong therapeutic partnerships. Nurse practitioners would visit patients regularly. About 70 percent of patient visits took place in homes or workplaces. The practice of making house calls had as much to do with placing interactions in a patient's zone of comfort as taking account of a patient's mobility impairment. One of the CMA nurse practitioners noted that in a traditional clinic setting, she saw up to 24 patients a day in 15-minute intervals, compared to an average of four patients a day at CMA. Relying heavily on nurses freed the physician to attend to urgent needs. Through concentrating on a single condition and contacting patients regularly, nurses became expert in caring for the person-with-the-condition.

The degree of familiarity that developed opened up opportunities for some exceedingly complex negotiations and a bit of arm-twisting, while serving as a barrier to crasser, more ethically objectionable forms of manipulation. For example, Master recommended that a patient with quadriplegia and muscular dystrophy check into the hospital for a two-to-four-week weight loss program to reduce his risk of developing pneumonia. An alliance between the nurse practitioner and the patient's girlfriend laid the groundwork, and the promise from the doctor of a clean bill of health for a vacation in Las Vegas was enough to motivate the patient to accept the weight-loss goal, but not the doctor's plan. Fearing that a hospital would pressure him to give up smoking, the patient came up with an alternative: CMA would pay for a nutritionist to visit once a week for one month, and the patient would try to lose 30 pounds. If this plan failed, he would go to the hospital. Master was willing to take the chance.

As for more conventional measures of success, patient satisfaction with CMA was consistently high, and departures from the plan from dissatisfaction were reported at less than one percent annually. Rates of potentially avoidable complications, such as inpatient days for pressure sores affecting persons with quadriplegia and admissions for pneumocystis pneumonia affecting persons with AIDS, fell dramatically.[96] Costs were low relative to the alternatives, although CMA would have been impossible without state guarantees against losses in the early years of the experiment and risk-adjusted capitation rates.

In 1997, CMA's monthly per patient costs were approximately $1,199, about $1,000 less than costs associated with caring for similar patients in fee-for-service plans. The lion's share of the savings came from decreased hospitalizations. To achieve these results, CMA willingly funded services that are often the subject of heated coverage disputes on the fee-for-service side. These include home health care, durable medical equipment, mental health services, augmentative communication devices such as voice amplifiers, and pioneering surgical treatments at national centers of excellence.

As an outgrowth of their work, Master and his colleagues have identified seven principles for designing care systems to meet the needs of people with disabilities: (1) develop new clinical roles that integrate true case management and clinical decision-making; (2) maximize the accessibility of clinicians who know the patient; (3) create environments that foster strong personal relationships between patients and clinicians; (4) help clinicians provide services in the most appropriate settings, deploying resources flexibly to support this activity; (5) employ clinicians with special knowledge of patients' conditions; (6) use early interventions aggressively to limit the complications of chronic illness; and (7) use risk-adjusted capitation to allow innovation in serving people at varying levels of need.[97]

The challenge is to sustain commitment to these principles in an environment in which successful small-scale experiments often expand too quickly and lose their distinctive character, or find themselves swallowed up by enterprises that care less. Mergers and acquisitions can contribute to organizational turbulence in the not-for-profit sector, as well as in the for-profit sector.[98]

Implications

If justice requires us to pay special attention to the plight of the least advantaged, and cooperative egalitarianism seconds the demand, then we will be unable to simply shrug off negative findings from the MOS and other studies. Steps to protect the vulnerable, such as oversampling of high-risk populations in quality assurance monitoring, and developing performance measures focused on conditions that disproportionately affect vulnerable groups, are clearly justified.[99] Yet once again, there are reasons to avoid broad-brush judgments.

In the MOS study, HMOs located in one study site organized mental health services in a manner that produced superior outcomes for the elderly. As the CMA example suggests, some forms of managed care may provide more comprehensive services and result in better outcomes for individuals with disabilities. In general, we can argue about whether it makes sense to posit a tight causal connection between payment structures abstractly considered and particular outcomes, good or bad.[100] One must observe how concepts work out in practice in particular situations, something statistics may hide.

Further, the concept of "outcome" is not straightforward. Morbidity and mortality are the most readily available outcome measures, but they may not be the most meaningful. The assumption that death and impairment of health are undesirable is generally a safe one, hence less death and less impairment will usually count as a good outcome. Still, patients' assessments of their own ability to function are arguably the best performance indicators. In any event, "outcomes evaluation" is only a tool. It yields information to assess in light of guiding purposes and principles.

Evaluating outcomes need not and should not translate into accepting health maximization as the only principle guiding the allocation of health care resources. Justice may require non-health-maximizing allocations by directing resources to those who have the most pressing needs. At the same time, those who care about the most needy will care about whether their needs are really being met. It would be a strange view of distributive justice that looked only at the aggregate dollar figure expended on the least advantaged, without regard to what the money accomplished.

More globally, much of what we care about *morally* is particular rather than general and resists quantification. We care that a statistically significant number of patients does better (or worse) under managed care. We also care that a particular patient was never told of a potentially beneficial treatment, treated with rudeness, or lied to, or that a particular physician was reprimanded for spending too much time with a distraught patient, or for recommending a potentially beneficial treatment not covered by the HMO.

We care that the health status of a particular patient cohort improved because the HMO put a great deal of thought, time, effort, and money into designing an effective health education and disease prevention program. We care that this particular patient felt better, even if he had no hope of getting better, because someone responded to his concerns and helped his family come to terms with the situation. We may want something more from persons, and organizations, than simple conformity to general requirements or an unexceptionable statistical profile.

Within the pragmatic framework, the considerations that count *against* specific managed care practices will include things like the potential to foster manipulative relations, paying too much attention to external goods and short-term results, and relying on a deficient understanding of human beings or organizations. Potential to promote a "creative" intelligence that takes the long- and wide-view and contributing to democratic community will both count in favor of a practice.

These criteria permit a strong endorsement of practices like cooperative care clinics, asthma outreach programs made feasible by capitated payment, and the various attempts at more participatory decision-making I discussed in Chapter 5. These criteria support a strong negative judgment concerning financial arrangements that reward individual clinicians for providing less care, or reward individual clinicians or provider organizations or insurers for avoiding people who need lots of care.

Using gatekeepers and guidelines, and relying on informed consent for legitimacy, are in a gray zone. These efforts can be good or bad, depending on the details. Gatekeepers as mentors, coordinators, judicious users of services and points of accountability are good. Gatekeepers as stern enforcers of "autonomous" choice, indifferent obstructionists, or demoralized middlemen are bad.

Guidelines as best practice advisories and as one of many tools for monitoring and improving quality of care are good. Guidelines as rules for saving money purporting to be best practice advisories, or objects of faith, are bad. Informed consent as a way of opening up communication, illuminating processes and enhancing accountability, is good. Informed consent as a legal formality, contributing to the erosion of personal responsibility ("don't look at me, you signed on knowing x"), or substituting for substantive protections of patient welfare, is bad. As always, the devil is in the details.

Ethicists and ethics committees, regulators, and pressure groups may figure as "guardian angels," but each form of oversight has its failings. Pragmatism as stereoscopic social criticism sees how the world might be made better, while acknowledging that remaking the world is a perilous project.

CONCLUSION

The Future of Managed Care

Many have linked managed care to the so-called "corporatization" of health care and would make of the corporation the locus of all the evil forces currently at work in society. It should be clear by now that such blanket indictments will not do. The truth in them—that corporations, particularly large corporations, pose certain dangers—is distorted by overbreadth.

Corporations have long been a part of health care. What is unprecedented is the consolidation among corporations and the extension of the corporate domain to include physicians. Also, while early forms of managed care were corporate in nature, such efforts were local and not-for-profit. National for-profit firms now dominate the field.

From a pragmatic perspective, we cannot equate change with decline. Neither can we take the increasing dominance of large corporations, and within that category, large for-profit corporations, as evidence of their superior efficiency, or desirability according to more strictly moral criteria. The work of Paul DiMaggio and Walter Powell suggests that pressures to conform may be as powerful among organizations as they are among teenagers.

I have cited the work of Eliot Freidson on the subject of professionalism. Freidson, in contrast to Paul Starr, does not see corporatization per se as a threat to health care. Rather, Freidson identifies the "industrialization" of health care as the development we must strenuously resist. He argues that fee-for-service payment to solo practitioners does not assure their independence, when reimbursement rates are low. Along the same lines, the mere fact of employment by large corporations, owned or directed by non-professionals, need not diminish professionalism.[1]

The industrial model, with its presupposition that all work can be segmented into tasks subject to external manipulation, and its disinterest in the effects of this transformation on producers and relationships, constitutes the real danger. The industrial model has become very influential in health care, but it is not clear that it will win the day.

In reflecting on organizations and health care in 1983, ethicist William F. May wrote, "We may be moving toward a period of duplex social organization in which we require both large-scale institutions, with the resources they can mobilize, and smaller, more informal communities, delivering services that supplement and experiment in ways unavailable to huge, more cumbersome institutions."[2] On occasion, these communities may even emerge within the confines of large corporations, as with Kaiser's cooperative care clinics.

There are some indications that managed care organizations, the new masters in health care, may soon be placed in a servant role. They may support the actual providers of health care services: physicians, other clinicians, hospitals, and health centers. This would not be the end of organizations in health care, but rather a reshaping of organizations to a more human scale.

EXPERIMENTS IN DIRECT CONTRACTING

What is arguably the next step in health care is beginning in Minnesota.[3] In 1995, approximately 80 percent of the insured individuals in the Minneapolis-St. Paul area were enrolled in managed care plans; three large plans alone accounted for nearly 78 percent of the managed care market. By state law, all plans operating in Minnesota must be not-for-profit.

An active group of business leaders contributed to the early dominance of managed care. But according to a spokesman for the group, they began to feel that networks had grown so large that data about quality of care was meaningless and premiums failed to reward efficient providers.[4] Many providers participated in multiple plans, and this overlap of providers in the major networks meant that quality and costs did not vary significantly among plans. The networks were mere aggregates put together to command market share.

Dissatisfaction gave rise to a new regime. Now the Buyers Health Care Action Group (BHCAG) contracts directly with competing sub-groups of providers within the large plans. Providers are assessed using standardized criteria of cost, quality, and service. The BHCAG has coined another catch-phrase for this purpose: the program is known as "Choice Plus." Employees of participating corporations can choose how much choice they want; the options offer different levels of cost and coverage. In the past, plans purchased the services of providers. Now provider groups purchase services such as information systems from plans.[5]

From an ethical perspective, it is important that the BHCAG has chosen a "blended" payment method that creates incentives for integration and efficiency, while limiting physician exposure to risk.[6] Another crucial component of this experiment in direct contracting by employers is the careful attention paid to confidentiality. Recognizing the temptations that would accompany unmediated access to employees' personal information, employers participating in Choice Plus have contracted with an independent organization to fulfill the role of "information trustee."

OTHER TRENDS

Other trends in health care run directly counter to the movement toward greater service integration. The preferred provider organization or PPO is the managed care form that seems to be growing most rapidly.[7] Generally, PPOs reduce costs by negotiating discounted fees with large numbers of providers, rather than through gatekeeping and other management techniques. By the same token, PPOs do not employ gatekeeping and other management techniques to monitor or improve the quality of care. They are not as tightly regulated as HMOs. They are usually not accredited.[8] And while many accounts suggest that we can attribute the resurgence of this looser form of managed care to consumer demand, consumers may find much to dislike once enrolled in these plans.

Consider the results of a study co-authored by Cathy Schoen and Pamela Davidson. Schoen and Davidson depart from the usual pattern of contrasting generic "fee-for-service" with generic "managed care." They constructed an organizational typology that differentiates among plans along dimensions of organizational cohesion, method of physician payment, and risk-sharing. They used this typology to analyze data from a 1994 survey of 3,300 adults in Boston, Los Angeles, and Miami. They found that differences among enrollees in different types of managed care plans were as great or greater than differences between enrollees in managed care and fee-for-service plans.

In particular, the newer, looser managed care forms, the network or mixed HMOs and the PPOs, consistently received lower ratings than group or staff HMOs and IPA HMOs. Concerning PPOs, Schoen and Davidson conclude: "Although PPOs may market their plans as combining positive aspects of FFS [fee-for-service] and managed care, in these three cities enrollee experiences are the opposite: responses indicate that PPO enrollees are encountering the negative features of both worlds, namely continued exposure to out-of-pocket costs, complex restrictions, and paperwork."[9]

Health care futurists are drawing attention to another trend counter to integration, the creation of nationwide chains of specialty hospitals and clinics.[10] While these narrowly focused facilities may improve care for specific conditions, they erode the precarious foundations of more comprehensive providers. Combining the old logic of maximizing reimbursement with the new logic of cream-skimming and cherry-picking, these enterprises provide the most profitable services to the most advantaged social groups. They mark a total break with a tradition that invested institutions in health care with a broad mission of serving the entire range of health care needs for the community. If managed care and the allied logic of integration have their difficulties, the balkanization of health care into separate specialty empires may be even more problematic.

New trends toward self-management and using information technology to diffuse knowledge and power are more promising, as the basis for more humane organizations and modes of medical practice. Technologies such as telemedicine, electronic medical records, and Internet-based decision support systems may remove some of the disadvantages of rural practice and support more decentralized organizational structures. This may create opportunities for greater responsiveness to local communities, for greater community participation and control. More general resources such as the "Community Toolbox," disseminated without charge via the Internet, provide detailed practical guidance for inclusive community problem-solving.[11] Consumers and patients may use the Internet to access information about health and disease and specific processes of care, as well as health plans and providers. E-mail, while less intimate than the office visit, allows for give-and-take with health care professionals and with others in similar circumstances. It also makes "just keeping in touch" manageable for both sides.[12]

Organizations such as the Health Commons Institute promote uses of computer technologies that foster equal partnerships between doctors and patients and better information at the point of decision making, with the ultimate goal of establishing a more effective and sustainable health care system.[13] The great irony here is that unequal access to new information technologies reproduces and reinforces unequal access to basic health care services. Possessing a home computer and Internet access are still marks of privilege.[14]

THE TAVISTOCK PRINCIPLES AND THE FUTURE OF HEALTH CARE

Is managed care destined to be another fad that leaves no trace? I think not. We will never return to the free-spending days of yore. Two basic social facts, the commitment to developing and diffusing new medical technologies, and the aging of the population, virtually guarantee that cost control will be a pressing concern for the next several decades. At the same time, appreciating the value of efficiency and economy in health care need not translate into accepting the business ideology as a sufficient account for health care.

Managing the resources available for health care prudently does not require the manipulation of the people who provide and receive health care. In time, an acquisitiveness without measure, ready to exploit any opportunity, will destroy the underpinnings of social trust and the internal goods of practices such as medicine and health care administration.[15] If the ideology of medicine is lacking, we need to do more than simply replace it with another that is equally flawed.

The story of managed care can be told as a story of heroes and villains and victims, high finance and low behavior. It can also be told as a story about facing problems and finding meaning. We grapple with the conflicts and confusions that arise as we seek to live with and understand ourselves and others.

Conclusion

We try to make sense of the structures and technologies that simultaneously liberate and oppress us.

The first tale is gripping; it evokes emotions of outrage and pity. The second demands that we put emotion to work in crafting a response to the problems created or exposed by managed care. I have moved from one stage to another: from exploring the ways in which the medicine-business dichotomy shapes and constricts the debate over managed care, to considering the value (and limits) of the stories of personal suffering and corporate intrigue that largely define managed care in the major media, to presenting the main features of a pragmatic framework focused on problems and organizational structures. I have offered a case study of a particular managed care organization, Kaiser Permanente.

I have attempted to reconstruct the ideologies of medicine and business, and I have made a plea for a recovery of the ideology of cooperative egalitarianism. Finally, I have undertaken an evaluation of certain practices characteristic of managed care. If I have stressed the importance of organizations, it has not been in order to minimize the importance of the personal relationships between the providers and the recipients of health care. Rather, I have been concerned with organizations as significant determinants of the quality of human relationships. If I have criticized the ideals and ideology of the medical profession, it has not been in order to minimize the importance of ideals, or to suggest that we might dispense with ideology (or physicians).

With the rise of managed care, many clinicians and patients have found themselves within molluscan organizations. It is possible that their dissatisfaction with managed care will move them to create organizations that are more flexible and humane, and yet employ many of the tools that have made managed care organizations so powerful: organization itself, and new approaches to payment, attention to the entire continuum of care, programs for quality assurance and quality improvement, the incorporation of the population health perspective, and sophisticated information management systems.

Further evolution will hinge upon a number of groups acting responsibly. It will require politicians and regulators who create room for innovation while providing the structure and visionary leadership on which socially beneficial innovation depends. It will require administrators ready to assess the character, policies, and practices of the organizations they manage, and ready to ask, "what kind of organization has this been, and what kind of organization should (shall) it be?" It will require clinicians conscious of their organizational affiliations and ready to dissolve them, if necessary.

Finally, the further evolution of health care will require citizens, consumers, plan members, patients, human beings ready to take responsibility for *their* organizational affiliations, ready to take responsibility for their health, and ready to share in directing health care as a corporate venture. Managed care as we know it is a bridge to something else. It has the virtue of forcing issues previously suppressed to the surface. We may hope to emerge with a social vision for health care informed by a deepened understanding of the domain of organizations.

Managed care may have served as the necessary catalyst for the first serious and sustained effort to arrive at a shared statement of ethical principles for those who shape and provide health care. An international group of fifteen, christened the "Tavistock Group" after an early meeting site, published a working draft of a statement of principles in 1999 in the *British Medical Journal*, and, somewhat ironically, a specialty journal, the *Annals of Internal Medicine*. The group included representatives from medicine, nursing, health care administration, ethics, law, economics, and philosophy.

It is a limitation of the project that it engages patients as audience, rather than as participants. Viewed as an attempt to put health care's own house in order, to establish an identity linked to a common vision before inviting wider public involvement, however, the project's structure is defensible.

Drawing on the work of the Tavistock Group, and drawing together the concerns and conclusions expressed in previous chapters, I would offer the following statements of conviction and commitment to those who care about the future of health care:

1. Health care ought to be conceived of as a human service—not business, and not philanthropy.

This principle has implications at the organizational and individual levels. Regarding organizations, the Tavistock Group declares, "Caring for sick people is a social obligation that extends beyond the commercial realm. Although ownership of health care delivery institutions or other organizations that deliver medical care may be appropriate, care itself cannot be owned and must be viewed as a service that is rendered and remunerated under the stewardship of those in the health care system rather than merely sold to individuals or communities."[16] As for individuals, those involved in providing health care benefit from extensive social subsidies. Where health care professionals claim the skills they possess as their exclusive property, they are displaying either näiveté or bad faith.

The judicious incorporation of certain business tools is simply good stewardship. Attention to customer service and information management are wonderful things. Yet in transferring them to health care, we must consider the special qualities of this singular endeavor. Customer service, yes, but without forgetting the nature of the service. Doctors and nurses should be more than dispensers of the most aggressively promoted pill upon demand. Information management, yes, but without forgetting the nature of the information, the trust in which it is given, and the many temptations for its misuse due to thoughtlessness, curiosity, or avarice.

As for philanthropy, it should be replaced, not with *caveat emptor*, but by the realization that *there is no substitute for working alongside* the people you serve.

Health care professionals should seek to stimulate rather than displace public involvement in the enterprise.

2. There is no magic in the market.

The authors of a recent study conclude that the "medical market is not rewarding quality and efficiency."[17] Theoretical and empirical work suggests that, at least in health care, organizational growth and dominance have little connection with superior management and performance manifested in delivering quality service at a reasonable cost. The medical market as currently structured rewards predatory competition and the avoidance of sick people. Competition of the right sort, however, can be a prod to a kind of excellence that embraces interdependence.

United Hospital in St. Paul, Minnesota, served as the catalyst for a broad-based campaign against violence on the part of its corporate parent, Allina Health System. Partnerships with local grassroots organizations and other non-profit social service agencies, and a partnership with a hospital in a rival network, greatly enhanced the campaign's effectiveness.

Regions Hospital, affiliated with Allina-competitor HealthPartners, agreed to perform specialized laboratory procedures for sexual assault victims seen at United Hospital at cost.[18] Competition of the right sort can advance important individual and social goals, but cooperation is an essential element in remaking and repairing the social fabric.

3. There are no miracles in management.

A scholar of business who has seen management fads come and go concludes, "Management is not a solution to seemingly intractable stresses. Rather, it is a means of coping with and sometimes improving only marginally tractable situations."[19] Sometimes all the options are bad. In any event, many factors are beyond the control of any single human being or project team. Acknowledging this reality does not amount to accepting management by muddling through. Exercising principled leadership and basing decisions on the core values of an enterprise have greater dignity than that.

When health care professionals assume management responsibilities, they can make an important contribution by using their special knowledge to make the business case for tempering short-term financial ends with longer-term, more inclusive ends.[20] In this project, they will find allies in the journalists, regulators, accreditation agencies, and public interest groups that can pressure organizations and expose the costs of cutting corners.

A major failing of managers in health care, as in other spheres, has been their excessive preoccupation with pay. Stanford Business School Professor Jeffrey Pfeffer, a voice in the wilderness, warns that focusing on extrinsic rewards such as money undermines intrinsic motivation, distorts judgment, and may actually diminish performance. Less tinkering with physician financial incentives, and more attention to the fundamentals of health care, would be in the interest of patients, physicians, and managed care organizations.

4. The ethic of health care must be broad enough to encompass individuals and populations.

The hard work for the future is to sustain the tension between what I have called encounter personalism and statistical rationalism, or more simply, individuals and populations. Statistical rationalism with its attention to the well-being of populations has arrived, and it is not leaving. Nor should it. This is the value dimension of developments in knowledge and technology. "Although the duty of individual health care workers is primarily to the individual patients whose care they assume, caregivers must be aware that the interrelationships inherent in a system make it impossible to separate actions taken on behalf of individual patients from the overall performance of the system and its impact on the health of society."[21]

Clinicians' primary duties are to their present patients, but even clinicians are obliged to consider those they affect (indirectly) by their actions. At a minimum, this means that clinicians should reflect on the broader effects of manipulating the system to secure benefits for patients.[22] Further, even clinicians are obliged to consider how to improve health care systems with the end in view of contributing to the welfare of the whole community. As in the Allina example, being aware of health problems in the immediate patient population should motivate clinician efforts to understand and address these problems through social action. Finally, even clinicians face a moral imperative to consider the harms of new technologies and to work toward a sustainable health care system.[23]

If the tension between encounter personalism and statistical rationalism is sustained, it may produce important insights. For example, "evidence-based medicine" is very appealing from the perspective of statistical rationalism. But developing a commitment to elderly persons through many clinical encounters will sharpen the clinician's awareness of the limitations of the "EBM" movement. A geriatrician defending the humanistic dimensions of medical practice writes, "This movement trusts only the products of randomized, controlled trials or, preferably, meta-analyses of those trials. But subjects over the age of 75 are rarely found in such trials, thus rendering this population invisible to scientific medicine. If we teach only what we know, and if we know only what we can measure in clinical trials, then we can say little of importance about the care of the elderly. The most important resources required in caring for the very old—sufficient time and empathy—are not included in the critical pathways of managed care."[24]

Of course, encounter personalism also has its characteristic oversights. Most proponents of evidence-based medicine are not so narrow in the evidence they admit, and supporters of evidence-based medicine within primary care see an opportunity to make clinical usefulness an object of and criterion for research.

Further, science tends to be self-correcting. Sweeping claims based on crude science will often be reined in by more refined science.[25]

5. System and service integration have moral importance.

Integration, whether actual or virtual, is crucial insofar as it ensures that people receive the full complement of services they require to exercise their rights and fulfill their responsibilities within their communities. Yet, over the past several decades, the mode of health care financing and organization utilized in the United States has favored institutional over community care. It has favored medical services over other kinds of social services that could contribute to health and well-being.

Perhaps even more significantly for the future, our mode of financing and organizing health care has served as a barrier to the full utilization of technologies that improve functioning by serving as (permanent) adjuncts to the body. For Boston's Community Medical Alliance, capitated payment at the plan level, and the moral and intellectual commitments of the medical director and the organization, combined to support the use of assistive technologies. When the voice of a plan member with multiple sclerosis weakened, the purchase of a voice amplifier did not turn on whether the device was truly a "medical" service. The provider justified the purchase by its potential to improve the plan member's quality of life through enhancing his capacity to communicate. One important aspect of the member's "enhanced capacity" was his greater ease in communicating with health care providers.[26]

6. Practices cannot survive without institutions.

Health care cannot survive without organizations. Yet organizations come with all the difficulties described in previous chapters. These include the difficulty of maintaining an appropriate balance between internal and external goods, the difficulty of resisting pressures to focus on short-term results, and so on.

As organizational ties become more visible in health care, commentators have focused on the problem of allegiance, asking whether physicians are becoming the agents of "corporate interests." Our growing entanglement with corporate interests is usually presented as an ominous development, and it can be, if it means that maximizing personal or shareholder wealth has become the primary end in view. On the positive side, corporate interests in another sense require us to put aside considerations of personal gain to further system improvement. In words chosen by the Tavistock Group, "Individual clinicians have the obligation to change practices that may serve their interests but are costly to the system as a whole."[27]

7. Openness is the foundation for accountability.

So many pressures internal and external to organizations foster defensiveness and concealment that people within the organizations must constantly strive to preserve a commitment to openness. Openness makes an important contribution to internal and external accountability; it serves to counter opacity in organizations and advances important projects in health care, like improving the quality of patient care.

It is alarming that many managed care organizations are unwilling to submit to scrutiny. Of the 359 managed care organizations that provided data to the National Committee for Quality Assurance (NCQA) in 1999, 112 asked that their data not be reported publicly, even in aggregate form. Many more organizations declined to participate in accreditation activities altogether.

8. Public involvement is essential and exceedingly difficult.

Deliberative democracy in forming sound health policy will require considerable change in the political culture. Lisa Disch describes how the 1994 health care reform debate was "depoliticized." With reference to the pro-reform forces, she observes that policy deliberations and choices were reserved for experts and carried out privately. Public events were staged spectacles that failed to equip citizens to evaluate alternative proposals critically.[28] As for the efforts of reform opponents, Darrell West and colleagues conclude, "The health care experience shows that outside strategies can work not just by targeting the public, but also by altering the impressions of news reporters and Washington elites. . . . If elites can be persuaded that the public does not approve of a particular proposal, that campaign is successful even if elite views are based on misperceptions."[29]

I find these interpretations of events persuasive and discouraging, but perhaps we can learn more from the 1994 experience. One lesson might be to begin at the local level to build understanding and trust, before attempting massive restructuring. Experiments at the city, county, or state level appear to be enjoying some modest success. For example, evidence is emerging that the Oregon health care reform failed as an experiment in rationing, but succeeded as an experiment in building support for social provision of a relatively generous package of health care services for disadvantaged groups.[30]

Regulators can also take steps to increase the consumer voice, and do what they can to transform bureaucracies in which sacrifice is parceled out according to rule into settings for collective reflection and mutual aid.[31] Under some conditions, participants may acknowledge that rights to demand financial support in pursuing health-related goals are tied to obligations of restraint. Under some conditions, participants may recognize that sharing financial resources does not exhaust the possibilities of human community.

Kaiser Permanente's experience with the HOCA/LOCA guideline illustrates some of the difficulties attending managed care's efforts at involving members (or the public). The Kaiser Permanente experience also affords some lessons for managed care organizations seeking to improve. Absent a massive increase in the social and private resources devoted to health care, allocation problems are bound to multiply. Superficial public relations strategies are unlikely to change the public perception that even corporate decisions aiming to improve care rather than ration it are in fact cost-driven.

I doubt that many people have gone to work for managed care organizations in the hopes of becoming society's rationing agents, perhaps the very definition of a thankless task; but that role has fallen to them by default. If they want help in the task, greater legitimacy, and greater public appreciation of the more positive role they can play in reinventing health care, they will have to apply themselves to the problem of involving members with the same seriousness they would bring to problems of comparable significance in medicine or business.

Given the stakes, investing substantially in research into the *process* of member involvement is warranted. Some on-going experiments appear to be bearing fruit. For example, California Health Decisions has worked with a large employer-purchaser, a physician group practice, and an HMO called Health Net, to conduct focus groups and assemble a project team of stakeholders to address areas of concern. The HMO has implemented various changes to practices as a result of these activities. One interesting finding has been that consumers who participated in focus groups assembled to elicit attitudes, concerns, and recommendations *and* in focus groups assembled to evaluate changes showed much stronger increases in satisfaction levels than a "control" group of consumers who experienced the same changes but participated in evaluation only.[32]

We should not occupy ourselves with longing for some prior golden age of freedom. We ought rather to face the future in the spirit suggested by May. "These difficulties . . . argue for critical reflection and experiment with alternative modes of organization, but they do not persuade one to join the nostalgic who yearn for the days of the free-lance entrepreneur, the private practitioner. . . . Men and women need community not merely for the instrumental purpose of producing greater things than they can achieve by themselves, but for the moral reason of helping them to be better than they can be by themselves."[33]

We have no guarantees concerning the future; indeed, we have some cause for pessimism. Yet in the venture of the imagination that displays what might be, and in the encounters that give meaning to the notion of common grace, we may find the nourishment we need to continue the project of reformation.

NOTES

INTRODUCTION

1. Macklin and Waymack have been selected because their work on managed care clearly shows the logic and limits of the dichotomizing framework. They represent the extremes, but the views they express in the vocabulary of bioethics are widely shared. This point is further developed in Chapter 2. The argument is not that either Macklin or Waymack is unusually dense; to the contrary, both have produced an extraordinarily rich body of work. Our misfortune is that the framework is a distraction preventing many exceptionally gifted philosophers and professionals from making important contributions to the managed care debate.

Note, too, that many of the issues raised by Macklin and Waymack can and must be explored once one moves beyond the medicine-business dichotomy. Mark Hall is a sophisticated proponent of a kind of contractual ethic for managed care, premised not on the total assimilation of health care to the standard business model, but rather on the development of the idea of informed consent and what he would describe as more adequate notions of beneficence and autonomy constrained by justice. For a discussion of Hall's argument, see Chapter 6, notes 39–43 and accompanying text.

2. Ruth Macklin, "The Ethics of Managed Care," *Trends in Health Care, Law & Ethics* 10, no. 1/2 (1995): 63–66. See also Ruth Macklin, *Enemies of Patients* (New York: Oxford University Press, 1993).

3. Mark Waymack, "Health Care as a Business: The Ethic of Hippocrates Versus the Ethic of Managed Care," *Business & Professional Ethics Journal* 9, no. 3/4 (1990): 69–78, 71, 74, 76.

4. Lynn Etheredge, Stanley Jonz, and Lawrence Lewin, "What Is Driving Health System Change?" *Health Affairs* 15, no. 4 (1996): 93–104. The picture changes a bit if one looks at *families*. A national household survey conducted in 1998-1999 found that 64 percent of families in which at least one family member was offered employer-sponsored insurance had a choice of plans. Sally Trude, "Who Has a Choice of Health Plans?" Issue Brief no. 27 (Washington, D.C.: Center for Studying Health System Change, 2000), available from the Center's website at www.hschange.com/issuebriefs/issue27.html (visited August 26, 2000). The survey found that 49 percent of families offered employer-sponsored insurance had a choice between an HMO and a plan with fewer restrictions.

5. Stephen L. Isaacs, "Consumers' Information Needs: Results of a National Survey," *Health Affairs* 15, no. 4 (1996): 31–41.

6. In a more subtle account, E. Haavi Morreim suggests that contractual justice must be supplemented by what she calls *contributive* justice. The argument is that in resolving ambiguities administrators must observe the implications of alternative interpretations for subscribers as a group. "[A]dministrators must look to the spirit of the agreement, the basic values governing health care and resource use that contractors

hoped to achieve in signing on. These are the expectations that subscribers held *ex ante*, at the time they chose their policy, not what a few now wish they had, after events have defined their needs more clearly." E. Haavi Morreim, "Moral Justice and Legal Justice in Managed Care: The Ascent of Contributive Justice," *Journal of Law, Medicine & Ethics* 23, no. 3 (1995): 247–65, 250. The problem with Morreim's discussion is her failure to recognize that values and expectations, as well as provisions in written contracts, may be ambiguous, unsettled, or in conflict.

7. In real life, it was "If you pay for a Chevrolet, don't expect a Cadillac." George Anders, *Health against Wealth: HMOs and the Breakdown of Medical Trust* (New York: Houghton Mifflin, 1996), 108.

8. This tentative conclusion rests on Macklin's strongly voiced distrust of any active role for administrators of managed care systems, and the polemical thrust of an earlier book. In "The Ethics of Managed Care," Macklin appears to dismiss all forms of utilization review as second guessing by distant "bureaucrats" (clearly a term of disdain), and she states that managed care systems are "run by business managers whose main objective is to minimize costs." Macklin, "The Ethics of Managed Care," 64. Hospital administrators are tarred with the same brush in *Enemies of Patients;* in many of the cases described in that text, administrators are among the enemies, the victimizers of patients. I do not believe my reading of the book is idiosyncratic. In a review, Stanley Reiser writes that institutional interactions are more complicated than Macklin's framework allows, and that "when she [Macklin] engages in this rhetoric of enemies and victims the author's analysis loses the nuanced excellence that she displays when she leaves the theme of enemies behind." Stanley Joel Reiser, "Complicated Interactions," *Hastings Center Report* 24, no. 3 (1994): 48. Macklin indicates that, under one scenario, the intrusion of administrators may be legitimate, if not welcome: "There is one circumstance that could justify placing some limits on the autonomy of patients and physicians: a societal agreement to ensure a more just system for delivering health care." Macklin, *Enemies,* 245. It appears she would reject Mark Hall's argument that if a lack of limits drives up the cost of insurance and increases the number of the uninsured, this dynamic by itself is sufficient to make limit-setting a matter of social justice.

9. E. Haavi Morreim, *Balancing Act: The New Medical Ethics of Medicine's New Economics* (Dordrecht: Kluwer Academic Publishers, 1991); Ezekiel J. Emanuel, *The Ends of Human Life* (Cambridge, Mass.: Harvard University Press, 1991).

10. Morreim, *Balancing Act,* 99.

11. Morreim, *Balancing Act,* 150.

12. Emanuel, *Ends of Human Life,* 158. Some of these themes, in particular, the status of the political model vis-a-vis other possible models, are further developed in Ezekiel J. Emanuel and Linda L. Emanuel, "Preserving Community in Health Care," *Journal of Health Politics, Policy and Law* 22 (1997): 147–84.

13. On this topic, see, e.g., *What Price Mental Health?: The Ethics and Politics of Setting Priorities,* ed. Philip J. Boyle and Daniel Callahan (Washington, D.C.: Georgetown University Press, 1995).

14. Sister Mary Loyola Hegarty, *Serving with Gladness: The Origin and History of the Congregation of the Sisters of Charity of the Incarnate Word, Houston, Texas* (Milwaukee: Bruce Publishing Co., 1967), 209. For other examples of early prepaid health plans, see Emily Friedman, "Capitation, Integration, and Managed Care: Lessons from Early Experiments," *JAMA* 275 (1996): 957–62.

15. Michael A. Shadid, *Crusading Doctor: My Fight for Cooperative Medicine* (Boston:

Meador Pub. Co., 1956; reprint, Norman: University of Oklahoma Press, 1992). The shortcomings of the "prevailing system" are discussed at pp. 63–81.

16. Donald Light has described the efforts of the profession to suppress "contract medicine," which involved competitive bidding for contracts to provide health care to the employees of large businesses. County and state medical societies conducted studies and reported on the (allegedly) awful conditions under which contract physicians labored, although published remarks of contract physicians stressed the advantages to physicians of guaranteed income and the opportunity to build a private practice. In addition, some medical societies sought to shame physicians who did contract work by putting their names on a list; the names of members who promised not to enter into competitive contracts were entered on an "honor roll." Others threatened to expel or censure those who signed contracts, a serious threat given that medical societies often controlled access to hospitals. Societies also lobbied for legislation prohibiting the corporate practice of medicine, i.e., the employment of physicians by non-physicians. Donald W. Light, "Reforming America's Health System: Origins and Dilemmas," transcript of lectures delivered November 14–18, 1994 at the University of Texas-Houston Health Science Center (HPI Discussion Paper No. 7) (Houston: Health Policy Institute, University of Texas-Houston Health Science Center, 1996), 13–14. Shadid, who was careful to distinguish his cooperative idea from contract medicine, recounted his many battles with the medical societies in *Crusading Doctor.* The story of how colorful Oklahoma governor "Alfalfa Bill" Murray saved Shadid's license to practice medicine is particularly entertaining. Shadid, *Crusading Doctor,* 116–22.

17. For a detailed analysis of the legislation and its effects, see Lawrence D. Brown, *Politics and Health Care Organization: HMOs as Federal Policy* (Washington, D.C.: The Brookings Institution, 1983).

18. Serious debate over the question of whether medical care makes any difference in the overall health of a society began in the mid-1970s. Paul Starr has a good, succinct discussion of the issues. Paul Starr, *The Social Transformation of American Medicine* (New York: Basic Books, 1982), 408–11. See also Donald W. Light, "Escaping the Traps of Postwar Western Medicine," *European Journal of Public Health* 3 (1993): 281–89. Of course, it may be that medical care is more than a technology for producing "health." As Eliot Freidson says, responsiveness and recognition may constitute (at least some part of) the service and its benefits. Eliot Freidson, *Doctoring Together* (New York: Elsevier, 1975), xii. We may still ask whether medical care as we currently have it is the best way of securing "responsiveness and recognition."

19. A good point of entry into the literature concerning the effects of managed care on health care expenditures is a report released by the Congressional Budget Office, *Trends in Health Care Spending by the Private Sector* (Washington, D.C.: CBO, 1997). Its strengths are also its weaknesses. The report provides a detailed analysis of the available data on private health care spending, but it tends to neglect the larger questions. For example, reduced expenditures for health care by employers may be associated with increased burdens on informal caregivers and community providers, e.g., public hospitals and programs, but information on these costs is not readily available. A KPMG Peat Marwick study finds significant cost-shifting to employees. U.S. Agency for Health Care Policy and Research, *Theory and Reality of Value-based Purchasing: Lessons from the Pioneers,* AHCPR Publication No. 98-0004, November 1997, 11. See also Eli Ginzburg, "Managed Care and the Competitive Market in Health Care: What They Can and Cannot Do," *JAMA* 277 (1997): 1812–13.

20. The percentage of workers in private firms who are enrolled in some form of managed care rose from 29 percent in 1989 to 70 percent in 1995. Etheredge et al., "Health System Change," 94. According to the *HMO Industry Report*, 80.8 million Americans were enrolled in HMOs as of July 1, 1999. Interstudy, *HMO Industry Report 10.1* (Minneapolis: InterStudy Publications, 2000).

21. In the *staff model*, physicians are typically employees of the HMO on a full-time salaried basis. In the *group model*, physicians are employed by a group practice, not the HMO. The HMO is usually responsible for marketing, enrollment, collections, and other aspects of plan administration. The staff and group models are also known as "closed panel" HMOs because the HMO is "closed" to physicians who are not on staff or part of a participating group. In the *network model*, the HMO contracts with multiple group practices to provide services to members. In the *IPA model*, as the term suggests, the HMO contracts with IPAs, associations of independent physicians or small groups of physicians formed for the purpose of contracting with HMOs. Many IPAs accept capitation payments from HMOs and "convert" these payments into (discounted) fee-for-service payments to individual participating physicians. A POS option allows individuals to retain some level of coverage when they seek services from providers with no contractual relationship to the HMO.

The PPO sits on the boundary between managed care and traditional fee-for-service medicine. Participating providers typically agree to abide by utilization management and other procedures and agree to accept the PPO's reimbursement structure and payment levels. In return, PPOs often limit the size of provider panels and provide incentives for their covered beneficiaries to use participating providers. In contrast to the traditional HMO, individuals are not restricted to providers on the PPO list, although there may be higher copayments or deductibles for "out-of-network" services. Recently the annual rate of growth in HMO enrollment has declined, partly due to a shift to PPOs. Even within the HMO "market," the trend is toward looser arrangements. See "Managed Care Shifts Direction," *Employee Benefit Plan Review* 54, no. 8 (2000): 22.

22. John K. Iglehart, "Managed Care," *New England Journal of Medicine* 327 (1992): 742–47 (emphasis added).

2. MANAGED CARE AND THE MEDICINE-BUSINESS POLEMIC

1. Council on Ethical and Judicial Affairs, American Medical Association, "Ethical Issues in Managed Care," *JAMA* 273 (1995): 330–35, 331 (emphasis added).

2. American Medical Association, "First Code of Medical Ethics," in *Ethics in Medicine: Historical Perspectives and Contemporary Concerns*, ed. Stanley J. Reiser, Arthur J. Dyck, and William J. Curran (Cambridge, Mass.: MIT Press, 1977), 26–34, 29. The philanthropic ethic is complemented by (and also stands in some tension with) what Albert Jonsen has dubbed the Lockean ethic of rights. Albert R. Jonsen, *The New Medicine and the Old Ethics* (Cambridge, Mass.: Harvard University Press, 1990). Both the philanthropic and Lockean ethics demand autonomy for the physician—the right to control the context of practice, the disease, and the patient. But in the Lockean ethic, autonomy is uncoupled from professional altruism and includes the freedom not to serve those in need. For another perspective on the fault lines in the ideology of medicine, see Deborah A. Stone, "The Doctor as Businessman: The Changing Politics of a Cultural Icon," *Journal of Health Politics, Policy and Law* 22, no. 2 (1997): 533–56.

The rudiments of a social ethic have from time to time made an appearance in organizational codes and policy statements, but this ethic has not been terribly robust. While public health concerns figure prominently in the 1847 Code of Ethics, only a general responsibility to participate in community improvement survives to 1996. In a most regrettable episode from the AMA's history, public health concerns were jettisoned in a bid to preserve autonomy. In the 1960s, the AMA opposed warning labels on cigarette packages, apparently as a quid pro quo for votes against Medicare from tobacco-state congressmen. See Edward A. Pont, "The Culture of Physician Autonomy: 1900 to the Present," *Cambridge Quarterly of Healthcare Ethics* 9, no. 1 (2000): 98–119, 106.

3. Eliot Freidson, *Doctoring Together* (New York: Elsevier, 1975), 124, 189–90.

4. Milton Friedman, "The Social Responsibility of Business Is to Increase Its Profits," *New York Times Magazine*, 13 September 1970, 33, 122–26. I use the term "classical" to distinguish this view from others in circulation within the business community, including the "stakeholder" conception with which Friedman is at war. For an in-depth analysis of the classical business ideology, see Francis X. Sutton, Seymour R. Harris, Carl Kaysen, and James Tobin, *The American Business Creed* (Cambridge, Mass.: Harvard University Press, 1956).

5. Robert Jackall, *Moral Mazes: The World of Corporate Managers* (New York: Oxford University Press, 1988), 200.

6. Friedman does not want corporate executives to pursue their own interests; he wants executives to fulfill their fiduciary obligations to owners. And even Friedman acknowledges that markets have a legal and social structure, although at times he speaks as if markets were natural rather than artificial. The picture for medicine is similarly complex. A profession as thoroughly organized as medicine cannot be individualistic in any simple sense. A physician can lament the power of managed care organizations and argue that the ultimate duty and power of decision rests with the individual physician, and then immediately turn around and state, "Realistically, however, no single physician or institution can stand up to the juggernaut of managed care." Randall J. Lewis, Letter to the Editor, *New England Journal of Medicine* 333 (1995): 1220.

7. Shortly after choosing this metaphor, I came across a piece by Mary Briody Mahowald entitled "On Treatment of Myopia: Feminist Standpoint Theory and Bioethics," in *Feminism & Bioethics: Beyond Reproduction*, ed. Susan M. Wolf (New York: Oxford University Press, 1996), 95–115.

8. Sam J. Sugar, M.D., Letter to the Editor, *New England Journal of Medicine* 333 (1995): 1220.

9. Lewis, Letter, 1220. The analysis of changes in health care in a more recent article in *JAMA* adopts the "two cultures" view, a variant of the business-medicine dichotomy with somewhat greater subtlety. John H. McArthur and Francis D. Moore, "The Two Cultures and the Health Care Revolution: Commerce and Professionalism in Medical Care," *JAMA* 277 (1997): 985–89.

10. Joanne Silberner, "Competition Threatens Survival of Catholic Hospitals," National Public Radio Morning Edition (March 12, 1996), 16–18, 17 (transcript).

11. The administrator of a Catholic hospital, a sister with an M.B.A., suggests a different model. She says that her hospital, which devotes about 11 percent of its budget to uncompensated care, is run like a business, but according to a different set of priorities. This means that "[b]ehind operating margins and all the other issues that are the business piece of health care is the patient, is the patient waiting for a pain medication, is

the person hoping to have their health restored, [are people] who are hoping not to die alone . . . , without anybody there to talk with them, to hold their hand, to care that they hurt, to care that they're scared." Silberner, "Competition," 17.

12. Arnold S. Relman and Uwe Reinhardt, "An Exchange on For-Profit Health Care," in Bradford H. Gray, ed., *For-Profit Enterprise in Health Care* (Washington, D.C.: National Academy Press, 1986), 209–23. (Relman and Reinhardt have made similar arguments in debating the benefits of managed care.) This exchange also caught the attention of Kenman Wong. Wong shares my view that much of the managed care discussion is less than helpful, and he suggests a way out of the impasse through stakeholder theory. See Kenman L. Wong, *Medicine and the Marketplace: The Moral Dimensions of Managed Care* (Notre Dame, Ind.: University of Notre Dame Press, 1998). For a review of reservations about stakeholder theory as a foundation for a new health care ethic, see John F. Peppin, "Business Ethics and Health Care: The Re-emerging Institution-Patient Relationship," *Journal of Medicine and Philosophy* 24, no. 5 (1999): 535–50, 544–45.

13. Albert Jonsen, "Barbarians at the Gates: Medicine, Money, and Morality," *Ophthalmology* 99 (1992): 162–64, 163.

14. Looking backward at the close of the progressive era, a prominent surgeon railed that "[o]ur charitable hospitals have become businesses and are . . . wolves in sheep's clothing." Ernest Codman, responding to a paper read by Robert L. Dickinson before a meeting of New York's Taylor Society and the Harvard Medical Club, quoted in David Rosner, *A Once Charitable Enterprise: Hospitals and Health Care in Brooklyn and New York, 1885–1915* (Cambridge: Cambridge University Press, 1982), 61. Rosner chronicles the transformation of Brooklyn hospitals from neighborhood institutions serving the worthy poor, without charge, into temples of science (and scientific management) accountable to central agencies and oriented toward the needs of paying patients and their physicians. The forces behind change included the "upstart" industrialists and businessmen who became trustees of the newer hospitals—such as the Jewish Hospital of Brooklyn founded in 1903—following the crisis in hospital financing that accompanied the depression of the 1890s. "[Abraham] Abraham and other trustees of this newest hospital did not feel that careful business management needed to conflict with the hospital's caring function. From their perspective, care could be provided only if the hospital were financially stable. But for many trustees reared in the older ideals of stewardship for the poor, the idea of a hospital that was not as poor as its clients was incongruous; hospitals were, by definition, in debt and dependent on charitable contributions." Rosner, *Charitable Enterprise*, 54.

Rosemary Stevens has traced the changing relation, sometimes supportive, sometimes antagonistic, between voluntarism and business throughout the 20th century. Stevens sees health care institutions as flexible and adaptive in serving an array of interests. She argues that the true voluntary ideal was only developed in the 1930s and represented an adjustment to the conditions of the Great Depression. The traditional ideal of voluntarism as charitable giving by benevolent elites (including wealthy capitalists, some of whom were the most ardent critics of any intrusion of business considerations into hospital operations) shifted mid-century and became more democratic and participatory. A major question in the 1960s was whether hospital administrators should train in business schools or schools of public health.

In the 1970s, "nonprofit" hospitals became "not-for-profit," a change that simultaneously acknowledged that hospitals were indeed making money (profit) and denied that they were "in it for the money." Government funding of hospitals and health care lessened the financial dependence of hospitals on local communities, including wealthy donors. Including capital costs in the reimbursable costs of patient care was especially momentous; between the late 1960s and the early 1980s, debt levels doubled, from approximately 40 percent of total capital financing to 80 percent. Stevens, *In Sickness and in Wealth: American Hospitals in the Twentieth Century* (New York: Basic Books, 1989), 299–300.

15. The sources are Erik Larson, "The Soul of an HMO," *Time*, 22 January 1996, 44–52; Michael A. Hiltzik, "Drawing the Line: HMO Dilemma," *Los Angeles Times*, 17 January 1996, Sec. A, p. 1; George Anders, *Health against Wealth: HMOs and the Breakdown of Medical Trust* (New York: Houghton Mifflin, 1996).

16. For evidence that coverage of the deMeurers case is representative, see Mollyann Brodie, Lee Ann Brady, and Drew E. Altman, "Media Coverage of Managed Care: Is There a Negative Bias?" *Health Affairs* 17, no. 1 (1998): 9–34. The article reports the findings of an exhaustive study of managed care reporting in the print and broadcast media between January 1, 1990 and June 30, 1997. Among other things, researchers observed a trend toward using anecdotes and identifying organizations as "the villain." For example, the use of anecdotal reference in all media climbed from 19 percent in 1990 to 29 percent in 1995. Further, only 7 percent of stories in 1990 portrayed a villain, while 21 percent of stories in 1995 portrayed a villain (17 percent portrayed a managed care plan or HMO as villain). There were significant differences between media.

"Managed care as problem for patients" was the big story in 33 percent of all special series stories and 19 percent of all broadcast stories (versus 4 percent for general newspapers and 2 percent for the business press). A patient and/or family was portrayed as victim in 50 percent of special series stories, 31 percent of broadcast stories, 12 percent of general newspaper stories, and 6 percent of business press stories. Regarding tone, researchers found that 69 percent of the stories were neutral, 25 percent were mainly critical, and 11 percent were mainly positive. However, the most visible media—special series and broadcast stories—had the most negative tone. Seventy-nine percent of all special series and 50 percent of all broadcast stories were negative, tied to themes such as "managed care backlash" or "managed care as a problem for patients."

For a discussion of the positive role anecdotes may play in the managed care debate—as catalysts for inquiry, sentinel events signaling system breakdowns, and vehicles for conveying the subjective and qualitative dimensions of experience and remedying gaps in "data"—see David Rochefort, "The Role of Anecdotes in Regulating Managed Care," *Health Affairs* 17, no. 6 (1998): 142–49. Rochefort also recognizes that anecdotes can be misused, as when they are taken at face value rather than verified. For evidence of this kind of sloppiness on the part of journalists and politicians, see Howard Kurtz, "Some Managed-Care Sagas Need Second Exam," *Washington Post*, 10 August 1998, A01. Of course, verification is complicated because medical records are confidential. HMO claims of unfairness may be legitimate where a patient accuses an HMO of wrongdoing and secures a "trial in the media," while refusing to allow the HMO to release information that might vindicate it.

17. When classified as Stage I, breast cancer is localized in the breast tissue. A lumpectomy or treatment with radiation may cure the disease at moderate cost; the ten-year survival rate is around 90 percent. At Stage IV, the most advanced stage, the cancer has

metastasized to other regions of the body. Standard chemotherapy may slow the progress of the disease, but the treatment itself often makes the patient violently ill, and it is not curative.

18. The high dose chemotherapy intended to destroy the cancer cells has a similar effect on the patient's immune system. Stored bone marrow or stem cells are then introduced in an attempt to rebuild the immune system.

19. A meta-analysis of the effectiveness of bone marrow transplants for advanced breast cancer concluded that transplants were of zero value, and possibly had negative effects on the length and quality of life. See Emergency Care Research Institute, *High Dose Chemotherapy with Autologous Bone Marrow Transplantation and/or Blood Cell Transplantation for the Treatment of Metastatic Breast Cancer,* Technology Assessment Custom Report Level 2 (Plymouth Meeting, Pa.: ECRI, March 1994). Large randomized clinical trials, expected to bring definitive answers concerning stem-cell transplantation (a more refined form of transplantation, often referred to as "bone marrow transplantation" or BMT for reasons of habit and convenience), are ongoing. Preliminary findings have been disappointing. See Joan Stephenson, "Opinions Divided on High-Dose Chemotherapy for Breast Cancer," *JAMA* 282 (1999): 119; Joan Stephenson, "Bone Marrow/Stem Cells: No Edge in Breast Cancer," *JAMA* 281 (1999): 1576–78; Joanne Zujewski, Anita Nelson, and Jeffrey Abrams, "Much Ado about Not . . . Enough Data: High-Dose Chemotherapy with Autologous Stem Cell Rescue for Breast Cancer," *Journal of the National Cancer Institute* 90, no. 3 (1998): 200–207; Joan Stephenson, "Researchers Struggle with Trials of Stem-Cell Transplants for Breast Cancer," *JAMA* 277 (1997): 1827–29.

The only trial with positive results was later exposed as a fraud. See Denise Grady, "Breast Cancer Researcher Admits Falsifying Data," *New York Times,* 5 February 2000, A9; Denise Grady, "More Deception Is Suspected in Cancer Study," *New York Times,* 10 March 2000, A13; Richard Horton, "After Bezwoda," *The Lancet* 355 (2000): 942–43. Investigators with the Philadelphia Bone Marrow Transplant Group recently published their results in a peer-reviewed journal; they found no improvement over standard therapy. Edward A. Stadtmauer et al., "Conventional-Dose Chemotherapy Compared with High-Dose Chemotherapy Plus Autologous Hematopoietic Stem-Cell Transplantation for Metastatic Breast Cancer," *New England Journal of Medicine* 342 (2000): 1069–76.

Information on coverage comes from E. Haavi Morreim, "Moral Justice and Legal Justice in Managed Care: The Ascent of Contributive Justice," *Journal of Law, Medicine & Ethics* 23 (1995): 247–65, 259, n. 26. Morreim points out that insurer willingness to cover such unproven treatments hampers the conduct of clinical trials that might establish their safety and effectiveness, or ineffectiveness. Relatively few women are willing to enter trials in which they may be assigned to a control group receiving standard treatment when their insurer will pay for an unproven treatment described by practitioners as "promising" or potentially curative. In 1997, Stephenson reported that breast cancer had become the most common indication for autotransplantation, with the number of procedures increasing six-fold between 1989 and 1995. Transplant units are considered moneymakers for medical centers.

20. The Health Net pamphlet containing coverage information listed bone marrow transplants as a covered treatment, with the exclusions for experimental or investigative procedures appearing many pages later. The company later modified the pamphlet to alert readers to the fact that covered items were subject to exclusions. See Anders, *Health against Wealth,* 119, 124.

21. Anders, *Health against Wealth*, 125.

22. The work of Renée Fox and Judith Swazey is instructive on this point, especially the chapter in *Courage to Fail* entitled "A Sociological Portrait of the Transplant Surgeon." Renée C. Fox and Judith P. Swazey, *The Courage to Fail: A Social View of Organ Transplant and Dialysis* (Chicago: University of Chicago Press, 1974), 109–21.

23. Larson, "HMO," 51.

24. Hiltzik, "Drawing the Line," A10.

25. Hiltzik, "Drawing the Line," A10.

26. Hiltzik, "Drawing the Line," A10.

27. Larson, "HMO," 46. The National Committee for Quality Assurance or NCQA was founded in 1979 by the Group Health Association of America and the American Managed Care Review Association, the major trade associations of the managed care industry (now merged into the American Association of Health Plans). In 1990, it was "spun off" as an independent not-for-profit. The chief activity of the NCQA has been developing and refining the performance measures which constitute the Health Plan Employer Data and Information Set (HEDIS). The NCQA is the managed care equivalent of the Joint Commission on Accreditation of Healthcare Organizations (JCAHO).

28. These figures do not reflect additional compensation in the form of stock or stock options, and other non-cash benefits.

29. " '[Rather than driving up the costs of health care, these pay packages are being financed by] the doctors and nurses and pharmaceutical companies on whom they put the squeeze . . . As long as the patients are happy, why should they care that Malik Hasan is going to be able to buy a new airplane every year?' " Quoted in Milt Freudenheim, "Penny-Pinching H.M.O.'s Showed Their Generosity in Executive Paychecks," *New York Times*, 11 April 1995, D1.

30. Frank Cerne, "Cash Kings," *Hospitals & Health Networks* 69, no. 7 (1995): 51–54, 54.

31. Michael A. Hiltzik, "HMO Deal Shows That Medicine Is Still Profitable," *Los Angeles Times*, 5 April 1995, Sec. D., p. 1.

32. Louise Kertesz, "Busted Merger with WellPoint Cost HSI $20.2 Million," *Modern Healthcare*, 19 February 1996, 13. A subsequent merger attempt with another giant managed care organization came to fruition. For a time, Hasan was the chief executive officer of the merged organization, Foundation Health Systems, Inc., the fourth largest publicly traded managed care organization in the United States, according to an October 1, 1996 news release. The company experienced some difficulties with integration, and in 1999 Hasan left the top post. Louise Kertesz, "Revolving Door Management," *California Medicine* (April/May 1999) at www.healthcarebusiness.com/archives /californiamedicine/0499/16.html (visited August 15, 2000). Foundation Health appears to be doing better financially—at least its stock price has been going up—and Health Net now boasts 5.3 million covered lives. Andrew Blankstein, "Health-Care Provider Makes Comeback; Renews Its Focus on Earnings," *Los Angeles Times*, 11 July 2000, B2.

33. Alicia Ault Barnett, "Do Health Plans Change Course When Doctors Take the Helm?" in *The 1996 Health Network & Alliance Sourcebook* (Washington, D.C.: Faulkner & Gray's Healthcare Information Center, 1996), C48–C51.

34. Robert Kuttner, "Columbia/HCA and the Resurgence of the For-Profit Hospital Business," *New England Journal of Medicine* 335 (1996): 446–51, 447. According to Kuttner, in 1992, thirty-three executives of Health Net purchased 20 percent ownership

of the post-conversion, for-profit company for $1.5 million. Roughly four years later, in April 1996, their shares were worth $315 million. The transaction was very complicated. Health Net (under Greaves) originally proposed to put $127 million into a foundation at the time of conversion. Thereafter, QualMed offered to pay $300 million for the company, with a commensurate increase in the foundation's endowment. When Health Net executives rejected QualMed's hostile takeover bid, QualMed sued. QualMed eventually triumphed. Anders, *Health against Wealth*, 71. Critics believe that Hasan and the Health Net executives still got a bargain. For more information on conversion transactions generally, see Lawrence E. Singer, "The Conversion Conundrum: The State and Federal Response to Hospitals' Changes in Charitable Status," *American Journal of Law & Medicine* 23(1997): 221–50.

35. Jack Beatty, "Combating Violence," *Foundation News & Commentary* 35, no. 3 (1994): 24–29.

36. Malik M. Hasan, "Let's End the Nonprofit Charade," *New England Journal of Medicine* 334 (1996): 1055–57, 1057. Hasan continued to take a leading role in the debate over the future of health care, at least to the point of his departure from Foundation Health. See, e.g., John K. Iglehart, "Listening In on the Duke University Private Sector Conference," *New England Journal of Medicine* 336 (1997): 1827–31.

37. Fitzhugh Mullan, "Sam Ho, MD: Idealist, Innovator, Entrepreneur, in Conversation with Fitzhugh Mullan, MD," *JAMA* 281 (1999): 947–51.

38. Of course, ethicists may still be dissatisfied with the employer's intrusion. For example, Wendy Mariner, a professor of health law, lists three practical problems with assuming that choice of plan satisfies the "requirements of choice": (1) employers choose plans; (2) patients rarely know what benefits their plans offer when they choose; and (3) many patients do not want to be bound by their contracts. The last is a little unusual. Mariner's point seems to be that, when someone is dying, contracts and such seem rather trivial, and patients do not find claims that their care must be limited due to scarcity credible when executives are raking in millions. Wendy K. Mariner, "Business vs. Medical Ethics: Conflicting Standards for Managed Care," *Journal of Law, Medicine & Ethics* 23, no. 3 (1995): 236–46.

39. A view expressed by Marc Rodwin, among others: "Unless they are already ill, . . . most people are unable to predict what services they will need—a fact that undermines meaningful choice among policies with different exclusions." Marc A. Rodwin, "Conflicts in Managed Care," *New England Journal of Medicine* 332 (1995): 604–607, 605.

40. In technology assessment, new procedures, drugs, and devices can be evaluated at three levels. At the first level, the only question is whether the new procedure is potentially beneficial, i.e., assessment concerns safety and efficacy. At the second level, one performs a cost-effectiveness analysis, asking where the new procedure stands relative to existing procedures in terms of benefit and cost. The third level is cost-benefit analysis; here the question is whether the benefit is worth the cost. See Mark A. Hall and Gerard F. Anderson, "Health Insurers' Assessment of Medical Necessity," *University of Pennsylvania Law Review* 140 (1992): 1637–62, 1659. Cost-effectiveness and cost-benefit analysis are discussed at Chapter 3, notes 18–22 and accompanying text.

41. As E. Haavi Morreim has pointed out, the emphasis on individuals, and the doctor-patient relationship, is a product of a specific history. Medical ethics as a discipline arose largely in response to revelations about the abuse of subjects in medical research and routine medical paternalism. Morreim, "Moral Justice," 248. Still, if the initial predisposition had not been to view such moral failures as problems of individual

judgment and action, medical ethics would not have taken the course it did. Change is underway. For example, Griffin Trotter offers an insightful analysis of the instability of dyadic relationships, and the limits of dyadic ethics, in *The Loyal Physician: Roycean Ethics and the Practice of Medicine* (Nashville, Tenn.: Vanderbilt University Press, 1997), 136–72.

42. For an extended consideration of what pragmatic liberalism might take away from MacIntyre, and what it must discard, see Gary Gutting, *Pragmatic Liberalism and the Critique of Modernity* (New York: Cambridge University Press, 1999).

43. Alasdair MacIntyre, *After Virtue*, 2nd ed. (Notre Dame, Ind.: University of Notre Dame Press, 1984), 23–24.

44. MacIntyre, *After Virtue*, 187. Practices also require obedience to certain rules. MacIntyre, *After Virtue*, 190.

45. MacIntyre, *After Virtue*, 196

46. MacIntyre, *After Virtue*, 194.

47. MacIntyre, *After Virtue*, 194–95.

48. Alasdair MacIntyre, "Why Are the Problems of Business Ethics Insoluble?" in *Moral Responsibility and the Professions*, ed. Bernard Baumrin and Benjamin Freedman (New York: Haven Publications, 1982), 350–59, 358.

49. Jeffrey Stout, *Ethics after Babel: The Languages of Morals and Their Discontents* (Boston: Beacon Press, 1988), 279.

50. Stout, *Ethics after Babel*, 280.

51. Stout, *Ethics after Babel*, 289.

52. See Robert Zussman, "The Contributions of Sociology to Medical Ethics," *Hastings Center Report* 30, no. 1 (2000): 7–11.

53. When I began writing the dissertation that would become this book, "limited" was an understatement. The volume of work devoted to organizational ethics is now increasing rapidly. A complete bibliography would include: Edmund D. Pellegrino and David Thomasma, *A Philosophical Basis of Medical Practice* (New York: Oxford University Press, 1981), especially Chapter 11, "The Social Ethics of Institutions"; volume 7, issue number 1 of *The Journal of Medicine and Philosophy*, 1982, devoted to the ethics of collective judgments in medicine and health care; *Integrity in Health Care Institutions*, ed. Ruth Ellen Bulger and Stanley Joel Reiser (Iowa City: University of Iowa Press, 1990); Leon R. Kass, "Practicing Ethics: Where's the Action?" *Hastings Center Report* 20, no. 1 (1990): 5–12; Dennis F. Thompson, "Hospital Ethics," *Cambridge Quarterly of Healthcare Ethics* 1, no. 3 (1992): 203–15; Susan M. Wolf, "Health Care Reform and the Future of Physician Ethics," *Hastings Center Report* 24, no. 2 (1994): 28–41; Stanley Joel Reiser, "The Ethical Life of Health Care Organizations," *Hastings Center Report* 24, no. 6 (1994): 28–35; Joan C. Callahan, "Professions, Institutions, and Moral Risk," in *Professional Ethics and Social Responsibility*, ed. Daniel E. Wueste (London: Rowman & Littlefield, 1994), 243–70; Dennis Brodeur, "Health Care Institutional Ethics: Broader Than Clinical Ethics," in *Health Care Ethics: Critical Issues*, ed. John F. Monagle and David C. Thomasma (Gaithersburg, Md.: Aspen Publishers, 1994); Ezekiel J. Emanuel, "Medical Ethics in the Era of Managed Care: The Need for Institutional Structures Instead of Principles for Individual Cases," *Journal of Clinical Ethics* 6, no. 4 (1995): 335–38; 358–65; Steven H. Miles and Ruth A. Mickelsen, "Introduction: Managed Care: New Institutions and Time-Honored Values," *Journal of Law, Medicine & Ethics* 23, no. 3 (1995): 221–22, and other articles in that volume devoted to the subject of managed care; Woodstock Theological Center, *Ethical Considerations in the Business Aspects of*

Health Care (Washington, D.C.: Georgetown University Press, 1995); Joan D. Biblo, Myra J. Christopher, Linda Johnson, and Robert Lyman Potter, *Ethical Issues in Managed Care: Guidelines for Clinicians and Recommendations to Accrediting Organizations* (Kansas City, Mo.: Midwest Bioethics Center, 1995); volume 12, issue number 1 of the Midwest Bioethics Center's *Bioethics Forum*, Spring 1996, devoted to managed care, and volume 12, issue number 2 of the Center's *Bioethics Forum*, Summer 1996, devoted to organizational ethics; Alycia C. Regan, "Regulating the Business of Medicine: Models for Integrating Ethics and Managed Care," *Columbia Journal of Law and Social Problems* 30 (1997): 635–84; volume 10, issue number 2 of *HEC Forum*, Summer 1998, devoted to organizational ethics; Rebecca D. Pentz, "Beyond Case Consultation: An Expanded Model for Organizational Ethics," *Journal of Clinical Ethics* 10, no. 1 (1999): 34–41; volume 24, issue number 5 of *The Journal of Medicine and Philosophy*, October 1999, devoted to managed care; volume 9, issue number 2 of *Cambridge Quarterly of Healthcare Ethics*, Spring 2000, devoted to issues in organization ethics and health care; James Lindemann Nelson, "Moral Teachings from Unexpected Quarters," *Hastings Center Report* 30, no. 1 (2000): 12–17; Patricia Illingworth, "Bluffing, Puffing and Spinning in Managed-Care Organizations," *Journal of Medicine and Philosophy* 25, no. 1 (2000): 62–76; Edward M. Spencer, Ann E. Mills, Mary V. Rorty, and Patricia H. Werhane, *Organization Ethics in Health Care* (New York: Oxford University Press, 2000); Robert M. Hall, *An Introduction to Healthcare Organizational Ethics* (New York: Oxford University Press, 2000). For an early effort to develop a code of ethics for for-profit providers of health care, see H. Tristram Engelhardt, Jr. and Michael A. Rie, "Morality for the Medical-Industrial Complex: A Code of Ethics for the Mass Marketing of Health Care," *New England Journal of Medicine* 319 (1988): 1086–89.

54. Kathryn Pyne Addelson, "Some Moral Issues in Public Problems of Reproduction," *Social Problems* 37, no. 1 (1990): 1–17; Susan M. Wolf, "Shifting Paradigms in Bioethics and Health Law: The Rise of a New Pragmatism," *American Journal of Law & Medicine* 20, no. 4 (1994): 395–415; Franklin G. Miller, Joseph J. Fins, and Matthew D. Bacchetta, "Clinical Pragmatism: John Dewey and Clinical Ethics," *Journal of Contemporary Health Law and Policy* 13, no. 1 (1996): 27–51; Glenn McGee, *The Perfect Baby: A Pragmatic Approach to Genetics* (New York: Rowman & Littlefield, 1997); Griffin Trotter, *The Loyal Physician: Roycean Ethics and the Practice of Medicine* (Nashville, Tenn.: Vanderbilt University Press, 1997); Lynn A. Jansen, "Assessing Clinical Pragmatism," *Kennedy Institute of Ethics Journal* 8, no. 1 (1998): 23–36 (critical perspective) and Joseph J. Fins, Franklin G. Miller, and Matthew D. Bacchetta, "Clinical Pragmatism: Bridging Theory and Practice," *Kennedy Institute of Ethics Journal*, 8, no. 1 (1998): 37–42 (response); *Pragmatic Bioethics*, ed. Glenn McGee (Nashville, Tenn.: Vanderbilt University Press, 1999); Christopher Tollefsen, "What Would John Dewey Do? The Promises and Perils of Pragmatic Bioethics," *Journal of Medicine and Philosophy* 25, no. 1 (2000): 77–106. Pragmatism has also turned up in the business ethics literature. J. Kevin Quinn, J. David Reed, M. Neil Browne, and Wesley J. Hiers, "Honesty, Individualism, and Pragmatic Business Ethics: Implications for Corporate Hierarchy," *Journal of Business Ethics* 16 (1997): 1419–30.

3. AN ETHIC FOR AN AGE OF ORGANIZATIONS

1. Jeffrey Stout concludes *Ethics after Babel* with a lexicon in which he defines the "superpower view of defense" as "Bernard Williams's name for the view that you have

adequately defended a position 'only if you can annihilate the other side'" (*Ethics and the Limits of Philosophy*, p. 84). Stout invites the reader to compare Robert Nozick's suggestion that philosophers hope for "arguments so powerful they set up reverberations in the brain: if the person refuses to accept the conclusion, he dies." Jeffrey Stout, *Ethics after Babel: The Languages of Morals and Their Discontents* (Boston: Beacon Press, 1988), 295.

2. Typically, approaches to ethics are classified as either *teleological/consequentialist* or *deontological*. Teleological or consequentialist approaches focus on the achievement of end-states—in utilitarianism, the end-state of welfare- or utility-maximization. Deontological approaches identify some acts as intrinsically wrong (or right) and hence, prohibited (or required) as a matter of duty. For deontologists, these duties function as inviolable "side-constraints." In another approach to classification, the contrast is between *rule-based* and *virtue-based* theories of ethics. Rule-based theories are concerned with the evaluation of acts or action-types. They tend to have a deductive structure in which principles produce more particular rules, which are then applied to particular situations. Virtue-based theories are concerned with character evaluation, employing concepts such as virtue or value to describe the ways in which character is formed and expressed.

3. Jean Porter makes this point in working out the implications of her agreement (with Hilary Putnam) that we cannot think exclusively in terms of "trade-offs" if we are to think morally. Jean Porter, *Moral Action and Christian Ethics* (Cambridge: Cambridge University Press, 1995), 53. I believe one could make the case that a limited set of moral absolutes can be accommodated within a mode of moral inquiry that does not claim access to (or aspire to) some kind of super-experiential knowledge. This is the point of Glen Stassen's interesting effort to refute the charge of moral relativism in relation to Michael Walzer's work on justice. Glen Stassen, "Michael Walzer's Situated Justice," *Journal of Religious Ethics* 22, no. 2 (1994): 375–399. If I were forced to attach one of the available labels to my own position, I suppose I would join William Frankena in the ambiguous middle territory of the "mixed deontological" theories. See William K. Frankena, *Ethics*, 2nd ed. (Englewood Cliffs: Prentice-Hall, 1973), especially 51–52.

4. Robert Nozick, *Anarchy, State, and Utopia* (New York: Basic Books, 1974), 29.

5. Onora O'Neill, *Towards Justice and Virtue* (Cambridge: Cambridge University Press, 1996), 192. ("Just institutions can aim to avert and mitigate many of the injuries to which characteristic and persistent vulnerabilities lay people open, but cannot generally avert or mitigate activity that exploits individuals' more variable and selective vulnerability.")

6. I am not suggesting that rules operate as mere guideposts, a view that would fail to make sense of the moral weight we attach to some kinds of rules. John Rawls argues that certain rules are definitive for practices: "If one wants to do an action which a certain practice specifies then there is no way to do it except to follow the rules which define it." John Rawls, "Two Concepts of Rules," *Philosophical Review* 64, no. 1 (1995): 3–32, 26.

One of the challenges of managed care is to identify the rules that are definitive for the practice of health care in this way. The rule that makes patient benefit the primary consideration in clinical decision-making seems a particularly weighty one; if there are qualifications they will need to be developed with some care. By way of contrast, the rules that govern payment seem to be customary or de facto rules that can be treated more freely.

7. Another approach to this complex area is through analyzing how emotion figures in moral reasoning and judgment. Ronald de Sousa offers a complex but highly persuasive articulation and defense of the role of emotion in the realm of axiology or value. Ronald de Sousa, *The Rationality of Emotion* (Cambridge, Mass.: MIT Press, 1987). Robert Solomon is the pioneer in the area. Robert C. Solomon, *The Passions* (New York: Anchor Press/Doubleday, 1976).

8. "The capacity of experts to store in memory tens of thousands of typical situations and rapidly and effortlessly to see the present situation as similar to one of these, suggests that the brain does not work like a heuristically programmed digital computer applying rules to bits of information. Rather it suggests, as some neuropsychologists already believe, that the brain—at times, at least—works holographically, superimposing the records of whole situations and measuring their similarity." Hubert L. Dreyfus and Stuart E. Dreyfus, "From Socrates to Expert Systems: The Limits of Calculative Rationality," in *Interpretive Social Science: A Second Look*, ed. Paul Rabinow and William M. Sullivan (Berkeley: University of California Press, 1987), 327–50, 341.

9. Heterarchy "suggests many partial systems working in parallel, with any one capable of taking over control according to need." De Sousa, *Emotion*, 74.

10. Along these lines, Alasdair MacIntyre has linked pragmatism with the view that "all problems are piecemeal and detailed" and the failure to criticize social wholes. (MacIntyre is referring to what he calls the "middle aged pragmatism" of proponents of the "end-of-ideology" thesis such as Edward Shils, Seymour Martin Lipset, and Daniel Bell.) Does the patient study of variables and contexts necessarily correlate with narrowness and complacency? John Dewey certainly did not share this belief: "The process of producing the changes will be, in any case, a gradual one. But 'reforms' that deal now with this abuse and now with that without having a social goal based upon an inclusive plan, differ entirely from effort at re-forming, in its literal sense, the institutional scheme of things." John Dewey, *Liberalism and Social Action* (New York: G. P. Putnam, 1935; reprint, LW 11:1–65), 45.

It may nevertheless be significant that later "pragmatists" were unable to sustain—or lost interest in—this broader vision and purpose. The lesson for those engaged in the process of retrieval is to beware of a tendency to become too cramped in outlook and forgetful of large ambitions. See Alasdair MacIntyre, "The End of Ideology and the End of the End of Ideology," in *Against the Self-Images of the Age: Essays on Ideology and Philosophy* (New York: Schocken Books, 1971), 3–11, especially 10–11.

11. The pragmatic recovery of experience must be distinguished from a phenomenological exploration of "lived experience." Pragmatists draw attention to the social and cultural formations that shape consciousness.

12. Timothy Kaufman-Osborn believes that ancient medicine offers a paradigm for resistance to the "subjugation" of experience. He writes that "within this domain there could be no supreme specialists whose assertion of expert wisdom so transcended the limitations of ordinary intelligence that it justified disregard for the claims of common sense or obviated the need for personal acquaintance with the matter at hand." Timothy V. Kaufman-Osborn, *Politics/Sense/Experience: A Pragmatic Inquiry into the Promise of Democracy* (Ithaca, N.Y.: Cornell University Press, 1991), 57. It is ironic that medicine evolved into a field of specialists and expertise over against "ordinary intelligence."

13. For example, Reiser introduces the idea of a corps of patient consultants who,

drawing on their experience as patients, would advise other patients and physicians. Stanley Joel Reiser, "The Era of the Patient: Using the Experience of Illness in Shaping the Missions of Health Care," *JAMA* 269 (1993): 1012–17.

14. According to Edith Wyschogrod, Dewey asserted that science must be anchored in experience or applied in two senses. First, science depends on the experiential context for its very intelligibility: "It may be necessary to formulate theories as free from particular existential reference but such theories are meaningless unless they become operational." Second, "human nature is as much part of the referential field of science as any other natural object," and hence, "a science which fails to become applied in a secondary sense, that is, to take human ends into account, has failed to fulfill its objective: It is science alienated from itself." Edith Wyschogrod, "The Logic of Artifactual Existents: John Dewey and Claude Lévi-Strauss," in *John Dewey: Critical Assessments*, ed. J. E. Tiles (London: Routledge, 1992), 4:158–73, 161–62.

Further, as Richard Bernstein observes, what Dewey admired in science and the scientific method was not the promise of certainty. "[I]t is crucial to look and see what he [Dewey] meant by 'scientific method.' . . . He did not mean a set of formal decision procedures or rules for advancing and justifying scientific hypotheses and theories. It is the openness of scientific inquiry, the imagination required for its successful practice, the willingness to submit hypotheses to public test and criticism, the intrinsic communal and cooperative character of scientific inquiry that Dewey highlighted when he spoke of 'scientific method.'" Richard J. Bernstein, "John Dewey on Democracy: The Task before Us," in *Philosophical Profiles: Essays in a Pragmatic Mode* (Cambridge: Polity Press, 1986), 260–72, 265.

15. John Dewey, *Freedom and Culture* (New York: G. P. Putnam, 1939), 171. We can make too much of the fact that Dewey and others unselfconsciously discuss the relative merits of various approaches to "social control." Robert Westbrook notes that, for those of Dewey's generation, the term signified opposition to laissez-faire market controls. Robert B. Westbrook, *John Dewey and American Democracy* (Ithaca, N.Y.: Cornell University Press, 1991), 189, n. 44. Hans Joas makes a similar point: "Dewey's program . . . is explicitly opposed to a 'naturalization' of the market and to a conception of it as a self-regulating, problem-solving mechanism. It is precisely the consequences of the interconnection of actions having economic ends that require a collective interpretation and assessment. In the specific way that the notion of 'social control' was used by this group of thinkers, this notion did not refer to a guarantee of social conformity but, rather, to conscious self-regulation, to the idea of self-government effected through the medium of communication and understood as the solving of collective problems. Thus, this concept of 'social control' was, in the theory of social order, the equivalent of the concept of 'self-control' in the theory of action." Hans Joas, *Pragmatism and Social Theory* (Chicago: University of Chicago Press, 1993), 25.

16. The following example may help to clarify my meaning. Let us say that I am a public health professional. I embark on this career with a burning desire to improve the well-being of African Americans. I propose to achieve this end by studying the natural course of syphilis, a disease prevalent in some African American communities. I do all I can to enlist the cooperation of potential subjects, even if this involves some compromise of the rules for ethical research; after all, my goal is to benefit this very group. Even when good treatments for syphilis become available, I do not offer them to subjects—nothing must be allowed to curtail the study. Because the means I chose was not

consistent with my considered end (e.g., the study compromised the well-being of its African American subjects), it undercut and displaced that end. The end it constituted, ultimately, in a manner that can scarcely be described as accidental, was a deep distrust of health care providers and the research enterprise among many African Americans.

17. As George Anders points out, the term functioned differently in its original context, the traditional indemnity insurance industry. There accountants used the term to describe the percentage of premium dollars paid out on medical claims. George Anders, *Health against Wealth: HMOs and the Breakdown of Medical Trust* (New York: Houghton Mifflin, 1996), 62. Insurance companies had no role in providing care, and they had little or no power to limit the quantity or quality of the health care services received by the people they insured. Their only real control over losses was the prospective adjustment of premiums to bring revenues in line with expenses. A slightly different problem has to do with the misunderstanding of this figure, which is evidenced in its use as a primary measure of organizational performance. See James C. Robinson, "Use and Abuse of the Medical Loss Ratio to Measure Health Plan Performance," *Health Affairs* 16, no. 4 (1997): 176–87.

18. In particular, "hypothetical bias" must be weighed against "strategic bias." Hypothetical bias refers to the weakness of the incentives respondents have to offer accurate information if they believe that questions have no relevance to their lives. Strategic bias refers to the incentive respondents have to strategically misrepresent their values if they believe that their responses will influence policy making that may affect them. Other forms of bias include starting point bias, vehicle bias, and information bias. See Donald Kenkel, Mark Berger, and Glenn Blomquist, "Contingent Valuation of Health," in *Valuing Health for Policy: An Economic Approach*, ed. George Tolley, Donald Kenkel, and Robert Fabian (Chicago: University of Chicago Press, 1994), 72–104, 72–73.

19. See George Tolley, Donald Kenkel, Robert Fabian, and David Webster, "The Use of Health Values in Policy," in *Valuing Health for Policy*, 345–91. For a thorough review of theoretical and methodological issues in connection with cost-effectiveness analysis, see Marsha R. Gold, Louise B. Russell, Joanna E. Siegel, and Milton C. Weinstein, ed., *Cost-Effectiveness in Health and Medicine* (New York: Oxford University Press, 1996).

20. For example, economists tend to equate moral with "moralistic," meaning moral language is an overlay that must be removed or recast in terms more congenial to their discipline. Such a translation project obviously assumes that nothing essential is being lost. To illustrate, economist Mark Pauly finds that, stripped of "moralistic overtones," statements that we as a society should meet the unmet needs of many people reduce to "some people do not consume as much medical care as some others would prefer to see them consume." Mark V. Pauly, *Medical Care at Public Expense: A Study in Applied Welfare Economics* (New York: Praeger, 1971), 52. See Evan M. Melhado, "Economic Theory, Economists, and the Formulation of Health Policy," *Journal of Health Politics, Policy and Law* 25, no. 1 (2000): 233–54.

21. Steven Kelman, "Cost-Benefit Analysis—An Ethical Critique," *Regulation* 5, no. 1 (1981): 33–40, 37–38.

22. For an analysis of the difference or "discrepancy" between consumer and citizen behavior, see Daphna Lewinsohn-Zamir, *Consumer Preferences, Citizen Preferences, and the Provision of Public Goods*, 108 Yale Law Journal 377 (1998). Lewinsohn-Zamir concludes with a two-pronged explanation for the discrepancy: people's preferences for public goods are more other-regarding than their preferences for private goods, and individuals fail to fully express their other-regarding preferences in daily life because

of the *perceived hopelessness* of realizing collective goals in private settings. Ibid., 406. For discussion of how social values might better be incorporated into the "effectiveness" side of economic analysis, see Paul Menzel, Marthe R. Gold, Erik Nord, Jose-Louis Pinto-Prades, Jeff Richardson, and Peter Ubel, "Toward a Broader View of Values in Cost-Effectiveness Analysis of Health," *Hastings Center Report* 29, no. 3 (1999): 7–15; Peter A. Ubel, *Pricing Life: Why It's Time for Health Care Rationing* (Cambridge, Mass.: MIT Press, 2000), 155–83.

23. Charles J. Dougherty, *Back to Reform: Values, Markets, and the Health Care System* (New York: Oxford University Press, 1996), 18. Dougherty's fuller explication of the concept is as follows: "Regarded naturally, values provide direction in life, driving humans toward goals and away from threats. No doubt they provide motives for behaviors that are linked to our survival as a species. Culturally, values provide standards for measuring success or failure, progress or decline. They are the content of our public symbols for the best and the worst in our social life. Existentially, values are a source of meaning in life. They provide individuals and groups with a sense of purpose that goes beyond the struggles or delights of the here and now. Values link the smallness, temporality, and incompleteness of all things human to grandeur, to permanence, and to the ideal." Ibid.

24. Dougherty, *Back to Reform*, 21.

25. For a more complete articulation of this perspective, the reader is referred to the work of feminist political philosopher Seyla Benhabib, e.g., "Afterword: Communicative Ethics and Current Controversies in Practical Philosophy," in *The Communicative Ethics Controversy*, ed. Seyla Benhabib and Fred Dallmayr (Cambridge, Mass.: MIT Press, 1990), 339–69, "The Generalized and the Concrete Other," in *Women and Moral Theory*, ed. Eva Feder Kittay and Diana T. Meyers (Totowa, N.J.: Rowan & Littlefield, 1987), 154–77, "The Methodological Illusions of Modern Political Theory: The Case of Rawls and Habermas," *Neue Hefte Für Philosophie* 21 (1982): 47–74, and *Situating the Self* (Cambridge: Polity Press, 1992).

26. Dewey, *Human Nature and Culture*, 202–3. This may be equivalent to saying that the meaning of life has something to do with the search for meaning. One reviewer asked if Dewey is imposing an undefended, comprehensive moral ideal—growth. This question requires a more thoughtful response than I am able to give it here and now. I do hope that the explorations that follow make the notions of widening horizons and giving self-command more concrete. At the very least, I hope they are sufficient to distinguish this goal from one of maximizing opportunities and promoting self-realization.

27. John Dewey, *The Quest for Certainty* (New York: Minton, Balch, 1929; reprint, *Later Works*, 4), 208 (reprint).

28. John Dewey and James Hayden Tufts, *Ethics*, rev. ed. (New York: Henry Holt, 1932; reprint, *Later Works*, 7), 227 (hereinafter "*Ethics II*").

29. For an analysis of the idea of community in the work of Josiah Royce and Dewey, see Mary Briody Mahowald, *An Idealistic Pragmatism* (The Hague: Martinus Nijhoff, 1972), 149–60 (a study of Royce), and John E. Smith, "The Value of Community: Dewey and Royce," *Southern Journal of Philosophy* 12, no. 4 (1974): 469–79. See Griffin Trotter, *The Loyal Physician: Roycean Ethics and the Practice of Medicine* (Nashville, Tenn.: Vanderbilt University Press, 1997), 76–86, for an account of mutual transformation through service and the formation of community through memory and hope. The influence of Dewey and the idea of community on contemporary sociology is demonstrated in the work of Philip Selznick and in the work of Robert Bellah and

his colleagues, e.g., Robert N. Bellah, Richard Madsen, William M. Sullivan, Ann Swidler, and Steven M. Tipton, *Habits of the Heart: Individualism and Commitment in American Life* (Berkeley: University of California Press, 1985) and Robert N. Bellah, Richard Madsen, William M. Sullivan, Ann Swidler, and Steven M. Tipton, *The Good Society* (New York: Alfred A. Knopf, 1991).

30. John Dewey, *The Public and Its Problems* (New York: Henry Holt and Company, 1927; reprint, Athens, Ohio: Swallow Press, 1980), 149 (reprint). The difference between this view of community and Jeremy Bentham's is striking. Bentham writes: "The community is a fictitious body, composed of the individual persons who are considered as constituting as it were its members. The interest of the community then is, what?— the sum of the interests of the several members who compose it." Jeremy Bentham, *An Introduction to the Principles of Morals and Legislation*, excerpted in *Utilitarianism and Other Essays*, ed. Alan Ryan (Hammondshire, England: Penguin Books, 1987), 65– 111, 65.

31. James Campbell, *Understanding John Dewey: Nature and Cooperative Intelligence* (Chicago: Open Court Publishing Co., 1995), 173–74. See also Giles Gunn, "Pragmatism, Democracy, and the Imagination: Rethinking the Deweyan Legacy," in *Pragmatism: From Progressivism to Postmodernism*, ed. David Depew (Westport: Praeger, 1995), 298–313.

32. John Dewey, *Democracy and Education* (New York: Macmillan, 1916; reprint, *Middle Works*, 9), 8–9 (reprint).

33. For all its dialogical properties, we may still criticize this way of describing things as overly individualistic in light of contemporary theories of communication. Thought itself is dialogical and social rather than monological.

34. Dewey and Tufts, *Ethics II*, 345.

35. ST II-II, Q. 61. Thomas Aquinas, *On Law, Morality and Politics*, ed. William P. Baumgarth and Richard J. Regan (Indianapolis: Hackett Publishing Co., 1988), 164–70.

36. See Michael Walzer, *Spheres of Justice: A Defense of Pluralism and Equality* (New York: Basic Books, 1983). Walzer's discussion of justice in relation to health care is at pp. 86–91.

37. It is interesting to note that Bentham was an early advocate of using financial incentives to ensure the performance of social duties. Some post-modernists have focused attention on the architecture of Bentham's "Panopticon," a prison design intended to permit total surveillance. Less has been written about Bentham's proposal for administration of the prison by contract. According to Elie Halévy, Bentham envisioned that an administrator-entrepreneur would take charge of the inmates. He would receive a fixed payment per head ("capitated" payment) plus the right to receive the returns from any convict labor. Under this scheme, the administrator would not be tempted to coddle the inmates or to waste money in running the prison.

Indeed, the administrator might be inclined to neglect the health and safety of his charges. Bentham recognized this and proposed certain measures to ensure that the administrator's duties toward the inmates were, in his words, " 'so bound up with his interest that he would be forced to do for his own advantage anything he was not inclined to do for theirs.' " Quoted in Elie Halévy, *The Growth of Philosophic Radicalism*, trans. May Morris (New York: Macmillan, 1928), 85. Halévy mentions imposing penalties for each death (a fixed dollar amount per life per year) and offering a reward for each life preserved or any reduction from expected mortality.

38. John Rawls, "The Basic Liberties and Their Priority," in Sterling M. McMur-

rin, ed., *Liberty, Equality, and Law: Selected Tanner Lectures on Moral Philosophy* (Salt Lake City: University of Utah Press, 1987; Cambridge: Cambridge University Press, 1987), 5.

39. And, in fact, while Walzer would reject the device of the original position in favor of a more hermeneutical approach, Rawls and Walzer share an underlying commitment to mutual respect and a shared self-respect, which motivate and inform the search for fair terms of social cooperation. See, e.g., Rawls, "Basic Liberties" (arguing that fair terms of cooperation must be such that all can acknowledge them without resentment or humiliation), Glen Stassen, "Walzer's Situated Justice" (arguing that Walzer's method of "deep interpretation" produces and demonstrates the persuasiveness of two principles, mutual respect for all persons and their communities and opposition to domination, an interpretation of his work Walzer has affirmed). Further, Rawls sometimes stresses the importance of interpretation in understanding justice, e.g., "the appropriate notion of fair terms of cooperation depends on the nature of the cooperative activity itself: on its background social context, the aims and aspirations of the participants, how they regard themselves and one another as persons, and so on." Rawls, "Basic Liberties," 15.

40. See Chapter 5, note 86 and accompanying text.

41. Robert Solomon, *A Passion for Justice: Emotions and the Origins of the Social Contract* (New York: Addison-Wesley Publishing, 1990), 33

42. Fear or insecurity (Bentham), mutual advantage (the Rawls of the original position), appreciation of excellence or merit (MacIntyre), and sympathy (Rawl's moral psychology and his idea of social union).

43. Robert Nozick and H. Tristram Engelhardt, Jr. argue this point to great effect. See Robert Nozick, *Anarchy, State, and Utopia,* and H. Tristram Engelhardt, Jr., *The Foundations of Bioethics,* 2nd ed. (New York: Oxford University Press, 1996). In the work of both philosophers, there is an interesting compound of libertarianism and communitarianism. (What is interesting is not really odd, given that these two lines intersect in anarchism.) In a more recent book, Nozick emerges as more strongly communitarian. See Robert Nozick, *The Examined Life: Philosophical Meditations* (New York: Simon and Schuster, 1989).

As for disagreement over the boundaries of the region of personal inviolability, one might regard a person's mind and body as inviolable in the sense that torture would never be permissible, without allowing that a person has a right to commit suicide and to enlist others in the effort. Those who argue in terms of respect for life will see a clear difference between the two cases, while those who argue in terms of property or control will see a distinction without a difference.

Likewise, one might regard certain forms of property as so closely bound up with personal identity that they share in the inviolability of mind-body, without allowing that there is an absolute private right of ownership extending to the means of production. Those who argue that the self is embedded in webs of relationships with other persons and things, with gradations of significance, will see a difference, while those who argue that the self is mixed with or extended into its products will not.

44. The "health tax expenditure" (i.e., tax foregone) for 1998 alone was an estimated $111.2 billion. The authors of the study that produced this figure note that tax preferences for health tend to favor higher income groups that have employer-sponsored coverage. Benefit varied from $2,357 per family with annual income of $100,000 or more to $71 per family with annual income of less than $15,000.

The authors conclude: "With more than forty-three million uninsured persons in the United States, most of whom are in relatively low income groups, it is important to ask ourselves whether it is appropriate that 68.7 percent of federal health benefits tax expenditures are going to the 36 percent of the population with the highest incomes ($50,000 or more)." John Sheils and Paul Hogan, "Cost of Tax-Exempt Health Benefits in 1998," *Health Affairs* 18, no. 2 (1999): 176–79. See also Uwe E. Reinhardt, "Wanted: A Clearly Articulated Social Ethic for American Health Care," *JAMA* 278 (1997): 1446–47.

45. Where a hospital is both provider and plan, as in a physician-hospital organization or PHO, there is a particularly strong temptation for the organization to use information available to it as a provider to cherry pick.

46. Walzer rules out a two-tiered system in his interpretation of justice in health care. With Beauchamp and Childress, I am skeptical that Walzer has made the argument that such a system would be *per se* unjust, either according to Walzer's basic framework and the notion of entailments, or with reference to the social meaning of health care in the United States. Tom L. Beauchamp and James F. Childress, *Principles of Biomedical Ethics,* 4th ed. (New York: Oxford University Press, 1994), 339.

47. Relative to cultural context, in that what is appropriate will depend on cultural conditions. In an agrarian society, each family might be enabled to grow its own food. In New York City, one might promote roof-top gardens, but it would probably be a good idea to focus on ensuring that each neighborhood has a clean, safe grocery store with a good selection of reasonably priced goods.

48. *Quadragesimo Anno* (1931), quoted in Dennis P. McCann, "Toward a Theology of the Corporation: A Second Chance for Catholic Social Teaching," in *Catholic Social Thought and the New World Order,* ed. Oliver F. Williams and John W. Houck (Notre Dame, Ind.: University of Notre Dame Press, 1993), 329–50, 342. Similar concerns have prompted Ivan Illich to decry the effects of industrial and technological growth on the autonomy of persons and communities. See Ivan Illich, *Medical Nemesis: The Expropriation of Health* (New York: Pantheon Books, 1982), especially 211–20.

49. In the pastoral letter on health and health care, the bishops affirm the value of pluralism, and they call for the creation of a comprehensive health system, drawing on the resources of the public and private sectors. National Conference of Catholic Bishops, "Pastoral Letter on Health and Health Care," *Origins* 11, no. 25 (1981): 400–2.

50. Kevin D. O'Rourke and Philip Boyle, *Medical Ethics: Sources of Catholic Teaching,* 2nd ed. (Washington, D.C.: Georgetown University Press, 1993), 8.

51. See Solomon, *Justice,* 90.

52. It would be even better to prevent strokes, but preventive measures cannot substitute for maintenance measures in the same way that restorative measures can.

53. Pragmatic democracy and justice do not require a leveling down: "It [equality] does not mean sameness; it is not to be understood quantitatively, an interpretation which always ends in ideas of external and mechanical equality. One person is morally equal to others when he has the same opportunity for developing his capacities and playing his part that others have, although his capacities are quite unlike theirs. When there is an equation in his *own* life and experience between what he contributes to the group activity and experience and what he receives in return in the way of stimulus and of enrichment of experience, he is *morally* equal." Dewey and Tufts, *Ethics II,* 346.

The central idea resembles Michael Walzer's notion of "complex" equality: "The aim of political egalitarianism is a society free from domination. This is the lively hope named by the word *equality:* no more bowing and scraping, fawning and toadying;

no more fearful trembling; no more high-and-mightiness; no more masters, no more slaves. It is not a hope for the elimination of differences; we don't all have to be the same or have the same amounts of the same things. Men and women are one another's equals . . . when no one possesses or controls the means of domination." Walzer, *Spheres of Justice,* xiii.

54. Another example would be the way in which attitudes about disability in the population at large—which are not shared by most people actually affected by disabilities—may influence valuations of health states. In one study, researchers found that nearly one-half of a sample of about 1,000 individuals felt that being confined to a wheelchair was as bad or worse than death. George Tolley, Donald Kenkel, and Robert Fabian, "State-of-the-Art Health Values," in *Valuing Health for Policy,* 323–44, 341. As I understand QALY analysis, this valuation would not result in a policy that people in wheelchairs should be denied care because they are "better off dead," but it could mean that treatments that could achieve no better outcome than wheelchair dependence might be ranked very low. See, e.g., Alexander Morgan Capron, "Oregon's Disability: Principles or Politics?" *Hastings Center Report* 22, no. 6 (1992): 18–20, 20.

55. In many cases, member-patients will have no direct contractual relationship with an HMO or other managed care organization. Rather, they will be beneficiaries under a contract between the managed care organization and their employer. While this fact is significant for the individuals involved, in that they are powerless to negotiate terms and may have trouble gaining access to the contract, it is still the case that the basic relationship is structured by contract.

56. Consider this example of pettiness. Many patients arrive at Bellevue Hospital in such severe distress that their identities cannot be immediately determined. Some are victims of accidents or violent crime. In nearly 100 such cases during a six-month span in 1995, managed care organizations refused to pay for treatment, on the grounds that Bellevue failed to notify them of the patients' status within 48 hours of admission. Anders, *Health against Wealth,* 146.

57. The consequences of routinization for ethical awareness is one of the themes in Daniel Chambliss's study of the moral lives of nurses and the "social organization" of nursing ethics. Daniel F. Chambliss, *Beyond Caring: Hospitals, Nurses, and the Social Organization of Ethics* (Chicago: University of Chicago Press, 1996), especially 58–60.

58. For an extended, and beautifully nuanced, treatment of character and contingency, see Nussbaum, *Fragility of Goodness,* especially 318–72 and 397–421.

59. See, e.g., Erik H. Erikson, *Identity: Youth and Crisis* (New York: W. W. Norton & Co., 1963), 91–141.

60. A similar view of character as closely linked to behavior and subject to change—over against Thomas Nagel's treatment of character as something substantial and unchangeable—is defended in Michele Moody-Adams, "On the Old Saw That Character Is Destiny," in *Identity, Character, and Morality: Essays in Moral Psychology,* ed. Owen Flanagan and Amélie Oksenberg Rorty (Cambridge, Mass.: MIT Press, 1990), 111–31.

61. John Dewey and James Hayden Tufts, *Ethics* (New York: Henry Holt, 1909), 368 (hereinafter *Ethics*). This analysis builds on the discussion at pp. 366–68.

62. A survey of 375 CEOs of hospitals and health systems found that 38 percent reported making sacrifices in their personal lives. Fewer than 50 percent reported regularly spending substantive time with their spouse or significant other, while 8 percent reported having no quality time at all. Eighty-one percent of respondents were men. Reported in Jan Greene, "Currents," *Hospitals & Health Networks* 71, no. 24 (1997): 10.

63. Or as Owen Flanagan puts it, "both countermoral and socially unindexed." Flanagan, *Moral Personality,* 259. I sidestep a definition of interests. Dewey and Tufts use the term in the simple sense of 'whatever someone happens to be interested in'. Interests are subjective in the sense that they are not fixed, but not in the sense of being arbitrary or "socially unindexed."

64. The research studies, conducted by Jerome Kagan and Daniel Stern among others, are discussed in Flanagan, *Moral Personality,* 108–109, and under the heading of intersubjectivity in Jessica Benjamin, *The Bonds of Love* (New York: Pantheon Books, 1988), 15–31.

65. Helen Haste suggests that we think in terms of a triangle consisting of "the *individual* (who has some agency in 'making sense'), the *interpersonal* network (within which meaning is constructed, negotiated, or merely transmitted through discourse and performance of shared tasks), and the *culture* (the sociohistorical context that constitutes the repertoire of available frameworks and schemata within which both interpersonal discourse and individual cognition are constrained and constructed)." Helen Haste, "Morality, Self, and Sociohistorical Context: The Role of Lay Social Theory," in *The Moral Self,* 175–208, 185 (emphasis added).

66. Dewey and Tufts, *Ethics,* 299.

67. Max Stackhouse, "Jesus and Economics: A Century of Reflection," in *The Bible in American Law, Politics, and Political Rhetoric,* ed. James Turner Johnson (Philadelphia: Fortress Press, 1985), 107–51, 113.

68. R. H. Tawney, *The Acquisitive Society* (New York: Harcourt, Brace & World, 1948), 49, 178.

69. Anders, *Health against Wealth,* 64–65. (This reminds me of a good piece of prudential advice: Little pigs get fat, big pigs get eaten.) Crowley eventually resigned his post as CEO after the merger of his company with HSI.

70. John Dewey, *Individualism, Old and New* (New York: Minton, Balch, 1930; reprint, *Later Works* 5:41–123), 68 (reprint).

71. In Reformed theology, common grace—contrasted with the special or saving grace which accompanies a certain type of religious experience—reflects God's favorable attitude toward creation in general. It provides a basis for human responsibility and for recognizing and appreciating what is good and beautiful in the world. Picking up this theme, Niebuhr suggests that we think of common grace as the gift of security, which frees the self of its self-preoccupation and enables one to reach out to others.

72. Reinhold Niebuhr, "Man's Selfhood In Its Self-Seeking and Self-Giving," in *Man's Nature and His Communities* (New York: Scribner, 1965), 106–25, 117.

73. Philip Selznick, *The Moral Commonwealth: Social Theory and the Promise of Community* (Berkeley: University of California Press, 1992), 233.

74. Those interested in pursuing the idea of community in contemporary management theory might begin with Fred Kofman and Peter M. Senge, "Communities of Commitment: The Heart of Learning Organizations," *Organizational Dynamics* 22, no. 2 (1993): 5–23.

75. Charles Perrow, *Complex Organizations: A Critical Essay,* 3rd ed. (New York: Random House, 1986).

76. My analysis takes a slightly different path than Christopher Stone's, but I follow Stone in proceeding pragmatically and putting the question of intelligibility first. See Christopher D. Stone, "Corporate Accountability in Law and Morals," in *The Judeo-*

Christian Vision and the Modern Corporation, ed. Oliver F. Williams and John W. Houck (Notre Dame, Ind.: University of Notre Dame Press, 1982), 264–91.

77. Kenneth E. Goodpaster and John B. Matthews, Jr., "Can a Corporation Have a Conscience?" in Kenneth E. Goodpaster, *Ethics in Management* (Boston: HBS Case Services, 1984), 145–54, 153 (commenting on the findings of management studies). Reprint from *Harvard Business Review* (January–February 1982).

78. Ibid.

79. This kind of concern seems to lie behind George Annas's statement that "[h]ospitals are corporations that have no natural personhood, and hence, are incapable of having moral or ethical objections to actions." George Annas, "Transferring the Ethical Hot Potato," *Hastings Center Report* 17, no. 1 (1987): 20–21.

80. I, for one, would reject the view, traceable to Otto von Gierke, that corporations are suprapersonal beings. The perspective defended here makes no such strong, ontological claims.

81. Another way of working through these issues would be to borrow from Anthony Giddens's theory of "structuration." One of Giddens's key concepts is the duality of structure. Giddens explains that "structure is both medium and outcome of the reproduction of practices" through action. Anthony Giddens, *Central Problems in Social Theory* (Berkeley: University of California Press, 1979), 5. It is both a property of social activity and its artifact.

Structure is instantiated in the form of rules and resources. (Giddens is a social rather than organizational theorist, and he does not distinguish between formal and informal structures.) Giddens is mainly concerned with preventing human subjects from disappearing altogether in social theory. As pictured in his work, persons are knowledgeable, with in-built capacities that they develop through learning, and they reflexively monitor their own conduct. Knowledgeable action both draws upon and reconstitutes structures, and therefore practices, institutions and social systems. At the same time, actions and consequences regularly escape intentions. Giddens's treatment of knowledge has an anti-elitist, emancipatory thrust, similar to that which characterizes Dewey's treatment of experience. Giddens writes that "all social actors, no matter how lowly, have some degree of penetration of the social forms which oppress them." Giddens, *Central Problems*, 72.

82. Richard Scott, *Organizations: Rational, Natural, and Open Systems*, 4th ed. (Upper Saddle River, N.J.: Prentice-Hall, 1998), 60.

83. Robert A. Scott, Linda H. Aiken, David Mechanic, and Julius Moravcsik, "Organizational Aspects of Caring," *Milbank Quarterly* 73, no. 1 (1995): 77–93.

84. Joint Commission on Accreditation of Heathcare Organizations, *1996 Comprehensive Accreditation Manual for Hospitals* (Oakbrook Terrace, Ill.: JCAHO, 1995), 95.

85. This is the conclusion of a comparative study of the experience with codes of ethics among health care and energy companies: "Despite relatively recent media attention focused on codes of ethics, our study indicates that the adoption of such codes is rarely accompanied by either a thorough development process or a system for assuring that the codes are known and used. As is indicated by existing literature, the absence of clear evaluation standards reflects a situation within which neither management nor employees know what to expect from a code of ethics. This situation holds from widely different sectors of the economy: *contrary to what might be expected, our health care facilities were less likely to develop or effectively implement codes than were our energy companies.*"

Isaac D. Montoya and Alan J. Richard, "A Comparative Study of Codes of Ethics in Health Care Facilities and Energy Companies," *Journal of Business Ethics* 13, no. 9 (1994): 713–17, 717.

Another study found few significant differences in the evaluation of ethically problematic advertisements by members of two groups, persons employed by an organization with a code of ethics and persons employed by an organization without such a code. The idea was to use the existence of a formal code of ethics (and degree of enforcement) to operationalize ethical organizational culture. The researchers concluded that the existence of an ethical code may actually lessen a sense of personal responsibility to make judgments of right and wrong. Ethical evaluation can become identified as somebody (else)'s job, and/or the tenets of the code of ethics can become a replacement rather than a support for individual moral judgment. Saviour L. S. Nwachukwu and Scott J. Vitell, Jr., "The Influence of Corporate Culture in Managerial Ethical Judgments," *Journal of Business Ethics* 16, no. 8 (1997): 757–76.

86. Selznick, *Moral Commonwealth,* 321.

87. Goodpaster and Matthews, "Conscience," 148. It is a little confusing to say that there are "differences in moral responsibility," since it suggests that corporations that have not institutionalized moral concern may be held to a lower moral standard. There is a bit of truth here. It makes more sense to hold an *institution* (in Selznick's sense) morally responsible, than it does to hold a pure organization, a rational tool, morally responsible. In the latter case, the connection with the individuals who use the organization as a tool is so clear and so tight that one might as well heap the whole of blame or praise on them. But one can imagine a corporation that is very much an institution, and yet has taken no steps to institutionalize moral concern. We have as much reason to hold this corporation morally responsible as we do the exemplary corporation described by Goodpaster and Matthews. It is less moral and less responsible, but not less morally responsible.

88. Selznick, *Moral Commonwealth,* 322–23. Integrity is a coherence notion. But to hold this virtue in high esteem one need not endorse a purely formal notion of morality. Quite the contrary.

In various fields of human endeavor, accounts of virtues and goods intrinsic to specific practices must be developed. For example, Stanley Reiser argues that health care institutions should be guided by the values of humaneness, reciprocal benefit, trust, fairness, dignity, gratitude, service, and stewardship, with each term having a particular meaning in the context of health care. Integrity would then entail fidelity to these values. Stanley Joel Reiser, "The Ethical Life of Health Care Organizations," *Hastings Center Report* 24, no. 6 (1994): 28–35. Also, integrity is not necessarily a solipsistic notion. Of integrity as a personal virtue, William May writes, "While referring to the self in its wholeness, integrity also points beyond the self toward the person, the ideal, the transcendent which gives shape to the person's life." William F. May, "The Virtues in a Professional Setting," *Soundings* 67, no. 3 (1984): 245–66, 259.

89. Philip Selznick, *TVA and the Grass Roots: A Study in the Sociology of Formal Organization* (New York: Harper Torchbooks, 1966), xiii (emphasis added). Originally published in 1949 by the University of California Press. Perrow would point out that in many cases there are villains, and organizations are frequently their tools. Perrow, *Complex Organizations,* 170.

90. The emphasis should be on the phrase "entirely neglects." For example, I would challenge the notion that not-for-profit organizations must literally "sell-out" to sur-

vive. An article describing the achievements of the Laurel Health System, one of the first integrated health networks in a rural area of the United States, notes that the system "reached its goals without much money." Claudia Coates, "Tucked Away in Rural Pennsylvania, an Advanced Medical Network," *Houston Chronicle,* 13 August 1995, 40A.

91. Selznick, *Moral Commonwealth,* 336.

92. Selznick, *Moral Commonwealth,* 350. For a helpful mapping of the many possible permutations of "community benefit" in health care, see Mark Schlesinger, Bradford Gray, Gerard Carrino, Mary Duncan, Michael Gusmano, Vincent Antonelli, and Jennifer Stuber, "A Broader Vision for Managed Care, Part 2: A Typology of Community Benefits," *Health Affairs* 17, no. 5 (1998): 26–49. Schlesinger and colleagues compare and contrast four approaches to (and ways of assessing) community benefit—the legal/historical perspective, the market-failures perspective, the community-health perspective, and the healthy-community perspective—before coming down in favor of a "balanced model" that requires some attention to each of the four.

93. The phenomenon of neutralization is portrayed, and then analyzed, in Murray Milner's case study of a community health center. Murray Milner, Jr., *Unequal Care* (New York: Columbia University Press, 1980), especially 165–67. See also Robert R. Alford, *Health Care Politics* (Chicago: University of Chicago Press, 1975), 221.

94. See Selznick, *Moral Commonwealth,* 353–54.

95. I know this from personal experience, but it is also documented in Robert Jackall, *Moral Mazes: The World of Corporate Managers* (New York: Oxford University Press, 1988). On the short tenure of many leaders in health care, see Louise Kertesz, "Revolving Door Management," *California Medicine* (April/May 1999) at www.healthcarebusiness. com/archives/californiamedicine/0499/16.html (visited August 15, 2000).

96. Wall Street, in the case of for-profit firms. Not-for-profits face their own version of the culture of short-sightedness. Donors increasingly demand demonstrations of effectiveness, "outcomes," within time frames that many administrators (in private) label unrealistic.

97. See Roger Friedland and Robert R. Alford, "Bringing Society Back In: Symbols, Practices, and Institutional Contradictions," in *The New Institutionalism in Organizational Analysis,* éd. Walter W. Powell and Paul J. DiMaggio (Chicago: University of Chicago Press, 1991), 232–63, 245. In a cruel parody of Adam Smith's notion of a hidden hand, it is possible for social *ills* to be attributable to no one's intentional action. Here is one such instance.

So long as they had a monopoly, the Nigerian railways and their customers fared well. When the railways had to compete with road transport, the situation deteriorated. Why? As a monopoly, the railways had not been disciplined by desertion, but they were still affected by protest. Competition did not deprive the railways of a random fraction of users; rather, it took away their most demanding customers. This example is discussed in Raymond Boudon, *The Unintended Consequences of Social Action* (New York: St. Martin's Press, 1982), 36–38.

98. Accounting rules may have effects other than the truncation of the time horizon. Accounting may have had a great deal to do with accelerating the trend toward managed care. Reducing health care expenditures became a priority for many large corporations because a change in the rules concerning accounting for retiree health benefits forced them to take multi-billion-dollar write-offs in 1989–1990. See Anders, *Health against Wealth,* 31.

99. Paul J. DiMaggio and Walter W. Powell, "The Iron Cage Revisited: Institutional Isomorphism and Collective Rationality in Organizational Fields," *American Sociological Review* 48 (1983): 147–60, 147, 152–53.

100. Isomorphism is defined as "a constraining process that forces one unit in a population to resemble other units that face the same set of environmental conditions." DiMaggio and Powell, "Iron Cage Revisited," 149. DiMaggio and Powell conclude that "[a]n understanding of the manner in which fields become more homogeneous would prevent policy makers and analysts from confusing the disappearance of an organizational form with its substantive failure." DiMaggio and Powell, "Iron Cage Revisited," 158. If the not-for-profit form of health care delivery is on the decline, this is not necessarily due to the greater "efficiency" of for-profit firms.

101. Nancy M. Kane, Nancy C. Turnbull, Cathy Schoen, "Markets and Plan Performance: Summary Report on Case Studies of IPA and Network HMOs" (Commonwealth Fund, January 1996), 13–14.

102. Anders, *Health against Wealth*, 62. Uwe Reinhardt has placed the collapse of the physician practice management industry in the context of a Wall Street investment community obsessed with short-term performance and climbing stock prices. One of the quickest and easiest ways to drive up earnings per share is to go on an acquisition binge. Portfolio managers for mutual funds reward these often illusory gains because they themselves are ranked on quarterly rates of return. Reinhardt concludes his analysis with a snipe at believers in the efficient markets hypothesis: "This imperative to achieve high short-run capital gains makes it attractive for fund managers to follow a Greater Fools strategy under which they knowingly purchase what they judge to be overvalued securities, in the hope that they can benefit from a further, unwarranted run-up in value and profitably unload the stock to the proverbial 'greater fool' sometime before its price ultimately collapses. From a human perspective, such a strategy of portfolio management is fully understandable, because with luck it can be profitable in the short run. Only Voltaire's Dr. Pangloss, however, would call playing the Greater Fools strategy 'efficient' pricing." Uwe E. Reinhardt, "The Rise and Fall of the Physician Practice Management Industry," *Health Affairs* 19, no. 1 (2000): 42–55, 54. On the pervasiveness of risky business, and regulators' efforts to rein it in, see Carol J. Loomis, "Lies, Damned Lies, and Managed Earnings," *Fortune*, 2 August 1999, 74–92.

103. The idea of institutions as agencies of character formation has also appeared in some recent writing on health care, e.g., Roger J. Bulger, "Covenant, Leadership, and Value Formation in Academic Health Center," in *Integrity in Health Care Institutions*, ed. Ruth Ellen Bulger and Stanley Joel Reiser (Iowa City: University of Iowa Press, 1990), 3–17, 6, and other essays in that collection, and Leon R. Kass, "Practicing Ethics: Where's the Action?" *Hastings Center Report* 20, no. 1 (1990): 5–12.

104. See Dewey and Tufts, *Ethics*, 355.

105. And the aesthetic virtues, such as sensitivity to beauty, should not be forgotten. James Haughton describes the corrosive effects of poor maintenance at Chicago's Cook County Hospital. Filth and disrepair expressed disrespect for patients and staff. They got the message and carried it into their dealings with one another. A thorough cleaning and a good paint job raised morale by affirming that the hospital's staff and clientele were worthy of a decent environment. James G. Haughton, "Determinants of the Culture and Personality of Institutions," in *Integrity in Health Care Institutions*, 141–47, 146.

106. Although I recognize faithfulness as an instrumental good, a precondition for the patient trust that in turn contributes to healing and "improved health outcomes," I

join M. Gregg Bloche in believing that the instrumentalist picture is incomplete. As Bloche writes, this picture "neglects, even denies, the affective experience of the victim of infidelity—the person who trusts and is betrayed and is thus intimately wounded by another person." M. Gregg Bloche, "Clinical Loyalties and the Social Purposes of Medicine," *JAMA* 281 (1999): 268–74, 272. Bloche considers whether faithfulness or fidelity to patients requires deception of third party payers in M. Gregg Bloche, "Fidelity and Deceit at the Bedside," *JAMA* 283 (2000): 1881–84.

107. This account is taken from Anders, *Health against Wealth,* 53–54. The extended quotation is from a personal essay by Peeno, "Going Beyond the Requirements," written in the spring of 1994.

108. The CEO of Barnes-Jewish Hospital, St. Louis, Peter Slavin, requires *all* hospital executives to spend at least one hour per week on the hospital floor visiting and talking to patients. They must do that because, as he tells a reporter for *Hospitals & Health Networks,* " 'That keeps us all grounded in terms of what we're here for.' " Chris Serb, "More Than Medicine," *Health & Hospital Networks* 73, no. 8 (1999): A-4–A-5. Slavin, an M.D./M.B.A., seems to share the world view of the nun/M.B.A. who told a reporter for National Public Radio that beyond "operating margins and all the other issues that are the business piece of health care is the patient." Joanne Silberner, "Competition Threatens Survival of Catholic Hospitals," National Public Radio Morning Edition (March 12, 1996), 16–18, 17 (transcript). Although the current generation of managed-care medical directors has clinical experience, and credits the experience with improving judgment and enhancing credibility, the trend is for administration-minded physicians to spend their preparatory years studying business rather than caring for patients. See Thomas Bodenheimer and Lawrence Casalino, "Executives with White Coats: The Work and World View of Managed-Care Medical Directors," *New England Journal of Medicine* 341 (1999): 1945–48, 1946.

109. The accountant hired to review the books at Allegheny Health, Education, and Research Foundation (AHERF) found that the nation's largest nonprofit health care failure was facilitated by organizational opacity. "According to Patrick Hurst, the 'chief forensic accountant' hired by creditors to sift through AHERF's finances, financial management was deliberately 'placed in boxes' so that each person or entity within AHERF could see only one piece of the overall financial position." Lawton R. Burns, John Cacciamani, James Clement, and Welman Aquino, "The Fall of the House of AHERF: The Allegheny Bankruptcy," *Health Affairs* 19, no. 1 (2000): 7–41, 23. The authors of this exhaustive case study also point to diffusion of responsibility, greed, and intimidation as factors in the quiescence of so many within and outside of the organization.

110. It is ironic that sociologists who have little to do with theologians and moral philosophers hold Niebuhr's judgments concerning corporate life in high esteem. The following quotation is taken from a footnote to Murray Milner's excellent case study of interorganizational relations in health care: "In dealing with individuals, the assumption of a clear preference for autonomy over interdependence is admittedly a problematic oversimplification, though probably more accurate than the opposite assumption. When, however, we are dealing with collectivities, such as organizations, the assumption is a much more tolerable one. While individuals may have some innate need for interdependence and a significant capacity to identify with the needs of others, these characteristics seem to be considerably weaker at the collective level. Probably the best discussion of this difference in individual and collective attributes is still Reinhold

Niebuhr's *Moral Man and Immoral Society.*" Murray Milner, Jr., *Unequal Care* (New York: Columbia University Press, 1980), 182, n. 12.

111. Scott, *Organizations,* 339–40.

112. Scott, *Organizations,* 340 (following James Coleman).

113. See Herman E. Daly and John B. Cobb, Jr., *For the Common Good* (Boston: Beacon Press, 1989), 184–85.

114. "[D]ifficulties that the large-scale organization of professionals faces in maintaining its drive for excellence argue for critical reflection and experiment with alternative modes of organization, but they do not persuade one to join the nostalgic who yearn for the days of the free-lance entrepreneur, the private practitioner. The nineteenth-century liberal myth saw people as better in isolation than in society. Even the realistic Reinhold Niebuhr fell prey to liberal innocence when he titled his work *Moral Man and Immoral Society. Men and women need community not merely for the instrumental purpose of producing greater things than they can achieve by themselves, but for the moral reason of helping them to be better than they can be by themselves.*" May, *Physician's Covenant,* 180–81 (emphasis added).

115. Dewey, *Democracy and Education,* 88–89.

116. The work of two contemporary institutional theorists, Roger Friedland and Robert Alford, offers some interesting parallels. See Friedland and Alford, "Bringing Society Back In," 248, 256, 232.

4. KAISER PERMANENTE

1. Approximately 58 percent of all managed care plans follow the independent practice association or IPA model. Approximately 73 percent of managed care plans are for-profit. Joseph W. Thompson, James Bost, Faruque Ahmed, Carrie E. Ingells, and Cary Sennett, "The NCQA's Quality Congress: Evaluating Managed Care in the United States," *Health Affairs* 17, no. 1 (1998): 152–58, 153. For a general review of the trends, see Jon Gabel, "Ten Ways HMOs Have Changed during the 1990s" *Health Affairs* 16, no. 3 (1997): 134–45. Recent surveys document an interesting shift in the way the public regards not-for-profit and for-profit health care organizations.

Historically, not-for-profits were rated more highly than for-profits in the area of community service, but rated less highly than for-profits in the areas of efficiency and quality. In a recent survey (January 1998) conducted by the Kaiser Family Foundation, not-for-profit hospitals and health plans scored more highly than their for-profit counterparts on responsiveness to customers and provision of quality care (a nearly complete reversal of the relative standings of the two forms of organization in March of 1997). Henry J. Kaiser Family Foundation, *For-Profit Health Care Companies: Trends and Issues* (Menlo Park, Calif.: Henry J. Kaiser Family Foundation, 1998).

2. "The Kaiser plan was the corporate product of a leading industrialist with a personal interest in health care and a conviction that the managerial techniques of private industry could furnish a solution to health care problems and therewith a private antidote to socialized medicine." Lawrence D. Brown, *Politics and Health Care Organization* (Washington, D.C.: The Brookings Institution, 1983), 104.

3. Lawrence Brown argues that current developments flow from the basic premise of the Nixon administration policy intended to encourage HMOs: that whatever strategy was adopted not cost too much money. Owing to this premise, any direct financial support to start-up ventures had to be very limited. This feature of the policy fa-

vored arrangements with low capital needs (such as independent practice associations) and/or other sources of capital (for-profit firms). Also, since little was offered, the requirements imposed on HMOs, as a quid pro quo for such advantages as there were, were minimal. Brown writes that the compromises incorporated in the HMO Act of 1973 left the HMO industry "widely and deeply depressed." The requirements were significant enough to disadvantage HMOs electing to become federally qualified vis-à-vis traditional health insurance, while the financial supports were insufficient to launch truly innovative ventures. Brown, *Politics,* 347.

4. Herman Weiner, "The Permanente Medical Groups: Organization and Responsibilities," in Anne R. Somers, ed., *The Kaiser-Permanente Medical Care Program* (New York: Commonwealth Fund, 1971), 91–96, 95.

5. "A capacity for reasonable negotiation is highly valued, indeed is thought to be as essential a quality in an administrator or physician-manager as managerial or medical expertise." Brown, *Politics,* 122.

6. Kaiser and other not-for-profit HMOs were not the only ones experiencing financial difficulties. Milt Freudenheim, "Weak Results for Oxford and Aetna: Signs of Trouble in Industry Seen," *New York Times,* 5 November 1997, National edition, C2; Ron Winslow and Scot J. Paltrow, "Ill-Managed Care," *Wall Street Journal,* 29 April 1998, A1.

7. See, e.g., Mark Hagland, "Dangling Modifiers," *Hospitals & Health Networks* 71, no. 7 (1997): 70–74. Similar changes are being experienced by other staff- and group-model HMOs, such as Harvard Pilgrim Health Plan and (for-profit) Prudential Health-Care, recently absorbed by Aetna-U.S. Healthcare. In some regions, Kaiser is also seeking to cut costs by contracting with independent hospitals. Anonymous, Regional News, *Modern Healthcare,* 22–29 December 1997, 36. For a general assessment of the prospects for socially-versus market-oriented models of managed care, see Robert Kuttner, "Must Good HMOs Go Bad?" (Parts I & II), *New England Journal of Medicine* 338 (1998): 1558–63, 1635–39.

8. Emily Friedman, "A Matter of Value: Profits and Losses in Healthcare," *Health Progress* 77, no. 3 (1996): 28–34, 48, 33–34. In the context of the labor dispute touched on below, the California Nurses Association issued a press release lambasting Kaiser for increasing Lawrence's salary 78 percent over a five year period, to $1,250,000 in 1997. CNA Press Release Page, "What's Behind Mass RN Strike July 17-18? Kaiser Seeks 13 Major Takeaways; RNs Have 1 Issue: Better Patient Care," 15 July 1997, www.cal-nurse.org/can/press/71597.htm (visited August 25, 2000). A 1998 *Wall Street Journal* article reported average earnings of $1.1 million in recent years, with Lawrence anticipating cuts in response to the financial bad news for 1997. Anders, "Kaiser's Red Ink," B19.

9. Unless otherwise indicated, all of the quotations that follow are taken from John K. Iglehart, "Changing Course in Turbulent Times: An Interview with David Lawrence," *Health Affairs* 13, no. 5 (1994): 65–77, 65–66. The text follows the flow of the interview, hence particular page citations are omitted.

10. At one time, Kaiser reportedly had plans to cut costs at least five percent per enrollee per year for five years. Louise Kertesz, "Kaiser Physicians Unhappy with Changes, Memo Says," *Modern Healthcare,* 19 February 1996, 12.

11. See, e.g., the exchange between Dr. Les Zendle of Kaiser and Drs. Grumbach and Bodenheimer published in *JAMA* in the Letters to the Editor section. "Controlling Costs: The Case of Kaiser," *JAMA* 274 (1995): 1135.

12. Annual payments on the order of $500 to $800 per employee were to be awarded if the Southern California operations met goals set for reductions in operating costs and increases in enrollment and member satisfaction. Editorial, "Nurses' Profit-Sharing Plan a Concept to Be Embraced," *Modern Healthcare*, 19 February 1996, 24. (The editors applauded Kaiser's move on more Darwinian, survival-of-the-fittest principles.)

13. J. Duncan Moore Jr., "Kaiser Nurse Pay May Be Tied to Early Patient Discharges," *Modern Healthcare*, 1 January 1996, 4.

14. Kaiser has joined a "renegade" group of HMOs (now a trio consisting of HIP Health Insurance Plans, the Group Health Cooperative of Puget Sound, and Kaiser) favoring legally enforceable standards to protect patient rights. Laurie McGinley, "All Sides Get Ready for Push to Regulate HMOs," *Wall Street Journal*, 17 November 1997, A28.

15. Indeed, in his skillful self-presentation, Lawrence calls to mind this description of the physician-leader of the future: "The goal is to develop physician leaders who understand patient care from a population-based perspective, who understand patients from a holistic perspective, who understand care delivery from a continuum of care perspective, who understand and are able to operate in teams and promote teamwork throughout the organization, and who understand how to use information systems to promote clinical integration work and to develop outcome measures for both continuous improvement and external accountability purposes." Stephen M. Shortell, Robin R. Gillies, David A. Anderson, Karen Morgan Erickson, and John B. Mitchell, *Remaking Health Care in America: Building Organized Delivery Systems* (San Francisco: Jossey-Bass, 1996), 187.

16. Kurt Eichenwald, "Doctors' Highest Paid Skill: Steering in Kidney Patients," *New York Times*, 5 December 1995, National edition, A1. This was apparently standard business practice for National Medical. The company that eventually acquired National Medical recently agreed to settle federal civil and criminal fraud charges for $486 million. According to the account of the settlement in the *New York Times*, three subsidiaries of National Medical were accused of charging for disputed intravenous feeding and blood tests deemed unnecessary and "violating anti-kickback laws by providing payments, discounts, yacht trips and bear-hunting excursions in Alaska to attract potential customers." Milt Freudenheim, "Dialysis Provider to Pay $486 Million to Settle Charges," *New York Times*, 20 January 2000, C8.

17. Kurt Eichenwald, "Making Incentives Work in Kidney Patients' Favor," *New York Times*, 6 December 1995, National edition, A1, C18.

18. David M. Eddy, "Applying Cost-effectiveness Analysis: The Inside Story," *JAMA* 268 (1992): 2575–82, at 2575. See also David M. Eddy, "Broadening the Responsibilities of Practitioners: The Team Approach," *JAMA* 269 (1993): 1849–55.

19. Eddy, "Cost-effectiveness Analysis," 2579.

20. "Although the focus groups provided good information about how our members thought about the risks and costs of contrast agents, they did not yield a clear answer to the questions of whether the lower reaction rates of LOCAs were worth the amount specified. For example, . . . they overwhelmingly indicated that they would not be willing to pay the higher costs of LOCAs in order to receive the lower risks. However, when members were asked to imagine themselves as healthy people who might some day need an IVP or CT scan and were asked whether they were willing to pay a slight increase in their monthly premium to receive LOCAs and their lower reaction rates (a mathematically equivalent but psychologically different question), they overwhelm-

ingly said they would be willing to pay for LOCAs. There are theoretical reasons to discount the answers to the second question because it involves numbers that are so small as to be nearly incomprehensible. Nonetheless, the inconsistency was disconcerting. More troublesome was the fact that when we examined some questions that were built into the process to determine whether the participants truly understood the issues, we discovered that many of them did not. For example, after they had read an information sheet saying that LOCAs cost about $82 more than HOCAs, they were asked which agent cost more money. Several participants answered 'HOCAs.'" Eddy, "Cost-effectiveness Analysis," 2579.

21. In his conclusion, Eddy writes that KPSC "has already initiated plans to reallocate resources to beef up our preventive activities such as cancer screening." Eddy, "Cost-effectiveness Analysis," 2580, 2582.

22. Eddy, "Cost-effectiveness Analysis," 2581.

23. Eddy, "Cost-effectiveness Analysis," 2581 (emphasis added). For confirmation that Eddy is a strict utilitarian (if any further evidence is required), see David M. Eddy, "Principles for Making Difficult Decisions in Difficult Times," *JAMA* 271 (1994): 1792–98.

24. Laurie Zoloth-Dorfman and Susan Rubin, "The Patient as Commodity: Managed Care and the Question of Ethics," *Journal of Clinical Ethics* 6, no. 4 (1995): 339–57, 344.

25. These deficiencies are discussed in greater detail in E. Haavi Morreim, *Balancing Act: The New Medical Ethics of Medicine's New Economics* (Dordrecht: Kluwer Academic Publishers, 1991), 53–58. On uncertainty and contingency in clinical decision making, see Eric B. Beresford, "Uncertainty and the Shaping of Medical Decisions," *Hastings Center Report* 21, no. 4 (1991): 6–11.

It is alarming that some have seized upon guidelines as a panacea. Guidelines, critical pathways, computerized medical information systems, and the like, are all for sale, and their promoters make extravagant claims for them. Their purchasers often seem to pin their hopes on these technologies or techniques alone, in lieu of the intelligent incorporation of selected items in the reorganization of practice to better meet the needs of individual patients and the population. David Blumenthal and Arnold M. Epstein, "The Role of Physicians in the Future of Quality Management," *New England Journal of Medicine* 335 (1996): 1328–31, 1330. The need for openness to adjustment may be greatest where guidelines are adopted exclusively as a cost control measure.

For example, guidelines may require a certain drug regimen because alternatives with fewer side-effects are more costly. Over time, the more expensive drugs may decline in price to the point where they are actually the least costly, in which case the guidelines make no sense. Or guidelines may have unintended effects, e.g., a Medicaid cap on the number of reimbursable drugs significantly increased non-pharmaceutical costs. See Scott Weingarten, "Practice Guidelines and Prediction Rules Should Be Subject to Careful Clinical Testing," *JAMA* 277 (1997): 1977–1978.

Mark Hall notes that guidelines developed by Milliman & Robertson seldom specify clinical features that may make the norm more or less appropriate in a particular case. Hall, *Medical Spending Decisions*, 85. Where detailed guidelines that truly provide guidance to clinicians have been developed, the process has been lengthy and expensive. For example, the fifteen or so practice guidelines sponsored by the Agency for Health Care Policy and Research (now the Agency for Healthcare Research and Quality, or AHRQ) consumed six years and tens of millions of dollars. Hall, *Medical Spending Decisions*, 86.

(Of course, that pales in comparison to the billion-dollar public and private budgets for development of new interventions.)

26. 1994 WL 718871 (9th Cir. 1994) (unpublished opinion), *cert. denied*, 514 U.S. 1110 (1995).

27. Freidson, *Professionalism Reborn*, 210–11. An amusing study showing the link between busy-ness and lack of moral concern may by relevant here: "In a truly mischievous experiment, . . . seminarians at Princeton Theological Seminary . . . were randomly assigned to prepare a short talk on either the parable of the Good Samaritan or the issue of job opportunities for seminary graduates. Subsequent to preparing the notes for their talks, each seminarian was sent from the preparation site ('Jerusalem') to the site where they were to give their talk ('Jericho'). Half the students in each group were told that they were running late and should hurry to the delivery site. A student confederate was slumped over in some distress along the route, and the dependent variable was simply whether the student stopped to help or not. Did the seminarians stop with any frequency? No. Was their stopping in any way related to the content of the talk they were about to give? No, not at all. The only variable of any significance was whether the seminarian was in a rush! The less the subjects were rushed, the more likely they were to help." Owen Flanagan, *Varieties of Moral Personality* (Cambridge, Mass.: Harvard University Press, 1991), 301–302.

28. For example, E. Haavi Morreim gives physicians the task of helping patients live with uncertainty. She writes, "Conversation, rather than technology, must become the greater tool for marginal reassurance." Morreim also expects a finer honing of skills in history taking, physical exams, and problem-solving following adoption of a new ethic of "diagnostic elegance and clinical parsimony." Morreim, *Balancing Act*, 100, 99. Gail Povar and Jonathan Moreno outline a similar approach, while acknowledging that time is also a cost. Gail Povar and Jonathan Moreno, "Hippocrates and the Health Maintenance Organization," *Annals of Internal Medicine* 109 (1998): 419–24.

29. Brown, *Politics*, 147.

30. Including demands for non-beneficial services. See Nancy S. Jecker and Albert R. Jonsen, "Managed Care: A House of Mirrors," *Journal of Clinical Ethics* 8, no. 3 (1997): 230–41, 232–33; Jerry Avorn and Daniel H. Solomon, "Cultural and Economic Factors That (Mis)Shape Antibiotic Use: The Nonpharmacologic Basis of Therapeutics," *Annals of Internal Medicine* 133 (2000): 128–35; Benjamin Schwartz, Arch G. Mainous III, and S. Michael Marcy, "Why Do Physicians Prescribe Antibiotics for Children with Upper Respiratory Tract Infections?" *JAMA* 279 (1998): 881–82, 882.

31. Kevin Lumsdon, "Working Smarter, Not Harder," *Hospitals & Health Networks* 69, no. 21 (1995): 27–31, 27. *Hospitals & Health Networks* is published by the American Hospital Association. On the link between managed care practice, decreased time with patients, and decreased job satisfaction, see Mark Linzer et al., "Managed Care, Time Pressure, and Physician Job Satisfaction: Results from the Physician Worklife Study," *Journal of General Internal Medicine* 15 (2000): 441–50, and Robyn S. Shapiro, Kristen A. Tym, Jeffrey L. Gudmundson, Arthur R. Derse, and John P. Klein, "Managed Care: Effects on the Physician-Patient Relationship," *Cambridge Quarterly of Healthcare Ethics* 9, no. 1 (2000): 71–81.

32. Actually, as one might expect, there are precedents. In England, chronic care clinics or "miniclinics" of a similar nature developed in the 1970s. See Edward H. Wagner, Brian T. Austin, and Michael Von Korff, "Organizing Care for Patients with Chronic Illness," *Milbank Quarterly* 74, no. 4 (1996): 522–44, 522.

33. Peter Boland, quoted in Lumsdon, "Working Smarter, Not Harder," 28.

34. Lumsdon, "Working Smarter, Not Harder," 29. The sense of community described by Strammel and participating patients is not unique to Kaiser's Denver operations. When a *Wall Street Journal* reporter visited a cooperative care clinic in Suitland, Maryland, participants expressed strikingly similar sentiments. Barbara Martinez, "Doctors Start Seeing Groups Of Patients to Save Time," *Wall Street Journal*, 21 August 2000, B1.

35. Arne Beck, John Scott, Patrick Williams, Barbara Robertson, Deborrah Jackson, Glenn Gade, and Pamela Cowan, "A Randomized Trial of Group Outpatient Visits for Chronically Ill Older HMO Members: The Cooperative Health Care Clinic," *Journal of the American Geriatrics Society* 45, no. 5 (1997): 543–49. Forty-nine percent of experimental patients rated the overall quality of care as "excellent," compared with twenty-seven percent of control patients. All of the physicians participating in the cooperative care clinics reported that they *greatly* enjoyed treating older patients and were *extremely* satisfied with their ability to treat this group of patients. Fewer than thirty percent of the physicians in the traditional care group reported greatly enjoying treating this group of patients, and fewer than five percent reported that they were extremely satisfied with their ability to treat this group.

36. Lumsdon, "Working Smarter, Not Harder," 29.

37. Lumsdon, "Working Smarter, Not Harder," 31.

38. Sheri Mycek, "Triage for Trouble Spots," *Hospitals & Health Networks* 72, no. 7 (1998): 40–41, 40.

39. Charlotte Huff, "Back-to-School Bonus," *Hospitals & Health Networks* 72, no. 20 (1998): 20.

40. For example, in March 1997, two investigators for the Texas Department of Insurance addressed an extremely damning report concerning the operations of Kaiser Foundation Health Plan of Texas to the state insurance commissioner. The report charged that Kaiser Texas failed to assure that health care services were provided in a manner that assured availability, accessibility and continuity of care; the HMO retroactively denied payment of emergency care services, has engaged in unfair settlement practices, and operated in contravention of its basic organizational documents and its health care plan. Texas Department of Insurance, *Report Concerning Kaiser Foundation Health Plan of Texas, Inc.*, by Olga Escobedo and Nancy Barbour (Austin, 1997), 1. The report details incidents of the following: refusals to pay for emergency room visits even when patients had been directed to the ER by Kaiser nurses, poor patient care, sloppy record-keeping, and failures in peer review and credentialing and the processing and investigation of quality of care complaints.

Dr. Bill Gillespie, the president of Kaiser Texas, disputed the charges, suggesting that the HMO made mistakes in the area of regulator-relations, not patient care. Kaiser agreed to pay a $1 million fine, infuse $80 million into its Texas operations, and take steps to improve patient care. Terrence Stutz, "Scathing State Report on Kaiser Made Public," *Dallas Morning News*, 23 April 1997, Sec. A, 1; Kathy Walt, "State Report Rips Health Care Giant," *Houston Chronicle*, 23 April 1997, Sec. A, 1. Kaiser has since sold its Texas operations.

41. Both cases that generated lawsuits against Kaiser's Georgia operations: the Adams case, described below, and *Janis O. Cummins et al. v. Kaiser Foundation Health Plan of Georgia Inc.*, pending in Georgia state court, described in George Anders, *Health against Wealth: HMOs and the Breakdown of Medical Trust* (New York: Houghton Mifflin, 1996), 140–41.

42. Anders, *Health against Wealth*, 133. (Citing Laurence C. Baker and Linda

Schuurman Baker, "Excess Cost of Emergency Department Visits for Nonurgent Care," *Health Affairs* 13, no. 5 (1994): 162–71.)

43. According to Anders, a Kaiser Permanente plan in California defines a covered emergency as "'medically necessary health services for unforeseen illnesses or injuries that require immediate medical attention as determined by Health Plan.'" Anders, *Health against Wealth*, 137.

44. The case resulted in a lawsuit and a $45 million damage award, $5 million to the parents and $40 million to the child. *Adams et al. v. Kaiser Foundation Health Plan of Georgia*, Case #93-VS-79895-E (Fulton County Court February 2, 1995). In April of 1995 the lawsuit was settled for an undisclosed amount. The case is discussed in Anders, *Health against Wealth*, 1–15.

45. *Engalla v. Permanente Medical Group*, No. 5048811 (Cal. June 30, 1997).

46. At that point, the Engallas went to court. When an ERISA preemption maneuver failed, Kaiser responded with a petition to compel arbitration; on that issue the case reached the California Supreme Court. The Court stated that petitions to compel arbitration are not granted when there are grounds such as fraud for rescinding the arbitration agreement. It found evidence to support a claim of fraudulent inducement in the record. In 1998, Kaiser terminated its existing arbitration system and hired a civil rights attorney to assemble a panel of arbitrators to handle claims.

47. Louise Kertesz, "Kaiser Physicians Unhappy with Changes, Memo Shows," *Modern Healthcare*, 19 February 1996, 12.

48. David R. Olmos, "Kaiser Told to Reveal Data on Patient Care," *Los Angeles Times*, 29 October 1997, D2. For more on the labor dispute, see Ilana DeBare, "Kaiser Nurses Buck the System," *San Francisco Chronicle*, 31 October 1997, B1. The rhetorical battle reflected a total breakdown in trust, with Kaiser nurses presenting themselves as protectors of quality of care and Kaiser administrators pointing to wages and benefits as the real issue. The dispute was settled in 1998, but implementation of an innovative "quality care liaison" program has been complicated by a climate of mutual distrust. Steve Ginsberg, "New Nursing Program Fails to Heal Rift at Kaiser," *San Francisco Business Times*, 14 July 2000, 21. Kaiser's relations with other unions have been friendlier. On November 9, 1999, Kaiser and the AFL-CIO announced an employment and job security agreement touted as the first of its kind in health care. On the occasion, John J. Sweeney, president of the AFL-CIO, told reporters the agreement insures that workers will be "'redeployed rather than laid off as a result of restructuring or other changes" and will "participate fully in joint problem-solving and planning without worrying that decisions we make will cause our members to forfeit employment or suffer cuts in pay." Lawrence talked about Kaiser's commitment to "attracting and retaining committed employees and making the best possible use of their knowledge" as "the key to meeting the challenges of the future in health care." "Collective Bargaining: Kaiser Permanente, Eight Unions Agree on Employment, Income Security for 60,000," *BNA's Health Care Daily Report*, 10 November 1999, 7.

49. David Mechanic and Mark Schlesinger, "The Impact of Managed Care on Patients' Trust in Medical Care and Their Physicians," *JAMA* 275 (1996): 1693–97, 1695.

50. Stutz, "Scathing Report Made Public," 9A; Walt, "State Report Rips Health Care Giant," 1A. Other embarrassments include a $1 million fine in connection with the death of a patient in 1996, a lawsuit charging that a policy applicable to Kaiser's Southern California operations permitted (or required) physicians to prescribe medications for patients they had never examined, and a lawsuit contending that many of Kaiser's

California facilities fail to meet the accessibility requirements of the Americans with Disabilities Act. See Julie Marquis, "Kaiser Fined $1 Million in Patient's Death," *Los Angeles Times*, 16 May 2000, A1; "Kaiser Drops San Diego Prescribing Practice in Response to Physician's Lawsuit," *BNA's Health Care Daily Report*, 9 May 2000, 13; John M. Glionna, "Suit Faults Kaiser's Care for Disabled," *Los Angeles Times*, 27 July 2000, A3.

51. See note 40 above for a list of some of the criticisms.

52. Researchers have suggested that physicians use natural anchoring bias to help patients understand medical risks by relating medical risks to known everyday nonmedical risks. Stanley T. Bogardus, Jr., Eric Holmboe, and James F. Jekel, "Perils, Pitfalls, and Possibilities in Talking about Medical Risk," *JAMA* 281 (1999): 1037–41, 1041. Similar strategies might be explored in the area of risk evaluation as an aspect of guideline development.

53. I owe these two Niebuhrean insights to Professor Elizabeth Heitman of the University of Texas School of Public Health.

54. Anders, *Health against Wealth*, 15, 37.

55. Per Leonard Abramson, the founder of U.S. Healthcare (now part of Aetna), "It doesn't count if you can't count it." Anders, *Health against Wealth*, 38.

56. Louise Kertesz, "Kaiser Ads: We're Not Like the Other HMOs," *Modern Healthcare*, 19 February 1996, 12.

57. Brown, *Politics*, 124.

58. E.g., "Kaiser management has benefited from its stubborn unwillingness to open its board of directors to elements that might paralyze or bully management. Whereas GHA [Group Health Association of Washington, D.C.] has always been constrained by the internal democratic norms of the consumer cooperative movement, norms that favor dominance of the organization by small bands of atypically interested and active elites with ideologies and axes of their own to grind, and HIP [Health Insurance Plan of Greater New York] by the 'interest group liberalism' incorporated in its board, the Kaiser program has been above all a business enterprise." "Few dispassionate students of the evolution of GHA and HIP will be inclined to deny that, unprogressive though it may seem, the Kaiser position, that an HMO should be run as a business and managed by men skilled and trained at management, has served the plan and its members well." Brown, *Politics*, 123–24. For more on the general issue, see Chapter 5, note 80 and accompanying text.

59. "[Our style of practicing] doesn't fit everyone. I don't think any one system is ever going to fit every patient." Weiner, "Permanente," 115.

5. THE MARKET, PROFESSIONALISM, AND COOPERATIVE EGALITARIANISM IN HEALTH CARE

1. For a complementary exercise in mapping health care with reference to three models of accountability (the professional, the economic, and the political), see Ezekial J. Emanuel and Linda L. Emanuel, "Preserving Community in Health Care," *Journal of Health Politics, Policy and Law* 22, no. 1 (1997): 147–84. Emanuel and Emanuel favor a hybrid "stratified" model in which the physician-patient relationship is governed by the professional model, the internal operations of managed care organizations are governed by the political model, and external relations are governed by the economic and political models.

2. For example, early capitalists used the law to ensure a ready supply of "free"

labor. Marx notes that "down to 1815, the emigration of mechanics employed in machine making was, in England, forbidden, under grievous pains and penalties." When, as a consequence of civil war in the United States, a majority of the workers in the Lancashire cotton industry lost their jobs, proposals were made for government support or voluntary contributions to enable the workers to emigrate, but the capitalists were not about to permit others to aid in the depletion of their reserve of workers desperate for employment. Karl Marx, *Capital*, vol. II, ch. 23 (London: Swan, Sonnenschein, Lowrey & Co., 1887), 586–88.

3. Bradford H. Gray, *The Profit Motive and Patient Care* (Cambridge, Mass.: Harvard University Press, 1991), 33, 37, 48–49.

4. See Christopher D. Stone, "Corporate Accountability in Law and Morals," in *The Judeo-Christian Vision and the Modern Corporation*, ed. Oliver F. Williams and John W. Houck (Notre Dame, Ind.: University of Notre Dame Press, 1982), 264–91. For a concrete example linking short-term profit maximization to large-scale financial failure and inefficiency, turn to Chapter 3, note 102.

5. We may pause to ask why the profit motive, and its twin, self-interest, have struck so many as appealing explanations of human conduct. On the face of it, these do not reveal a particularly engaging view of human nature. The attractions include the promise of a containment of forces, calculability, and even harmony. See Albert O. Hirschman, *The Passions and the Interests: Political Arguments for Capitalism before Its Triumph*. (Princeton, N.J.: Princeton University Press, 1977).

6. Charles W. Anderson, *Pragmatic Liberalism* (Chicago: University of Chicago Press, 1990), 26.

7. Jeffrey Stout, *Ethics after Babel: The Languages of Morals and Their Discontents* (Boston: Beacon Press, 1988), 281–82. The Advisory Commission on Consumer Protection and Quality in the Health Care Industry appointed by President Clinton endorsed the following "Statement of Purpose" for the United States health care system: "The purpose of the health care system must be to continuously reduce the impact and burden of illness, injury and disability, and to improve the health and functioning of the people of the United States." This is translated into a number of aim statements, including reducing the underlying causes of illness, injury, and disability, expanding research on treatments and effectiveness, assuring appropriate use of services, reducing errors, addressing areas of over- and undersupply, and increasing patients' participation in their care. Advisory Commission on Consumer Protection and Quality in the Health Care Industry, *Quality First: Better Health Care for All Americans* (Washington, D.C.: U.S. Government Printing Office, 1998).

8. Anderson, *Pragmatic Liberalism*, 27.

9. Bradford Gray notes that an AMA survey found that physicians practicing in for-profit hospitals were two-to-four times more likely to report that the hospital had policies meant to "discourage admissions" of uninsured, Medicare, or Medicaid patients. Gray, *Profit Motive*, 105–6. On the question of price competition or allocative efficiency: "Research on the theoretically interesting question of whether for-profits are indeed more efficient than nonprofits has produced answers that range from equivocal to negative. Research making the more practical comparison of the direct cost to purchasers of care shows clearly that it has cost more to buy hospital services from for-profit hospitals than from nonprofit hospitals." Gray, *Profit Motive*, 92.

10. David U. Himmelstein, Steffie Woolhandler, Ida Hellander, and Sidney M. Wolfe, "Quality of Care in Investor-Owned vs Not-for-Profit HMOs," *JAMA* 282 (1999): 159–

63; Elaine M. Silverman, Jonathan S. Skinner, and Elliott S. Fisher, "The Association Between For-Profit Hospital Ownership and Increased Medicare Spending," *New England Journal of Medicine* 341 (1999): 420–26. Significantly, the quality of care study found the greatest discrepancy on the two indicators most relevant to patients with serious medical illness: beta-blocker prescription filled for patients discharged after a myocardial infarction with no evidence of contraindication, and patients with diabetes who are receiving insulin or oral hypoglycemic agent and who had an eye examination in the past year. In a third study, the researchers found that for-profit dialysis facilities in the U.S. have higher mortality rates and lower rates of listing for renal transplantation than not-for-profit facilities. Pushkal P. Garg, Kevin D. Frick, Marie Diener-West, and Neil R. Powe, "Effects of the Ownership of Dialysis Facilities on Patients' Survival and Referral for Transplantation," *New England Journal of Medicine* 341 (1999): 1653–60.

11. Jeffrey Pfeffer, "Six Dangerous Myths about Pay," *Harvard Business Review* 76, no. 3 (1998): 109–19, 112. Pfeffer notes that incomplete theories can appear more powerful than they really are because they shape the behavior they purport to explain. For example: "If we believe people will work hard only if specifically rewarded for doing so, we will provide contingent rewards and thereby condition people to work only when they are rewarded. If we expect people to be untrustworthy, we will closely monitor and control them and by doing so will signal that they can't be trusted—an expectation that they will most likely confirm for us." Ibid., 113.

12. Ibid., 119.

13. Reinhold Niebuhr, "The Christian Faith and the Economic Life of Liberal Society," in *Faith and Politics,* ed. Ronald H. Stone (New York: George Braziller, 1968), 139–64, 140.

14. See Hirschman, *The Passions and the Interests,* note 5 above.

15. This is not simply because health care is a complex good, but because health care is more like a can of tuna than a dress. I can look at a dress and even try it on before I buy it. I can only learn how good the tuna is by consuming it. So a seller of tuna could conceivably put a low quality product in an attractive package and do quite well—for a time. To the extent that the seller desired repeat business, however, there would be an incentive not to pull this kind of trick. The problem in the health care case is that a failure on one occasion may be sufficient to end the consumer's life.

More generally, the losses patients experience while the system works itself out may be intolerable. Such losses would include not only the physical and emotional toll on specific patients and their families, but also a potentially irremediable loss of social trust. On the distinction between "search" qualities and "experience" qualities, see Edward R. Trubac, "Economic Guidelines for Corporate Decision-Making," *Judeo-Christian Vision,* 33–54 at 40. David Mechanic cites Kenneth Arrow's work in making the same point. David Mechanic, "Trust and Informed Consent to Rationing," *Milbank Quarterly* 72, no. 2 (1994): 217–223.

16. Mark Schlesinger, "Countervailing Agency: A Strategy of Principaled Regulation under Managed Competition," *Milbank Quarterly* 75, no. 1 (1997): 35–87, 44–46.

17. James Boyd White, "How Should We Talk about Corporations? The Languages of Economics and Citizenship," *Yale Law Journal* 94 (1985): 1416–25, 1424, 1418.

18. Philip Selznick, *The Moral Commonwealth: Social Theory and the Promise of Community* (Berkeley: University of California Press, 1992), 280.

19. Reinhardt is something of a contrarian on this point, since he credits bureau-

crats, and government bureaucrats no less, with introducing several innovations in health care administration that have been taken up by the private sector. Uwe E. Reinhardt, "A Social Contract for 21st Century Health Care: Three-Tier Health Care with Bounty Hunting," *Health Economics* 5 (1996): 479–99, 496.

20. In what may be the ultimate technocratic verdict on the utility of bureaucratic hierarchy, Richard Scott and a colleague conclude that "formal hierarchies aid the performance of tasks requiring the efficient coordination of information and routine decision making, but they interfere with tasks presenting very complex or ambiguous problems." Richard Scott, *Organizations: Rational, Natural, and Open Systems*, 3rd ed. (Englewood Cliffs, N.J.: Prentice-Hall, 1992), 161.

21. On "patrimonial bureaucracy," see Robert Jackall, *Moral Mazes: The World of Corporate Managers* (New York: Oxford University Press, 1988), 11–12.

22. Selznick, *Moral Commonwealth*, 285–86.

23. Mitchell T. Rabkin, "The Hospital-Academic Health Center Interface: The Community of Practice and the Community of Learning," in *Integrity in Health Care Institutions*, ed. Ruth Ellen Bulger and Stanley Joel Reiser (Iowa City: University of Iowa Press, 1990), 130–40, 137–38. See also Mitchell T. Rabkin and Laura Avakian, "Participatory Management at Boston's Beth Israel Hospital," *Academic Medicine* 67, no. 5 (1992): 289–294.

A post-bureaucratic managed care organization would restore much discretion to physicians, but some reform of the hierarchical structures which have long been a part of medicine would also be required. "Hierarchical structures" denotes physician dominance over nurses, specialist dominance over primary care physicians, the strict observance of a chain of command to the detriment of patient care, and, in some settings, a concern with pecking order that may strike other professionals as absurd. It is interesting to note that some business authors have linked the new organizational styles to the principle of subsidiarity. See Charles Handy, "Balancing Corporate Power: A New Federalist Paper," *Harvard Business Review* 70, no. 6 (1992): 59–72; Thomas W. Malone, "Is Empowerment Just a Fad? Control, Decision Making, and IT," *Sloan Management Review* 38, no. 2 (1997): 23–35.

24. Ruth Macklin offers a most distressing example in *Mortal Choices* (New York: Pantheon Books, 1987), 163–64.

25. Paul Wallich, "Not So Blind After All: Randomized Trials—the Linchpin of Medicine—May Often Be Rigged," *Scientific American* 274 (May 1996): 20–22.

26. Eliot Freidson, *Medical Work in America* (New Haven: Yale University Press, 1989), 71.

27. Freidson, *Medical Work*, 73 (emphasis added).

28. David Mechanic, another eminent sociologist, makes the connection between the distancing effects of bureaucratic control and a vicious cycle of manipulation: "Administrative authority frequently becomes insensitive to the human dilemmas and variabilities so obvious at the clinical level. Physicians and patients seek to manipulate and evade rules they view as irrational, and often such adaptive responses bring about subterfuge, perverse outcomes, and inequities in distribution." David Mechanic, "Rationing of Medical Care and the Preservation of Clinical Judgment," *Journal of Family Practice* 11 (1980): 431–33, 432.

29. On gaming the system, see E. Haavi Morreim, *Balancing Act: The New Medical Ethics of Medicine's New Economics* (Dordrecht: Kluwer Academic Publishers, 1991), 71–87.

30. Freidson, *Medical Work*, 246. In good pragmatic fashion, William Sullivan writes that "if the experiential context of life rewards cooperation and trust, the individual will come to accept these attitudes as normal and rational responses to reality. If, on the other hand, experience validates a social context of distrust and threat, defensive self-interest will come to seem to such persons the obviously reasonable stance toward life." William M. Sullivan, *Work and Integrity: The Crisis and Promise of Professionalism in America* (New York: HarperCollins, 1995), 205.

31. Eliot Freidson, *Professionalism Reborn* (Chicago: University of Chicago Press, 1994), 186.

32. Steven Miles describes a particularly egregious example: "Recently surgeons told a colleague of mine that they never withdrew futile or unwanted life-support within thirty days of cardiac transplantation in order to defer deaths beyond the peri-operative period so as to not adversely affect their eligibility for Medicare reimbursement." Steven H. Miles, "New Business for Ethics Committees," *H.E.C. Forum* 4, no. 2 (1992): 97–102, 98.

33. Administrators tended to ignore the fact that "[m]any factors, even the inclination to rationally calculate economic self-interest, are variables rather than constants, so that if they change so will the aggregate results." Freidson, *Medical Work*, 6.

34. Freidson, *Medical Work*, 196 (emphasis added). Bradford Gray gives many examples of what he calls the logic of distrust and its malign consequences. As a researcher involved in a number of physician surveys, he reports that many physicians "express scorn for UMOs [utilization management organizations], because it is so easy to manipulate them by telling them something that is clinically significant but difficult to verify from afar." Gray, *Profit Motive*, 310. Unfortunately, because some UMOs rely on retrospective reviews for verification, erroneous information may be entered into the patient's permanent medical record, with possible effects on subsequent care or insurability. Further, suspecting manipulation, UMOs have begun to request additional documentation such as copies of lab reports and x-rays, increasing the paperwork burden that so frustrates physicians. The same logic may extend to relations between providers and payers. Gray writes that third-party payment "has become a cops-and-robbers game in which the individuals and organizations that provide health services probe for weaknesses and gaps in payment and monitoring systems, and payers strive to catch up." Gray, *Profit Motive*, 330.

35. If another example of subversion is necessary, Bradford Gray describes how a rule change to discourage referrals for unnecessary testing was followed by an increase in physician office testing, with the additional unfortunate consequence that routine quality assurance monitoring became much more difficult. Gray, *Profit Motive*, 201.

36. For example: "The director of a public tuberculosis hospital was instructed to improve efficiency by following a plan of management by quantitative objectives. The director was instructed to define the hospital's objective, develop a measurable index of success in attaining that objective, and to evaluate all activities and personnel in terms of their measured contribution to that goal. Stating the goal was easy: restoring TB patients to health. A measurable index of success was more difficult, but not impossible. TB victims cough a lot. As they get better they cough less. Little microphones were placed by each pillow to record the coughs of each patient. Soon the staff and even the patients realized the significance of those tiny microphones. The frequency of coughing fell dramatically as prescriptions of valium and codeine increased. Relaxed patients cough less. Patients who cough less must be getting healthier, right? Wrong. They were

getting worse, precisely because they were not coughing and spitting out the congestion. The cough index was abandoned."

Herman E. Daly and John B. Cobb, *For the Common Good* (Boston: Beacon Press, 1989), 148–49.

37. Freidson, *Medical Work*, 245–46.

38. Robert Kuttner, "The Corporation in America: Is It Socially Redeemable?" *Dissent* 40, no. 1 (1993): 35–49, 42–43.

39. "[T]he greater the number of plans, the less likely it is that any one plan will consider itself responsible for the broader health needs of the community." Mark Schlesinger, "Paradigms Lost: The Persisting Search for Community in U.S. Health Policy," *Journal of Health Politics, Policy and Law* 22, no. 4 (1997): 937–92, 955. Unfortunately, Schlesinger's monopolist is the kind of corporate Goliath economists like least. James Robinson argues that different types of organizational growth have different economic implications. Of the five types he reviews, he argues that the case of horizontal integration within one market is the least important, but also the strongest candidate for regulation. James C. Robinson, "The Dynamics and Limits of Corporate Growth in Health Care," *Health Affairs* 15, no. 2 (1996): 155–69.

40. Leading to the term "casino capitalism." Paul Hirst, *Associative Democracy: New Forms of Economic and Social Governance* (Amherst: University of Massachusetts Press, 1994), 143. On the trend toward consolidation in health care, see Victor R. Fuchs, "Managed Care and the Merger Mania," *JAMA* 277 (1997): 920–21. The reader is no doubt waiting for the concluding caution, the "on the other hand." The hazards posed by large organizations scarcely render smaller ones risk-free. Hirst cites the sweatshop as evidence that small enterprises can be as exploitative as large ones. Hirst, *Associative Democracy*, 128–29.

41. See Charles Perrow, *Complex Organizations: A Critical Essay*, 3rd ed. (New York: Random House, 1986), 47.

42. Donald A. Barr, "The Effects of Organizational Structure on Primary Care Outcomes under Managed Care," *Annals of Internal Medicine* 122 (1995): 353–59.

43. Robinson, "Dynamics," 165.

44. See Lawrence D. Brown, *Politics and Health Care Organization: HMOs as Federal Policy* (Washington, D.C.: The Brookings Institution, 1983), 76–78.

45. Freidson, *Medical Work*, 237.

46. In particular, Freidson found that the rules of etiquette blocked transmission of information about abusive behavior toward patients, negligence and fraud. Freidson, *Doctoring Together* (New York: Elsevier, 1975), 165.

47. Stephen M. Shortell, Robin R. Gillies, David A. Anderson, Karen Morgan Erickson, and John B. Mitchell, *Remaking Health Care in America: Building Organized Delivery Systems* (San Francisco: Jossey-Bass, 1996), 5–6. See also *To Err Is Human: Building a Safer Health System*, ed. Linda T. Kohn, Janet M. Corrigan, and Molla S. Donaldson (Washington, D.C.: National Academy Press, 2000); Lucien L. Leape, David D. Woods, Martin J. Hatlie, Kenneth W. Kizer, Steven A. Schroeder, and George D. Lundberg, "Promoting Patient Safety by Preventing Medical Error," *JAMA* 280 (1998): 1444–47; Lucian L. Leape, "Error in Medicine," *JAMA* 272 (1994): 1851–57.

48. Tawney, *Acquisitive Society*, 95. The Institute of Medicine (IOM) report on for-profit health care delivers the same message: "Ideals, even if imperfectly realized, may affect where the balance is struck, as may the way care is organized and paid for." In-

stitute of Medicine, introduction to *For-Profit Enterprise in Health Care*, ed. Bradford H. Gray (Washington, D.C.: National Academy Press, 1986), 14.

49. Tawney believed that industry, as well as the traditional professions, could provide good work. He saw no sharp line between industries such as footwear manufacturing or construction and professions such as teaching and medicine: "The work of making boots or building a house is in itself no more degrading than that of curing the sick or teaching the ignorant. It should be at least equally bound by rules which have as their object to maintain the standards of professional service. It should be at least equally free from the vulgar subordination of moral standards to financial interests." Tawney, *Acquisitive Society*, 96.

Some would object that one cannot have a professional without a client. I favor a more general definition of profession, in keeping with the concept of practice. For example, a professional can be defined as one who displays four attributes: "(1) training in a systematic body of knowledge ('professed' social knowledge); (2) dedication to values that will enhance the common good; (3) voluntary adherence to norms of practice established and enforced by colleagues; and (4) participation in a system of rewards, monetary and honorary, which acknowledge excellence in performance." Williams and Houck, *Judeo-Christian Vision*, 260. (Somewhat ironically, the more business takes Friedman's view of the manager as an agent for the stockholder as its ideal, the more nearly it satisfies the client-centered definition of profession.)

50. Some of the parallels between the two fields are striking: "In 1992, Sears, Roebuck & Company was inundated with complaints about its automotive service business. Consumers and attorneys general in more than 40 states had accused the company of misleading customers and selling them unnecessary parts and services. In the face of declining revenues, shrinking market share, and an increasingly competitive market . . . Sears management attempted to spur the performance of its auto centers by introducing new goals and incentives for employees. The company increased minimum work quotas and introduced productivity incentives for mechanics. The automotive service advisers were given product-specific sales quotas . . . and paid a commission based on sales. Under this new set of organizational pressures, with few options for meeting their sales goals legitimately, some employees' judgment understandably suffered. *Management's failure to clarify the line between unnecessary service and legitimate preventive maintenance, coupled with customer ignorance, left employees to chart their own courses through a vast gray area* . . . " Lynn Sharp Paine, "Managing for Organizational Integrity," *Harvard Business Review* 72 (March–April 1994): 106–17, 107–108 (emphasis added). My auto mechanic has a Code of Ethics posted on his wall.

51. In the areas of retail sales and literary production, practitioners might follow the example of the Hafetz Hayim, the keeper of a general store and author: "He refused to handle any merchandise except that which was fresh and perfect. He always added a little over the amount ordered and paid for by his customers to be sure that he had not failed to give them full measure. In order to avoid committing *hassagat gevul*—the sin of competing against his neighbors unfairly and depriving them of income that they needed and were entitled to—he closed his store early every day, so that some of the people who might have patronized his establishment would go to those of his competitors. And when his books were published, he personally checked the conditions of employment at the printing plant to be sure that the employees of the printer were treated justly and fairly—that they received proper wages, that the conditions of their employ-

ment were safe and healthful, and that they enjoyed all the fringe benefits to which they were entitled by the laws of the Torah." Burton M. Leiser, "The Rabbinic Tradition and Corporate Morality," in *Judeo-Christian Vision*, 141–58, 156.

MacIntyre believes much industrial and service work is organized to exclude the defining features of practices, owing to the moral deficiencies of modernity rather than business. John Dobson, "MacIntyre's Position on Business: A Response to Wicks," *Business Ethics Quarterly* 7, no. 4 (1997): 125–32. See also Kathryn Balstad Brewer, "Management as a Practice: A Response to Alasdair MacIntyre," *Journal of Business Ethics* 16, no. 8 (1997): 825–33; Robert C. Solomon, *Ethics and Excellence: Cooperation and Integrity in Business* (New York: Oxford University Press, 1992).

52. The professional organization for health care administrators, the American College of Healthcare Executives, has devoted considerable attention to ethics. American College of Healthcare Executives, *Code of Ethics* (Chicago: American College of Healthcare Executives, 1994) (including appendices), American College of Healthcare Executives, *Ethical Decision Making for Healthcare Executives* (Chicago: American College of Healthcare Executives, 1997) (policy statement).

53. Tawney, *Acquisitive Society*, 95–96.

54. Freidson, *Professionalism Reborn*, 176.

55. William M. Sullivan develops this theme in *Work and Integrity*. Sullivan's thesis is that "[t]he vital mission of professional work is to infuse economic activity with opportunities for individuals to develop themselves through contributing to public values." Sullivan, *Work*, 149. The public dimension means that issues of trust, equity, and civic cooperation, and not technical competence alone, should be objects of concern for professionals. For physicians this would mean training in mutual understanding and compromise, as well as history-taking and differential diagnosis and the mechanics of their particular specialty or subspecialty. For a clear-eyed review of lapses in medical professionalism antedating managed care, and a hard but simple set of principles for improving matters, see David J. Rothman, "Medical Professionalism: Focusing on the Real Issues," *New England Journal of Medicine* 342 (2000): 1284–86.

56. Chapter 2, note 33 and accompanying text. Whether for good or ill, there are also signs that occupational solidarity expressed as reluctance to question the conduct of colleagues may give way when there is money at stake. Physicians with a medical group that terminated its contract with Aetna U.S. Healthcare apparently cited Aetna's refusal to share claims information as the major source of dissatisfaction. According to newspaper accounts, the group was paid on a capitated basis and wanted the information to identify colleagues who were overusing expensive tests and drugs. See Phil Galewitz, "Doctor Defections from HMOs Grow," *AP Online*, 20 October 1998, accessible via the Westlaw ALLNEWS database at 1998 WL 21174068. For a short, trenchant essay on money and the professions, see William F. May, "Money and the Medical Profession," *Kennedy Institute of Ethics Journal* 7, no. 1 (1997): 1–13.

57. At a press briefing, Randolph D. Smoak Jr., chairman of the AMA's Board of Trustees, stated: "Our objective here is to give America's physicians the leverage they now lack to guarantee that patient care is not compromised or neglected for the sake of profits." Steven Greenhouse, "A.M.A.'s Delegates Vote to Unionize," *New York Times*, 24 June 1999, A1. The AMA has dubbed its new collective bargaining unit "Physicians for Responsible Negotiations."

58. See Michael M. Weinstein, "If Doctors Win Right to Organize, Patients Could Lose," *New York Times*, 8 July 1999, C2. Were the benefits to patients from an antitrust

exemption clearer, a boycott exploiting physicians' power to prescribe might have been easier to take. According to the *New York Times*, hundreds of doctors stopped writing prescriptions for drugs manufactured by Merck & Company in order to pressure Merck into ending its anti-antitrust-exemption lobbying efforts. Robert Pear, "Doctors in Antitrust Fight Boycotting Merck Products," *New York Times*, 23 May 2000, A23. While boycott organizers said no patient would be harmed because substitutes are available, it is not unheard of for patients to have different responses to different drugs in the same therapeutic class. Indeed, physicians have vociferously objected to drug substitution policies and formulary changes that force them to switch a patient from one drug to another, policies and changes managed care organizations defend with claims of therapeutic equivalence.

59. I was very struck by the following passage from a report on a managed care summit convened by the United States Chamber of Commerce and the AMA: "Leaders from business and doctor groups deeply divided over proposals to regulate HMOs found little to agree on after spending part of the week together at a Florida resort. . . . The only major players missing from the meeting were consumer advocates, though the AMA said it was speaking on behalf of patients." Laura Meckler, "AMA, Chamber Discuss HMO Rules," *AP Online*, 18 February 1999, accessible via the Westlaw ALLNEWS database at 1999 WL 12931242.

60. E.g., Ruth Macklin, *Enemies of Patients* (New York: Oxford University Press, 1993); George Annas, "A National Bill of Patients' Rights," *New England Journal of Medicine* 338 (1998): 695–99.

61. For example, some physicians and some members of the general public consider the self-inflicted nature of an illness relevant to allocation decisions, but this view is much more pronounced among physicians. Einer Elhauge, *Allocating Health Care Morally*, 82 Calif. L. Rev. 1449, 1524 (1994). A related concern is that physicians have or will tend to adopt a utilitarian approach to justice, setting priorities in terms of cost-effectiveness, cost-benefit, or some understanding of efficiency. In my own contact with physicians, I have not found any general commitment to utilitarianism, and indeed the traditional ethic with its focus on the needs of the presenting patient seems to work against it. Studies of physician behavior when intensive care units are crowded reveal that doctors use reasonable rationing criteria, screening out less serious cases.

In a different kind of study, physicians presented with hypothetical resource allocation problems favored the efficient (health-maximizing) use of scarce resources, but deviated from strictly utilitarian criteria in response to concerns over equity. Hall, *Medical Spending Decisions*, 121. Of course, this may be changing due to the increasing prominence of population-centered values. In any event, cost-effectiveness analysis does not rule out large expenditures to meet pressing needs. See, e.g., Tom L. Beauchamp and James F. Childress, *Principles of Biomedical Ethics*, 4th ed. (New York: Oxford University Press, 1994), 295–296.

Further, if one adopts the Rawlsian approach, it is hard to imagine rational contractors designing a health care system that is maximally inefficient in the sense that it pours massive resources into marginal improvements in the condition of persons with truly devastating impairments. So even a Rawlsian such as Daniels can find reason for some consideration of utility and efficiency. Indeed, "value for money," in terms of clinical efficacy, is one of the ten benchmarks of fairness promoted by Daniels and others. Norman Daniels, Donald W. Light, and Ronald L. Caplan, *Benchmarks of Fairness for Health Care Reform* (New York: Oxford University Press, 1996).

62. This is the central thesis of Carl E. Schneider, *The Practice of Autonomy: Patients, Doctors, and Medical Decisions* (New York: Oxford University Press, 1998). See also Mark A. Hall, *Making Medical Spending Decisions: The Law, Ethics, and Economics of Rationing Mechanisms* (New York: Oxford University Press, 1997), 37–38; Howard Brody, *The Healer's Power* (New Haven: Yale University Press, 1992), 89.

63. "Patients indeed get better because of specific cures worked through the application of medical science, and they get better because the natural history of the disease process tends toward spontaneous recovery, but they also get better, a good deal of the time, because of the symbolic aspects of the healing encounter and because the meaning of the experience of being ill has been rendered more positive and less frightening. This occurs, in turn, when the patient receives a satisfactory explanation of the illness, when those around him respond with care and support, and when he regains a sense of mastery or control over the illness [citation omitted]. A skilled healer can facilitate all these changes, but she can best do so if she has a fair amount of cultural, charismatic, and social power in addition to pure Aesculapian power." Brody, *Healer's Power*, 34.

64. Brody writes that some critics of physicians (particularly in the role of case manager) insist that "patients' rights and autonomy must be protected at all costs, even if it means that what could have been a humane and compassionate relationship is replaced by an adversarial and bureaucratic one." "The goal of medical ethics is seen as defanging the powerful physician, even if he then is not the sort of person from whom we wish to seek help when we are ill." Brody, *Healer's Power*, 201.

65. Hall, *Medical Spending Decisions*, 150.

66. See Chapter 6, notes 38–42 and accompanying text.

67. Hall reviews the results of three surveys. The content of the surveys varied, but the consistent results were high rankings for family doctors or panels of medical professionals as rationing agents (with one survey also finding strong support for decision making about coverage by a committee of patients), and extremely low rankings for bureaucrats (government officials, judges, insurers and employers) as rationing agents. Hall, *Medical Spending Decisions*, 65. Curiously, none of these surveys seems to have offered respondents the option of cooperative decision making by a panel of health care professionals and laypeople.

68. Another physician, Howard Brody, argues: "The challenge for physicians (and other experts) is to find ways to make their patients feel genuinely more powerful to control their own lives and health; to be more aware of the actual ends of their social and cultural power, not only the ends that bear the most benign interpretation; and to be willing to accept responsibility for the use of power with a realistic understanding of all its facets." Brody, *Healer's Power*, 229.

69. E.g., Freidson, *Professionalism Reborn*, 124. Freidson favors the "analytical" model of professionalism, which is cool not only toward medicine's traditional claims to moral superiority, but toward moral language in general. For a provocative analysis of the relation between the social sciences and morality, see Alan Wolfe, *Whose Keeper? Social Science and Moral Obligation* (Berkeley, Calif.: University of California Press, 1989).

70. I do not think the following observation by Freidson, which strikes me as very shrewd, undermines my argument: "[The ideology of professionalism] may also be used to motivate workers in the *absence* of occupational control over work. Indeed,

those working under the direction of professionals may very well manifest greater de-votion to serving others than do professionals themselves." Freidson, *Professionalism Reborn*, 124. My impression is that nurses have a better claim than physicians to moral heroism. No doubt there are certain psychological compensations for the nurse-heroes, given that they lack the satisfactions associated with controlling their work; no doubt it has suited others to have nurses dedicating themselves to an ideal of service and de-manding little in the way of pay or power. What I mean to deny is that power games and psychological mechanisms explain (away) the use of moral language, and contests over values, without remainder.

71. See, e.g., Jackall, *Moral Mazes*.

72. Daniel F. Chambliss, *Beyond Caring: Hospitals, Nurses, and the Social Organiza-tion of Ethics* (Chicago: University of Chicago Press, 1996). Andrew Jameton has also called attention to the neglect of power and organization in mainstream medical ethics. Andrew Jameton, "Dilemmas of Moral Distress: Moral Responsibility and Nursing Practice," *AWHONNS Clinical Issues in Perinatal and Women's Health Nursing* 4, no. 4 (1993): 542–51. Jameton says he has chosen to study the situation of nurses because, in most areas of life, most of us are similarly situated—we are neither omnipotent nor entirely powerless. The paradigm questions for nursing ethics include the scope of one's responsibility (especially in the face of others' failures to meet their obligations), the extent of the personal risks to be taken on behalf of patients (career risks as well as health risks), and assessment of moral complicity.

73. Several case studies of whistle-blowing by nurses (in Australia) are presented in Debra Jackson and Maree Raftos, "In Uncharted Waters: Confronting the Culture of Silence in a Residential Care Institution," *International Journal of Nursing Practice* 3, no. 1 (1997): 34–39. The nurses interviewed, relative newcomers to the institution, first went to management expecting that the abuses they reported would appall administra-tors and lead to swift corrective action. They were quickly disabused of this notion. The organization was oriented to satisfying the paperwork requirements of payers rather than the actual care needs of patients/residents. The nurses were also ostracized by colleagues, who had, after all, been complicit in the substandard care for years. Rosamond Rhodes and James Strain use the case of a senior physician who combines clinical brilliance with a total want of humanity to anchor their account of whistleblow-ing. Rosamond Rhodes and James J. Strain, "Trust and Transforming Medical Institu-tions," *Cambridge Quarterly of Healthcare Ethics* 9, no. 2 (2000): 205–17.

74. William F. May, "Code, Covenant, Contract, or Philanthropy?" *Hastings Center Report* 5, no. 6 (1975): 29–38; William F. May, *The Physician's Covenant: Images of the Healer in Medical Ethics* (Philadelphia: Westminster Press, 1983).

75. In this respect, David Mechanic may be a better guide than Freidson, for Me-chanic has devoted a great deal of thought and attention to trust. E.g., David Mechanic and Mark Schlesinger, "The Impact of Managed Care on Patient's Trust in Medical Care and Their Physicians," *JAMA* 275 (1996): 1693–1697; David Mechanic, "Managed Care as a Target of Distrust," *JAMA* 277 (1997): 1810–11. His concern with trust influences Mechanic's advice to managed care organizations: "In the longer range, man-aged care can better gain public legitimacy by building the kind of collaboration with physicians that allows patients' trust in their physicians to generalize to the plan." Me-chanic, "Managed Care," 1811.

76. "It is organization which gives birth to the domination of the elected over the

236

Notes to Pages 128–129

electors, of the mandatories over the mandators, of the delegates over the delegators. Who says organization says oligarchy." Robert Michels, *Political Parties* (Glencoe, Ill.: Free Press, 1949), 401.

77. See Benjamin R. Barber, *Strong Democracy: Participatory Politics for a New Age* (Berkeley: University of California Press, 1984).

78. Selznick, *Moral Commonwealth*, 247.

79. See Chapter 4, note 58 and accompanying text.

80. I am raising what Alan Ryan, in his writing on Dewey, labels the "central puzzle" of participatory democracy—what does it look like? "Dewey did not suppose that the American public was longing for a world in which the average worker would come home from work at six in the evening, grab a sandwich, and rush off to a town meeting to decide whether his block should purchase its electricity from Con Edison or brew its own. Oscar Wilde had complained that socialism was all very well but would eat rather painfully into one's evenings, and Dewey was not so attached to head-in-the-air abstraction that he could not see the point. But what is it to be like? Every clear answer is a negative answer." Alan Ryan, *John Dewey and the High Tide of American Liberalism* (New York: W. W. Norton & Company, 1995), 311. Although I admire Ezekiel Emanuel's work, I think Emanuel, like his mentor, Michael Sandel, envisions a world in which working men and women attend a lot of evening meetings.

The work of Michael Walzer has strongly influenced my views. In a short piece on civil society, Walzer looks at four common answers to the question of the good life. The first, the "left" political, holds that the preferred setting for the good life is the political community, and "[i]f politics is our highest calling, then we are called away from every other activity (or, every other activity is redefined in political terms)." But, says Walzer, the political ideology is not "real," as the rule of the *demos* is in significant ways illusory, and "despite the singlemindedness of republican ideology, politics rarely engages the full attention of the citizens who are supposed to be its chief protagonists."

Ordinary folk must worry about earning a living. Further, although republican theorists tend to disdain non-political activity, a more generous—and less aristocratic—view will allow that work, family, etc. have their own value. The other three answers to the question of the good life are the Marxist, capitalist, and nationalist. Walzer favors a fifth option, "civil society," which is "part alternative, part incorporation" of the others. Civil society is less . . . political than the political conception of the good life seems to allow: "A democratic civil society is one controlled by its members, not through a single process of self-determination, but through a large number of different and uncoordinated processes." Such a society is not relentlessly democratic (in the political sense), "for we are likely to be members of many associations and we will want some of them to be managed in our interests, but also in our absence." Michael Walzer, "The Idea of Civil Society," *Dissent* 38 (1991): 293–304, 294–95.

81. Barber, *Strong Democracy*, 272. This would also be the response to Mark Hall's concern that lay people may not want responsibility for making significant decisions affecting their care. Although there are good reasons for skepticism concerning universal participation in governance, we must also factor in the effects of a culture that tends to disable people for roles other than that of consumer.

Hall's other reservations concerning democratic processes of decision-making mostly relate to the stance that whatever emerges from "democratic" processes is definitive of what is moral, i.e., not subject to moral criticism, a stance not defended here. Hall, *Medical Spending Decisions*, 91–101. Hall also sees major practical problems with democratic rationing decisions *as an alternative* to bedside rationing: How detailed will the rules be? What of the general weaknesses of rules as moral guides?

Since I am arguing for more participation across the board as a goal, not a principle to be taken to its logical extreme regardless of other considerations, I can accept that there are limits to representative democracy as a mechanism for rationing decisions. For suggestions on how to improve community decisions programs and increase consumer voice in the direction of health care delivery, see Jack H. Nagel, *Combining Deliberation and Fair Representation in Community Health Decisions,* 140 University of Pennsylvania Law Review 1965, 1980–85 (1992); Leonard M. Fleck, *Just Health Care Rationing: A Democratic Decisionmaking Approach,* 140 University of Pennsylvania Law Review 1597 (1992); Jane Perkins, Kristi Olson, Lourdes Rivera, and Julie Skatrud, *Making the Consumers' Voice Heard in Medicaid Managed Care: Increasing Participation, Protection and Satisfaction* (Washington, D.C.: National Health Law Program, 1996); Kristi Olson and Jane Perkins, *Recommendations for Making the Consumers' Voice Heard in Medicaid Managed Care: A Guide to Effective Consumer Involvement* (Washington, D.C.: National Health Law Program, 1999); and California Health Decisions, *Partners in Healthcare: Consumer Input, Consumer Impact* (Orange, Calif.: California Health Decisions, 1999).

82. While we tend to think of participation in terms of participation qua policy maker in macro decision making, the possibilities are broader. Broadening our vision of participation is equivalent to (and related to) broadening our vision of democracy to include social democracy as well as political democracy. For a useful framework that classifies participation along three dimensions (decision making domain, role perspective, and level of participation), see Cathy Charles and Suzanne DeMaio, "Lay Participation in Health Care Decision Making: A Conceptual Framework," *Journal of Health Politics, Policy and Law* 18, no. 4 (1993): 881–904.

83. For example, as noted by Laurie Zoloth-Dorfman and Susan Rubin, the care which has been exercised in reforming Medicare, and the protections which have been established for Medicare recipients, contrast sharply with the haste in turning Medicaid beneficiaries over to managed care organizations—with any problems to be worked out later. They point to the existence of an effective lobbying organization for the elderly, the American Association of Retired Persons, as the crucial distinguishing factor. Laurie Zoloth-Dorfman and Susan Rubin, "The Patient as Commodity: Managed Care and the Question of Ethics," *Journal of Clinical Ethics* 6, no. 4 (1995): 339–57.

84. For more on these themes, see Arthur Brownlea, "Participation: Myths, Realities and Prognosis," *Social Science and Medicine* 25, no. 6 (1987): 605–14; John McKnight, *The Careless Society: Community and Its Counterfeits* (New York: Basic Books, 1995); John P. Kretzmann and John L. McKnight, *Building Communities from the Inside Out: A Path toward Finding and Mobilizing a Community's Assets* (Evanston, Ill.: Institute for Policy Research, 1993). Although the term "community empowerment" is trite from overuse, Brownlea correctly points out that "[p]articipation requires as much self-help as it does input into other people's systems," while McKnight develops the idea that communities possess assets as well as needs. For a short history of participation as an outgrowth of U.S. health policy, see John W. Hatch and Eugenia Eng, "Community Participation and Control: or Control of Community Participation," in Victor W. Sidel and Ruth Sidel, editors, *Reforming Medicine: Lessons of the Last Quarter Century* (New York: Pantheon Books, 1984), 223–44.

85. Einer Elhauge reaches a similar conclusion in his analysis of resource allocation in health care: "Efficiency—here understood as maximizing health improvements out

of a given set of resources—is thus not in 'tension' with equity as commonly thought. Rather, each different measure of efficiency or equity implies a given measure of its counterpart, and any choice of efficiency or equity is part and parcel of a single decision: what should our health priorities be?" Elhauge, *Allocating Health Care*, 82 Calif. L. Rev. 1449, 1513.

A more detailed argument, without particular reference to health care, is presented in Julian LeGrand, "Equity versus Efficiency: The Elusive Trade-Off," *Ethics* 100, no. 3 (1990): 554–568. LeGrand makes three points: (1) the concept of efficiency can refer to *value* or *production* and the two meanings must be kept distinct; (2) if efficiency refers to society's ability to attain its primary objectives, the notion of a trade-off between equity and efficiency is incoherent; and (3) even if efficiency is given a value meaning, economic growth, and made a primary objective, there are serious problems in describing what is being traded off against what.

86. Norman Daniels and James Sabin, "Limits to Health Care: Fair Procedures, Democratic Deliberation, and the Legitimacy Problem for Insurers," *Philosophy & Public Affairs* 26, no. 4 (1997): 303–50, 318–21. It is worth stressing that all important trade-offs do not fit neatly into the category of "efficiency (or utility) versus equity." Some choices are between different kinds of equity or equity at different points in time. For example, researchers gave three groups of subjects a choice between two scenarios. In the first, a crude but inexpensive screening test for colon cancer is offered to all people at low risk for the disease, preventing 1000 deaths. In the second, a better, more expensive test is offered to half the low risk people, randomly selected, preventing 1100 deaths. The second approach clearly wins in terms of efficiency, but it is also equitable viewed prospectively, since everyone in the low risk group has an equal chance of being selected for the test. On the other hand, the first approach treats everyone equally at the point of testing. Peter A. Ubel, Michael L. DeKay, Jonathan Baron, and David A. Asch, "Cost-Effectiveness Analysis in a Setting of Budget Constraints," *New England Journal of Medicine* 334 (1996): 1174–77.

87. Robert Veatch thinks utility and equity should be weighted nearly equally, and he makes an interesting proposal: "Given the wide range of intuitions about how to balance utility and equity, I suggest that the two be given equal moral status for purposes of health policy. That would mean that both utility and equity determinations have to be made in order to make an allocation decision. Once each determination has been made, they would have to be compared on some standardized scale. For example, one might strive to maximize the function: net utility divided by standard deviation." Robert M. Veatch, "Allocating Health Resources Ethically: New Roles for Administrators and Clinicians," *Frontiers of Health Services Management* 8, no. 1 (1991): 3–29, 17.

88. Veatch, "Allocating Health Resources," 18 (emphasis added).

89. Research suggests that most people can make sense of health plans that specify one or two parameters in their benefit provisions. As the number of parameters increases, comprehension falls off sharply. See M. Susan Marquis, "Consumers' Knowledge about Their Health Insurance Coverage," *Health Care Financing Review* 5 (1983): 65–80.

90. Rocky Mountain Center for Healthcare Ethics, *Code of Ethics for Managed Care in Colorado: Working Document* (Denver, Colo.: Rocky Mountain Center for Healthcare Ethics, 1997), 1. Information concerning the process derives from this document and from a presentation given by the Executive Director and Senior Consultant to the Rocky Mountain Center, Elizabeth M. Whitley and Gerard F. Heeley, "Values, Voices and Vi-

sion: A Code of Ethics for Managed Care," at the annual meeting of the American Association of Bioethics, the Society for Bioethics Consultation, and the Society for Health and Human Values, Baltimore, Md., November 6, 1997.

91. Rocky Mountain Center, *Code,* 7.

92. Issues raised during the question and answer period at the November 6 presentation. It may now be clear why I would partially agree with and partially dissent from the conclusions reached by Susan Dorr Goold in her analysis of "informed democratic decision making" as a process for making rationing decisions. Susan D. Goold, "Allocating Health Care: Cost-Utility Analysis, Informed Democratic Decision Making, or the Veil of Ignorance," *Journal of Health Politics, Policy and Law* 21, no. 1 (1996): 69–98. Goold rejects a "grass roots" model that relies on self-selection in favor of selected representation, because people cannot be relied upon to self-select in a manner that ensures the balanced representation of interest groups. I take her criticism (largely directed at Oregon) as correct, but I would argue that the problem should be addressed with at least two strategies.

First, follow the example of the Rocky Mountain Center and combine means of recruitment. This can be done so long as participation or membership is unrestricted. Second, break up power and policymaking. It may be best that some decisions be made by a board with restricted membership, and selected representation may be the best avenue for ensuring balance on this board. Nevertheless, the limitation on participation is an evil, and it should be mitigated by moving as many projects and policies as possible into more open forums or structures. As noted in Chapter 3, interest group-style representative democracy sits uneasily with social democracy. (Goold proposes selection of board members from among the representatives of established advocacy groups for the elderly, poor, disabled, etc. She views their close identification with the interests of defined constituencies as an advantage.) Reinhold Niebuhr would name it in two ways to register its ambiguous moral status: group selfishness, and the effective use of power against power by disenfranchised groups.

93. Norman Daniels and James Sabin, "Last Chance Therapies and Managed Care: Pluralism, Fair Procedures, and Legitimacy," *Hastings Center Report* 28, no. 2 (1998): 27–41, 32. Patient-centered concerns include giving proper attention to (urgent) patient needs, avoiding harms that can arise from adversarialism, and managing uncertainties and risks through collaborative treatment planning. Population-centered concerns include prudent use of shared resources (stewardship) and promotion of public goods such as knowledge about efficacy and safety. For other perspectives on resource allocation cases, see the cases and commentaries collected in *Ethical Challenges in Managed Care,* ed. Karen G. Gervais, Reinhard Priester, Dorothy E. Vawter, Kimberly K. Otte, and Mary M. Solberg (Washington, D.C.: Georgetown University Press, 1999).

94. As of March 1999, Group Health had 608,714 enrollees, 39,000 of whom were voting members. In order to apply for a voting membership, one must be at least 18 years old. There is no charge, but there is a commitment: "by becoming a voting member, you are stating that you understand, support, and will assist in the shaping and implementation of Group Health's mission, goals, and policies." See "About Group Health," www.ghc.org/about_gh/facts.html (visited September 8, 1999). For the history of Group Health, see Walt Crowley, *To Serve the Greatest Number* (Seattle: University of Washington Press, 1996).

95. Daniels and Sabin, "Limits to Health Care," 340–41. As Daniels and Sabin note, democratic deliberation is not tied to large, public votes, nor even to grassroots or town-

meeting democracy. In the tradition arising out of the work of Tocqueville and Dewey, democracy happens whenever and wherever people come together to work out their problems and celebrate their achievements on terms of moral equality. Of course, the ideal is still the health care cooperative in which democratic deliberation occurs at multiple levels and in multiple venues.

96. Daniels and Sabin, "Last Chance Therapies," 33–34. In fact, between 1994 and 1996, only six out of the 2.5 million members asked for an independent consultation. Ibid.

97. If the policy does nothing more than ensure consistency, it will be an advance over business as usual in the insurance industry. A study covering the period from 1989 to 1993 found significant heterogeneity between insurers in frequency of approvals. Further, many companies approved some requests but not others (the variability not being attributable to patients' clinical characteristics or the design of the protocol in which the patient was enrolled). The investigators concluded that "insurers do not generally make decisions related to coverage for complicated research therapies in a consistent or medically relevant manner." William P. Peters and Mark C. Rogers, "Variation in Approval by Insurance Companies of Coverage for Autologous Bone Marrow Transplantation for Breast Cancer," *New England Journal of Medicine* 330 (1994): 473–77.

98. As noted in Chapter 2, insurer willingness to fund HDC/ABMT for advanced breast cancer outside clinical trials—as a result of public relations concerns, threats of litigation, and legislation—is arguably a major factor discouraging women from enrolling in trials. And given that transplants are very lucrative, providers are scarcely disinterested judges of need. See Chapter 2, note 19.

99. Overwhelmingly negative accounts of the breast cancer research findings were soon followed by accounts emphasizing differing interpretation and division over clinical relevance. Contrast, for example, Joan Stephenson, "Bone Marrow/Stem Cells: No Edge in Breast Cancer," *JAMA* 281 (1999): 1576–78 and Joan Stephenson, "Opinions Divided on High-Dose Chemotherapy for Breast Cancer," *JAMA* 282 (1999): 119. (On the tendency to believe more must be better, and the tendency to reject data at odds with this belief, see Elliot S. Fisher and H. Gilbert Welch, "Avoiding the Unintended Consequences of Growth in Medical Care: How Might More Be Worse?" *JAMA* 281 (1999): 446–53.) Attended by less media fanfare have been advances in the underlying technology. See, e.g., Daniel Q. Haney, "Drug Helps Bone Marrow Transplants," *AP Online*, 3 June 1999, accessible via the Westlaw ALLNEWS database at 1999 WL 17810099.

For an insightful analysis of the social construction of the debate over HDC/ABMT at earlier stages, see Susan E. Kelly and Barbara A. Koenig, "'Rescue' Technologies following High-Dose Chemotherapy for Breast Cancer: How Social Context Shapes the Assessment of Innovative, Aggressive, and Lifesaving Medical Technologies," in Philip J. Boyle, ed., *Getting Doctors to Listen: Ethics and Outcomes Data in Context* (Washington, D.C.: Georgetown University Press, 1998), 127–52. Among other things, Kelly and Koenig discuss the factors that led to the rapid dissemination of HDC/ABMT, and they hone in on Western individualism, differences between transplant specialists and medical oncologists, and uncertainty and responses to it as key aspects of the problem of HDC/ABMT for breast cancer. They also note that naturalism set up an expectation that findings from clinical trials, then only beginning, would end uncertainty—an expectation doomed to disappointment.

100. Andrew Jameton argues that "[t]he medical and nursing roles are divided in a

way that is inefficient, morally problematic, and ultimately burdensome to those who must play its parts." Jameton, "Dilemmas of Moral Distress," 549. Jameton's proposed modifications include: (1) redistribution of decisional power, toward an ideal of shared decision making, (2) increased appreciation of the value of the relational, supportive, caring aspects of relationships with patients, expressed through accountability and reward structures (see Chapter 3, note 33 and accompanying text), and (3) equalization of income and status. Empirical studies confirm that collaborative relationships between physicians and nurses result in better patient care. See, e.g., April A. Lassen, Donna M. Fosbinder, Stephen Minton, and M. Mureno Robins, "Nurse/Physician Collaborative Practice: Improving Health Care Quality While Decreasing Cost," *Nursing Economics* 15, no. 2 (1997): 87–91, 104; Claire M. Fagin, "Collaboration between Nurses and Physicians: No Longer a Choice," *Academic Medicine* 67, no. 5 (1992): 295–303; Judith Gedney Baggs, Sheila A. Ryan, Charles E. Phelps, J. Franklin Richeson, and Jean E. Johnson, "The Association between Interdisciplinary Collaboration and Patient Outcomes in a Medical Intensive Care Unit," *Heart & Lung* 21, no. 1 (1992): 18–24.

101. A physician's account of a bad experience in an HMO in the 1980s begins with "the office." Dr. Henry Scovern writes: "A low pay scale for the nonprofessional staff attracted applicants with little training or experience. The orientation given to the nonprofessional personnel was minimal, and their general organization was poor. Those who acquired competence on the job tended to leave for better positions shortly thereafter. The administrative and personnel shortcomings resulted in inept telephone reception and patient scheduling, difficulty in communicating with consultants by telephone, and the virtual absence of secretarial assistance. The patients' charts were frequently unavailable, and the filing of laboratory and consultants' reports was delayed by as much as several weeks. In the patients' minds, the administrative confusion fostered an impression of shoddy health care." Henry Scovern, "Hired Help: A Physician's Experiences in a For-Profit Staff-Model HMO," *New England Journal of Medicine* 319, no. 12 (1988): 787–90, 787.

102. Paulo Freire, *Pedagogy of Hope: Reliving Pedagogy of the Oppressed,* trans. Robert R. Barr (New York: Continuum, 1994), 130. One bar to meaningful education is the belief that certain persons (especially persons in lower income groups) lack interest. A recent study found that while low-income patients were more likely to say they received too much advice on health risk behaviors (compared to affluent patients), the *overwhelming majority* of patients in the low-income group reported receiving too little advice. Further, of those who reported receiving too much advice, most reported changing or trying to change risky behavior due to their physician's advice. Deborah A. Taira, Dana Gelb Safran, Todd B. Seto, William H. Rogers, and Alvin R. Tarlov, "The Relationship between Patient Income and Physician Discussion of Health Risk Behaviors," *JAMA* 278, no. 17 (1997): 1412–17.

103. Jay Katz, *The Silent World of Doctor and Patient* (New York: Free Press, 1984), 103. Beyond the intrinsic appeal of more equal relationships characterized by greater mutuality, there are narrowly utilitarian grounds for pursuing this ideal. Research findings indicate that patients who take more responsibility for their treatment experience better (lower) mortality rates and (higher) quality of life. Richard L. Street and Becky Voigt, "Patient Participation in Deciding Breast Cancer Treatment and Subsequent Quality of Life," *Medical Decision Making* 17 (1997): 298–306, Sheldon Greenfield, Sherrie Kaplan, and John E. Ware, "Expanding Patient Involvement in Care: Effects on Patient Outcomes," *Annals of Internal Medicine* 102 (1985): 520–28.

104. "Partners in Policymaking: How to get connected and make a difference in the lives of people with developmental disabilities," http://thearc.org/misc/pip.html (visited September 8, 1999).

105. Dewey, *Freedom and Culture*, 166–67.

106. This was the conclusion reached by Dewey and Tufts. Dewey and Tufts, *Ethics*, 521.

107. Dewey, *Freedom and Culture*, 159–61.

108. See, e.g., Benedict M. Ashley and Kevin D. O'Rourke, *Health Care Ethics: A Theological Analysis*, 4th ed. (Washington, D.C.: Georgetown University Press, 1997), a text that combines a strong emphasis on community with a powerful universalism.

109. As in a number of the case studies published in Eileen Connor and Fitzhugh Mullan, eds., *Community Oriented Primary Care: New Directions for Health Services Delivery* (Washington, D.C.: National Academy Press, 1983).

110. Schlesinger, "Paradigms Lost," 952. As a point of information, Schlesinger opts for geographic proximity as the chief factor in the definition of community.

111. Dave Lindorff, *Marketplace Medicine: The Rise of For-Profit Hospital Chains* (New York: Bantam Books, 1992), 67.

112. An instance of manipulative pseudo-Gemeinschaft if ever there was one. Among the listed benefits: (1) "Childbirth is a natural event and an early homecoming is a celebration of such." (2) "Bonding with an infant is an intimate pleasure which can best be pursued in the privacy of one's own home." (3) "Unlimited visitors at home." Still, the list also included such seldom-discussed truths as "Hospital food is not tasty" and "Less risk of nosocomial [hospital-acquired] infections when hospital stay is brief." Cited in Laurie Zoloth-Dorfman and Susan Rubin, "The Patient as Commodity: Managed Care and the Question of Ethics," *Journal of Clinical Ethics* 6, no. 4 (1995): 339–57, 346.

113. The results of a public opinion survey indicate distrust of communities as mechanisms for the allocation of health care resources. Analyzing the findings in light of the history of community in health care, Mark Schlesinger concludes "community-based programs may be feasible only in an era when the federal government itself has greater legitimacy." Schlesinger, "Paradigms," 986. The survey of public opinion was conducted by telephone in July and August of 1995. The response rate was 69 percent, yielding 1,527 interviews.

6. MAKING SENSE OF MANAGED CARE

1. These facts are derived from *Shea v. Esensten*, 107 F.3d 625 (8th Cir. 1997), *cert. denied*, 522 U.S. 914 (1997). Mrs. Shea sued for malpractice and lost but continued to pursue other claims. *Shea v. Esensten*, 208 F.3d 712 (8th Cir. 2000).

2. An HMO in San Antonio, Texas, allegedly adopted this payment scheme to reduce length-of-stay. E. Haavi Morreim, *Balancing Act: The New Medical Ethics of Medicine's New Economics* (Dordrecht: Kluwer Academic Publishers, 1991), 38. Another example Morreim cites is an HMO that (allegedly) raised its fee of $1200 per delivery, with a 30 percent withhold, to $1700 per delivery—but with the costs of any sonograms, fetal monitoring, or stress tests deducted directly from the fee. The idea, clearly, was to discourage use of these tests. These kinds of payments may run afoul of federal law (for Medicare and Medicaid) and state laws affecting provider incentives.

3. For a catalogue of some possible variations, for bonuses and for other features

of managed care incentive schemes, see Thomas S. Bodenheimer and Kevin Grumbach, "Capitation or Decapitation: Keeping Your Head in Changing Times," *JAMA* 276 (1996): 1025–31.

4. Tony Dreyfus and Richard Kronick, "Paying Plans to Care for People with Chronic Illness," in *Making Managed Care Work for the Chronically Ill*, ed. Richard Kronick and Joy de Beyer (Chicago: Health Administration Press, 1999), 27–66, 32. This volume provides a thorough overview of risk-adjustment. See also Mita Giacomini, Harold S. Luft, and James C. Robinson, "Risk Adjusting Community-Rated Health Plan Premiums: A Survey of Risk Assessment Literature and Policy Applications," *Annual Review of Public Health* 16 (1995): 401–30. For a more summary treatment, see Bodenheimer and Grumbach, "Capitation or Decapitation," 1028.

5. Comprehensive data on the payment arrangements between physicians and managed care organizations was published in 1995. Marsha R. Gold, Robert Hurley, Timothy Lake, Todd Ensor, and Robert Berenson, "A National Survey of the Arrangements Managed-Care Plans Make with Physicians," *New England Journal of Medicine* 333 (1995): 1678–83. A 1996 survey of primary care physicians in California found that roughly 30 percent had bonus arrangements with managed care plans. Grumbach et al., "Primary Care Physicians' Experience," note 11 below.

6. Stephen R. Latham, "Regulation of Managed Care Incentive Payments to Physicians," *American Journal of Law & Medicine* 22, no. 4 (1996): 399–432.

7. Latham identifies two reasons for the effect, the "psychological tendency for people to weigh immediate concerns more heavily than those that are distant," and the "impact of the physician's uncertainty, at the beginning of any given year, as to whether she will experience a high- or low-cost year." As to the second factor, he comments that "[a]ny sophisticated physician (and especially one who is paid according to an incentive scheme) will keep track of her costs, and as the end of the fiscal year approaches, she will have much better information about what kind of cost-year she has been having." She may find "her entire annual bonus amount riding on her ability to save substantial costs in the relatively few cases left for her to manage." Latham, "Regulation," 424.

8. Latham, "Regulation," 411.

9. The empirical evidence concerning the effects of incentives is limited. See Katherine Swartz and Troyen A. Brennan, "Integrated Health Care, Capitated Payment, and Quality: The Role of Regulation," *Annals of Internal Medicine* 124, no. 4 (1996): 442–48, 444 (literature review). A recent study suggests that utilization does not vary systematically as between physicians paid on a fee-for-service (or fee-for-production of service) basis and physicians paid by salary. Douglas A. Conrad, Charles Maynard, Allen Cheadle, Scott Ramsey, Miriam Marcus-Smith, Howard Kirz, Carolyn A. Madden, Diane Martin, Edward B. Perrin, Thomas Wickizer, Brenda Zierler, Austin Ross, Jay Noren, and Su-Ying Liang, "Primary Care Physician Compensation Method in Medical Groups," *JAMA* 279 (1998): 853–58.

10. Donald M. Berwick, "Payment By Capitation and the Quality of Care," *New England Journal of Medicine* 335 (1996): 1227–31, 1227–28. Berwick concludes that the research literature confounds these variables. The study of utilization by Alan Hillman and colleagues supports the conclusion that factors besides direct financial incentives are at work. Although the investigators found that capitation was associated with lower rates of hospitalization than fee-for-service payment, salary was associated with even lower rates, a statistic that leads to speculation about the effects of peer review. Also, a finding of no direct association between placing physicians at financial risk as individu-

als and hospitalization rates might be explained by bias in patient selection, another complicating factor. Alan L. Hillman, Mark V. Pauly, and Joseph J. Kerstein, "How Do Financial Incentives Affect Physicians' Clinical Decisions and the Financial Performance of Health Maintenance Organizations?" *New England Journal of Medicine* 321 (1989): 86–92. Hillman has commented on "the important role of the context or organizational culture in which financial incentives are used." Alan L. Hillman, "Health Maintenance Organizations, Financial Incentives, and Physician's Judgments," *Annals of Internal Medicine* 112 (1990): 891–93, 892.

11. Kevin Grumbach, Dennis Osmond, Karen Vranizan, Deborah Jaffee, and Andrew Bindman, "Primary Care Physicians' Experience of Financial Incentives in Managed-Care Systems," *New England Journal of Medicine* 339 (1998): 1516–21.

12. Ibid., 1521. A complementary study focused on the relationship between basic payment method and patient trust. Audiey C. Kao, Diane C. Green, Alan M. Zaslavsky, Jeffrey P. Koplan, and Paul D. Cleary, "The Relationship between Method of Physician Payment and Patient Trust," *JAMA* 280 (1998): 1708–14. Nearly one-third of 2086 respondents were incorrect in identifying their physician's payment method, and just over one-third were don't knows. Most respondents (84 percent) completely or mostly trusted their physicians, but trust varied among groups: 94 percent of patients actually in the fee-for-service indemnity group said they trusted their physician to put their health and well-being above keeping down the health plan's cost, versus 85 percent in fee-for-service managed care, 83 percent in capitated managed care, and 77 percent in the salaried physician group.

However, patients of salaried physicians who correctly identified their physician's method of payment had higher levels of trust than others. The power of perception seems clear. Further, analysis revealed a statistically significant difference in trust between patients in capitated plans and patients in fee-for-service indemnity plans even after controlling for patients' perceptions of how their physicians were paid. As noted in the accompanying editorial, "physician payment mediates patient trust both directly (how patients feel about their perceptions of how their physicians are paid) and indirectly (through patients' responses to their physicians' responses to these factors)." Alan L. Hillman, "Mediators of Patient Trust," *JAMA* 280 (1998): 1703–1704, 1704.

The finding that patients of salaried physicians report the lowest levels of trust is startling, but then a study of base method of payment alone does not account for other pay features such as bonuses or equity stakes, let alone non-payment-related contextual factors that may influence physician behavior and patient trust. Because the study was confined to a single large insurer operating in the Mid-Atlantic states, it would not have included members of established staff or group model HMOs that tend to use salary, such as Kaiser.

13. A study of care for elderly patients with myocardial infarction found that patients admitted to the hospital by primary care physicians had fewer cardiac procedures and medications than those admitted by cardiologists, and were 12 percent more likely to die within one year. James G. Jollis, Elizabeth R. DeLong, Eric D. Peterson, Lawrence H. Muhlbaier, Donald F. Fortin, Robert M. Califf, and Daniel B. Mark, "Outcome of Acute Myocardial Infarction According to the Specialty of the Admitting Physician," *New England Journal of Medicine* 335 (1996): 1880–87.

The key factor may be experience rather than specialty; a study of primary care physicians caring for patients with AIDS found that the median survival of patients of physicians with the least experience with AIDS was 14 months, compared with 26 months for patients of physicians with the most experience. Mari M. Kitahata, Thomas D. Koepsell, Richard A. Deyo, Clare L. Maxwell, Wayne T. Dodge, and Edward H. Wagner, "Physicians' Experience with the Acquired Immunodeficiency Syndrome as a Factor in Patients' Survival," *New England Journal of Medicine* 334 (1996): 701–706. In a recent survey, a significant proportion of primary care physicians with gatekeeping responsibilities reported that the scope of care they were expected to provide was greater than it should be. Robert F. St. Peter, Marie C. Reed, Peter Kemper, and David Blumenthal, "Changes in the Scope of Care Provided by Primary Care Physicians," *New England Journal of Medicine* 341 (1999): 1980–85.

The evidence also suggests that permitting direct access to specialists does not increase expenditures for physician services. In fact, erecting barriers to access may be counterproductive in economic terms. Kanika Kapur, Geoffrey F. Joyce, Krista A. Van Vorst, and Jose J. Escarce, "Expenditures for Physician Services under Alternative Models of Managed Care," *Medical Care Research and Review* 57, no. 2 (2000): 161–81.

14. Latham, "Regulation," 423.

15. Robert A. Berenson, "A Physician's View of Managed Care," *Health Affairs* 10, no. 4 (1991): 106–19, 112.

16. "Research has shown that financial incentives change clinical behavior in the aggregate. However, . . . their impact in specific clinical circumstances is much more difficult to measure than is the impact of rules." Alan L. Hillman, "Managing the Physician: Rules Versus Incentives," *Health Affairs* 10, no. 4 (1991): 138–46, 141.

17. Researchers interviewed medical directors of capitated health plans participating in the Oregon Medicaid managed care system and staff within the Office of Medical Assistance Programs, the oversight agency. They learned that there were few patient requests for agency arbitration of denials of care, a finding that generated this comment: "That few appeals ever reached the Office of Medical Assistance Programs was not surprising, because almost every medical director stated that capitated care incentives minimize the number of cases formally reviewed and, hence, formally denied. Therefore, patients may not have been aware that services were refused even if they were entitled to them under the defined benefits package." Peter A. Glassman, Peter D. Jacobson, and Steven Asch, "Medical Necessity and Defined Coverage Benefits in the Oregon Health Plan," *American Journal of Public Health* 87 (1997): 1053–58, 1056.

18. See Chapter 5, note 74 and accompanying text.

19. In a fairly recent survey, only 8 percent of managed care plans responding (n=108) reported paying primary care physicians by salary with no withholding or bonus. A total of 60 percent (84 percent, in the case of IPA-type HMOs) reported some sharing of risk with primary care physicians, and 37 percent (56 percent of IPA HMOs) reported using capitation as the predominant method of payment. Capitation numbers for specialists were slightly lower. Gold et al., "National Survey," 1681.

20. Council on Ethical and Judicial Affairs, American Medical Association, "Ethical Issues in Managed Care," *JAMA* 273, no. 4 (1995): 330–35. For a vigorous critique of the AMA report, see Steven H. Miles and Robert Koepp, "Comments on the AMA Report 'Ethical Issues in Managed Care,'" *Journal of Clinical Ethics* 6, no. 4 (1995): 306–11. Numerous bioethicists and policy experts have weighed in on financial incentives as well. One of the more recent entries is Steven D. Pearson, James E. Sabin, and Ezekial J. Emanuel, "Ethical Guidelines for Physician Compensation Based on Capitation," *New England Journal of Medicine* 339 (1998): 689–93. See also Morreim, *Balancing Act*, 124; Ezekiel J. Emanuel, "Medical Ethics in the Era of Managed Care: The Need for Insti-

tutional Structures Instead of Principles for Individual Cases," *Journal of Clinical Ethics* 6, no. 4 (1995): 335–38; Ezekiel J. Emanuel and Nancy Neveloff Dubler, "Preserving the Physician-Patient Relationship in the Era of Managed Care," *JAMA* 273, no. 4 (1995): 323–29; and Swartz and Brennan, "Integrated Health Care," 447.

21. One study demonstrated a significant (two- to three-fold) increase in the prescription of two drugs among physicians who attended expense-paid seminars introducing the drugs. In informal interviews, the physicians who accepted invitations to attend the seminars, both held at luxury resorts, insisted (and, in the investigators judgment, sincerely believed) that such inducements would not affect their prescribing patterns. James P. Orlowski and Leon Wateska, "The Effects of Pharmaceutical Firm Enticements on Physician Prescribing Patterns," *Chest* 102, no. 1 (1992): 270–73.

In a study to test the influence of advertising, physicians were asked to state the properties of certain drugs and their appropriate uses. Answers revealed beliefs that did not correspond to published medical reports but did reflect the claims made in advertisements. Again, the physicians studied insisted that they based their assessment of medical products only on scientific evaluations, literature, and experience. Two studies found that pharmaceutical companies' sponsorship of continuing medical education influenced the attitudes of instructors and participants in the courses. Instructors assessed the drug made by their sponsoring firm more favorably, and participating physicians increased their use of the sponsor's drug the most. These biases emerged even though the host institution, Georgetown University School of Medicine, followed guidelines that required disclosure of the sponsorship and affiliation of speakers, and even though drugs were only referred to by their generic names. These studies are cited in Marc A. Rodwin, *Medicine, Money, and Morals: Physicians' Conflicts of Interest* (New York: Oxford University Press, 1993), 109–10. For more on pharmaceutical company largesse, and its influence on physicians' prescribing practices, see Ashley Wazana, "Physicians and the Pharmaceutical Industry: Is a Gift Ever Just a Gift?" *JAMA* 283 (2000): 373–80; Letters to the Editor, "Gifts to Physicians From the Pharmaceutical Industry," *JAMA* 283 (2000): 2655–58.

Other empirical work suggests that commercial sponsorship significantly affects the outcomes of clinical research. An analysis of 107 clinical trials found that those with pharmaceutical company support were much more likely to favor the new therapy than those with general support. Roger J. Porter, "Conflicts of Interest in Research: The Fundamentals," in *Biomedical Research: Collaboration and Conflict of Interest*, ed. Roger J. Porter and Thomas E. Malone (Baltimore: Johns Hopkins University Press, 1992), 121–34, 131. Although direct financial benefit to the investigators may be a factor, a more general desire for career advancement and continued funding for one's work may be all that is required. As a final example of susceptibility to influence, consider physicians' willingness to prescribe antibiotics they know to be ineffective in response to patient demands.

22. "Requirements for Physician Incentive Plans in Prepaid Health Care Organizations," 61 Fed. Reg. 13430, 13432 (1996) (codified at 42 C.F.R. pts. 417, 434). Other provisions require plans to conduct an annual survey of beneficiaries and those who disenroll (if plans put physicians at substantial financial risk), and to disclose general features of physician incentive arrangements to enrollees who ask. A section of the Health Care Financing Administration's website is devoted to "Physician Incentive Plan (PIP) Regulation Guidance," www.hcfa.gov/medicare/physincp/pip-info.htm (visited September 8, 1999). Items available via the website include suggested language for

communications with beneficiaries. Additional regulations respecting financial incentives have been issued under the Balanced Budget Act of 1997, with no significant departures from the initial regulatory approach.

23. It is not uncommon for legislation to target yesterday's abuse. Latham traces the single-patient rule back to the controversy provoked by the Paracelsus Healthcare Corporation when it offered to split the difference between the Medicare prospective payments and the actual costs of hospitalization with admitting physicians. Latham, "Regulation," 419. On the Paracelsus controversy, see Bradford H. Gray, *The Profit Motive and Patient Care: The Changing Accountability of Doctors and Hospitals* (Cambridge, Mass.: Harvard University Press, 1991), 136–37.

24. Berwick, "Payment by Capitation," 1228 (emphasis added).

25. Berwick, "Payment by Capitation," 1229.

26. This suggestion is made in Stephen M. Shortell, Robin R. Gillies, David A. Anderson, Karen Morgan Erickson, and John B. Mitchell, *Remaking Health Care in America: Building Organized Delivery Systems* (San Francisco: Jossey-Bass, 1996), 109.

27. The favorable initial results of a pilot program using community-based lay workers as part of a coordinated approach to the care of 23 low-income children with moderate to severe asthma are described in James W. Stout, Lisa C. White, La Tonya Rogers, Teresa McRorie, Barbara Morray, Marijo Miller-Ratcliffe, and Gregory J. Redding, "The Asthma Outreach Project: A Promising Approach to Comprehensive Asthma Management," *Journal of Asthma* 35, no. 1 (1998): 119–27. Client satisfaction with the program was very high, and utilization review showed a reduction in hospitalizations, emergency department visits, and unscheduled clinic visits, in conjunction with an increase in follow-up clinic visits.

28. The description of the Harvard Pilgrim program comes from Michael L. Millenson, *Demanding Medical Excellence: Doctors and Accountability in the Information Age* (Chicago: University of Chicago Press, 1997), 329–32. Millenson's account is derived from interviews and review of internal reports, rather than articles in peer-reviewed journals. (Millenson's reliance on non-peer-reviewed accounts elicited a scold in a book review by Steffie Woolhandler and David Himmelstein in the *New England Journal of Medicine*.)

29. See Berenson, "A Physician's View of Managed Care," 115.

30. The managed care organization is United HealthCare Corp. Initial data revealed widespread failure to adhere to standards for good practice, including annual glucose-monitoring tests for diabetics, and prescription of beta blockers for heart-attack survivors and ACE inhibitors for patients with chronic heart failure. Thomas M. Burton, "An HMO Checks Up On Its Doctors' Care and Is Disturbed Itself," *Wall Street Journal*, 8 July 1998, A1. Physicians may be prescribing drugs without adequate attention to warnings about toxic side-effects and interactions, as well as failing to prescribe drugs where indicated. Chris Adams, "The Fine Print: Are Too Many Doctors Missing Safety Alerts on Drugs?" *Wall Street Journal*, 24 March 2000, B1. Recent research suggests that computer-based guidelines may be particularly effective in changing physician behavior. The introduction of computer-based guidelines for treatment of occupational exposures to body fluids improved quality of care according to five outcome measures: documentation of essential items in patient history and aftercare instructions (increased by 42 percent and 62 percent, respectively), compliance with testing and treatment guidelines (increased by 20 percent and 13 percent, respectively), and total per-patient charges (decreased from $460 to $384). David L. Schriger, Larry J. Baraff, William H.

Rogers, and Shan Cretin, "Implementation of Clinical Guidelines Using a Computer Charting System: Effects on the Initial Care of Healthcare Workers Exposed to Body Fluids," *JAMA* 278 (1997): 1585–90. The Agency for Healthcare Research and Quality (formerly the Agency for Health Care Policy and Research), the American Association of Health Plans, and the American Medical Association have collaborated to create an on-line National Guideline Clearinghouse at www.guideline.gov (visited September 8, 1999). Any physician, or person, with access to the Internet can now review the most current information on treatments for a range of conditions free of charge. Also, the American Cancer Society is "translating" detailed clinical guidelines for common cancers into laypersons language.

Milliman & Robertson is the best-known purveyor of guidelines for cost-conscious plans and providers. Guidelines recommending 24-hour maternity stays and outpatient mastectomies for women with breast cancer have captured the attention of the public, and, in the case of the former, provoked federal legislation. The legislation was a response to the perception that in practice these guidelines operated as inflexible rules. In a report on the firm's development of guidelines for pediatric care, a physician-administrator remarked, "If I get 100% adherence to a pathway, I'm terrified because it means that no one paid attention to the actual patients." George Anders and Laurie McGinley, "Medical Cop: Actuarial Firm Helps Decide Just How Long You Spend in Hospital," *Wall Street Journal*, 15 June 1998, A1, A16.

31. The breast cancer guidelines are described in Dean C. Coddington, Keith D. Moore, and Elizabeth A. Fischer, *Making Integrated Health Care Work* (Englewood, Colo.: Center for Research in Ambulatory Health Care Administration, 1996), 89–90.

32. George Anders looks at subcontracting for cardiac care in great detail in George Anders, *Health against Wealth: HMOs and the Breakdown of Medical Trust* (New York: Houghton Mifflin, 1996), 92–111. Laboratory services are a frequent item for subcontracting. Consider, then, these comments from the chief actuary of a major California HMO in 1994: "'I marvel at the kinds of deals we're able to get from medical labs. It's literally impossible for labs to make money at the rates we're getting.'" If the labs are making money, is there any question that corners are being cut?

The case of Karin Smith, a young woman who died of cervical cancer which repeated pap smears and biopsies failed to disclose, illustrates the potential weaknesses of quality control measures. Smith's test results had been analyzed at a lab affiliated with her HMO. A reporter, Edward Dolnick, pinpointed the system failure. The lab followed industry practice in reinspecting one in every ten slides for quality control. But a technician testified in a sworn deposition that the lab reinspected only those slides with a code number ending in two and this system was known among the technicians. As Dolnick observed, "'A technician could race along to her heart's content so long as she remembered to slow down and pay extra attention to those special slides.'" Ibid., 240. For a primary care physician's personal narrative of frustration with selective contracting, see Thomas Bodenheimer, "Selective Chaos," *Health Affairs* 19, no. 4 (2000): 200–5.

33. James E. Sabin and Carlos Neu, "Real World Resource Allocation: The Concept of 'Good-Enough' Psychotherapy," *Bioethics Forum* 12, no. 1 (1996): 3–9, 4. The article title refers to Sabin and Neu's adaptation of D. W. Winnicott's concept of "good-enough mothering" to the practice of psychotherapy in the managed care context. I think their effort to develop an ethic adapted to the managed care environment out of the resources of their own discipline (practice) is to be commended.

34. Kevin Grumbach, Joe V. Selby, Cheryl Damberg, Andrew B. Bindman, Charles Quesenberry, Jr., Alison Truman, and Connie Uratsu, "Resolving the Gatekeeper Conundrum: What Patients Value in Primary Care and Referrals to Specialists," *JAMA* 282 (1999): 261–66.

35. Henry Scovern, "Hired Help: A Physician's Experiences in a For-Profit Staff-Model HMO," *New England Journal of Medicine* 319, no. 12 (1988): 787–90, 788–89. (This particular problem has likely ceased to exist with the introduction of DRGs and other prepaid or global fee arrangements for hospital care.)

36. Scovern, "Hired Help," 789–99.

37. The researchers conclude that "[o]veremphasis of primary care gatekeepers as agents of cost control threatens to undermine primary care in the United States." Grumbach et al., "Resolving the Gatekeeper Conundrum," 266; on physician attitudes, see St. Peter et al., supra note 13, Ethan A. Halm, Nancyanne Causino, and David Blumenthal, "Is Gatekeeping Better Than Traditional Care? A Survey of Physicians' Attitudes," *JAMA* 278 (1997): 1677–81.

38. Howard Brody, *The Healer's Power* (New Haven, Conn.: Yale University Press, 1992), 191–201. Another way of framing this is to say that, under appropriate system and organizational conditions, modest rationing of resources by physicians as a means of balancing obligations to the presenting patient with obligations to other patients is an instance of *dual* rather than *divided* loyalties. Beauchamp and Childress argue that while divided loyalties can only be reconciled by abandoning or seriously modifying one set of obligations, dual loyalties can be sustained through specification and balancing. Tom L. Beauchamp and James F. Childress, *Principles of Biomedical Ethics*, 4th ed. (New York: Oxford University Press, 1994), 431.

39. Mark A. Hall, *Making Medical Spending Decisions: The Law, Ethics, and Economics of Rationing Mechanisms* (New York: Oxford University Press, 1997), 88.

40. Appealing ideas that seem to avoid the moral tension, such as Robert Veatch's proposal for rationing by patient advisory groups supported by medically trained agents insulated from pressures of the plan and clinicians, might be difficult to implement. Robert M. Veatch, "Allocating Health Resources Ethically: New Roles for Administrators and Clinicians," *Frontiers of Health Services Management* 8, no. 1 (1991): 3–29, Robert M. Veatch, "Who Should Manage Care? The Case for Patients," *Kennedy Institute of Ethics Journal* 7, no. 4 (1997): 391–401. If insulation is to be achieved by ceding actual control of the bulk of an organization's assets or income to these groups (or, where an organization sponsors multiple plans, dividing resources up among groups), there may be significant legal and administrative problems.

41. Hall's complete analysis of the trade-offs between rules (which allow for rationing decisions to be made by professionals, patients, bureaucrats, or a combination of these) and discretion (which points to a physician making rationing decisions "at the bedside") is roughly as follows. Rules save time and they serve the cause of justice by ensuring uniform treatment. On the other hand, because rules generalize, they are inexact (a point made by Aristotle): "The complexity of human affairs dictates that a limited set of factors will rarely, if ever, capture perfectly the background justification that motivates the rule. . . . The exceptional case can form the basis for subsequent amendment of the rule, but to deviate on the spot is to exercise discretion, not rule-based authority." Hall, *Medical Spending Decisions*, 77. Also, the judgment of rulemakers may be distorted by bias. Further, the efficiency advantage of rules depends on tak-

ing them at face value, and the habit of taking the rules at face value may blunt a sense of responsibility.

Discretionary decision making has complementary strengths and weaknesses. It is case specific, and therefore attentive to relevant differences. It promotes justice by allowing for a review of the particulars of the case. On the other hand, there is a loss in terms of efficiency, decision making is less public and less accountable, and space is created for the operation of individual dishonesty and incompetence as well as bias.

Hall's preference is for a mixture of rules and discretion: "Rules might best establish which treatments are entirely excluded, when dramatic and high-stakes treatment can be withheld, and what the broad parameters are for ordinary items of care. . . . The undefined spheres of medicine or those where patient values vary widely could then be shaped by financial, professional, and liability incentives, in combination with physicians' conversations with their patients." Hall, *Medical Spending Decisions*, 81.

42. For a summary of some of the existing evidence, see Chapter 5, footnote 61 and accompanying text.

43. "[I]ndividuals may or may not agree to their physicians making cost/benefit trade-offs on their behalf, but we should not presume their desires when it is possible to ask them." Hall, *Medical Spending Decisions*, 142–43.

44. Morreim, *Balancing Act*, 108.

45. The AMA itself has been accused of less than adequate disclosure in its report on ethics and managed care. In the late 1970s, the Federal Trade Commission investigated charges that the AMA was conspiring to inhibit the growth of HMOs, in part through its pronouncements on ethics. In 1979, the federal agency imposed a "cease and desist" order on anticompetitive use of ethics standards. The AMA Report is nearly silent on these events (and the constraints that resulted). See Miles and Koepp, "Comments on the AMA Report," 306–307.

46. American Association of Health Plans (AAHP), "Philosophy of Care" (Washington, D.C.: AAHP, 1996); Advisory Commission on Consumer Protection and Quality in the Health Care Industry, *Consumer Bill of Rights and Responsibilities* (Preamble), November 20, 1997, available at http://www.hcqualitycommission.gov/cborr/ (visited September 8, 1999). The President's Advisory Commission states that consumers should receive information on: (1) benefits, cost-sharing, and dispute resolution (e.g., limits on coverage, drug formularies, how drugs, devices, and procedures are deemed experimental, and dispute resolution procedures); (2) health plan characteristics and performance (e.g., licensing, certification and accreditation status, consumer satisfaction measures, clinical performance measures, service performance measures, and disenrollment rates); (3) network characteristics (e.g., aggregate information on numbers, types, board certification status, and geographic distribution of providers, with the same information in detail for PCPs plus openness to new patients, languages/translation services, accessibility, compensation methods, and policies concerning out-of-network, urgent care, and specialist access); and (4) upon request, care management (e.g., preauthorization and utilization review procedures, any guidelines pertinent to the consumer's clinical circumstances, programs for persons with disabilities, inclusion of particular drugs in the formulary, and qualifications of reviewers).

There are also information items that would relate to the health professionals and facilities under consideration by a particular consumer. For a review of legal and policy considerations, see Tracy E. Miller and William M. Sage, "Disclosing Physician Financial Incentives," *JAMA* 281 (1999): 1424–30; William M. Sage, "Regulating Through

Information: Disclosure Laws and American Health Care," 99 Columbia Law Review 1701 (1999).

47. Several commentators note that disclosure mandates and other consumer protection-style laws are not substitutes for more substantive protections that take account of the special vulnerabilities of people seeking health care. See Sage, "Regulating through Information"; Wendy Mariner, "Standards of Care and Standard Form Contracts: Distinguishing Patient Rights and Consumer Rights in Managed Care," *Journal of Contemporary Health Law and Policy* 15, no. 1 (1998): 1–55; Carl E. Schneider, *The Practice of Autonomy: Patients, Doctors, and Medical Decisions* (New York: Oxford University Press, 1998), 198–227 (elaborating on the distinction between consumer choice and consumer welfare models).

48. E. Haavi Morreim, "To Tell the Truth: Disclosing the Incentives and Limits of Managed Care," *American Journal of Managed Care* 3 (1997): 35–43, 41.

49. Howard Brody suggests a similar strategy for disclosing serious but very low-probability risks. "In a reasonable and realistic medical conversation, we cannot disclose this remote risk [in Brody's example, the one-in-40,000 chance of dying from intravenous pyelograms] without at the same time conveying additional messages that are both unintended and confusing. It therefore seems that we have done our duty by relating the general existence of remote risks; and that unless the patient asks, explicit inclusion of those risks makes the conversation less useful, not more so, from the patient's perspective." Brody, *Healer's Power*, 99. Brody does believe that more detail may be appropriate in printed forms.

50. Cleary and Edgman-Levitan, "Health Care Quality," 1610. Government agencies are also making greater use of new technologies. Currently, Medicare beneficiaries can access a HCFA database to generate comparisons of premiums and basic benefits for Medicare managed care plans, via the Internet. Such efforts should become increasingly sophisticated, as the databases grow and the technology is refined. Recent focus group research suggests that comprehension, attitudes toward specific kinds of financial incentives (e.g., salary), desire for information, and preferences concerning source of disclosure are all highly variable. In one study, agreement was limited to two areas. First, there was a clear preference for written materials with some opportunity to ask follow-up questions, versus video. Second, focus group participants expressed "strong reluctance" to raise the issue with their physician, for reasons ranging from a fear of embarrassing or angering the physician to a desire to devote precious time to clinical matters, but agreement evaporated when participants were asked whether they would welcome a discussion *initiated by* their physician. Tracy E. Miller and Carol R. Horowitz, "Disclosing Doctors' Incentives: Will Consumers Understand and Value the Information," *Health Affairs* 19, no. 4 (2000): 149–55. These findings support efforts to tailor disclosure to the needs and preferences of the individual.

These data also buttress claims that information on plan structure and performance may be most useful to group purchasers, plans, health care providers, and citizens (versus consumers). See, e.g., Sage, "Regulating through Information"; Martin N. Marshall, Paul G. Shekelle, Sheila Leatherman, and Robert H. Brook, "The Public Release of Performance Data," *JAMA* 283 (2000): 1866–74. For example, Sage writes that while mandated disclosure is often justified as a corrective for information asymmetry, the assumption that plans and providers know what they are doing is often unjustified. "An underappreciated attribute of mandatory disclosure laws is their ability to help, or perhaps force, the health care system to figure it out." As a corollary, resistance to disclosing management practices "may reflect unwillingness to reveal ignorance or arbitrariness rather than protection of competitive advantage." Sage, "Regulating through Information," 1771, 1791.

51. Sabin and Neu, "Real World Resource Allocation," 6.

52. Hall reviews the results of several studies establishing that HMO advertisements aim to persuade consumers that they provide generous and unlimited services, and that consumers believe. Mark A. Hall, *A Theory of Economic Informed Consent*, 31 Georgia Law Review 511, 520 (1997).

53. In 1996, Humana, not atypically, paid sales people $9,400 a month for enrolling seven or eight elderly people a week; Foundation Health offered up to $190,000 a year in perquisites and bonuses to those who could bring in fifty new recruits in a month. Managed care plans participating in TennCare, Tennessee's Medicaid managed care program, offered free turkeys, credit cards, life insurance deals, and other inducements to attract members. TennCare officials originally regarded such gimmicks as benign, but changed their views when critics pointed out that giveaways were diverting funds from health care. HMOs were also allowed to pay "per-head" commissions to door-to-door sales workers. One enterprising salesperson signed up prison inmates, who were already receiving free care. Door-to-door salespeople were sometimes given explicit instructions on whom to avoid—such as pregnant women. Anders, *Health against Wealth*, 66, 198–99.

54. "It is more difficult for doctors to inform patients that economic considerations are influencing clinical decisions when patients do not perceive this to be normal practice. When physicians do not meet patients' expectations (as influenced by marketing), or are the first to break the news that there are limits on the members' benefits, the doctor-patient relationship suffers." Susan Dorr Goold and Howard Brody, "Rationing Decisions in Managed Care Settings: An Ethical Analysis," in *Health Care Crisis? The Search for Answers*, ed. Robert I. Misbin, Bruce Jennings, David Orentlicher, and Marvin Dewar (Frederick, Md.: UPG, 1995), 135–64, 145–46. Of course, there is also a problem when patients bring extremely low expectations to the relationship. Physicians in focus groups suggested that the central ethical issue for them was not actual conflicts of interests in seeking to serve patients and health plans, but rather patient perception that they were serving two masters. Nancy S. Jecker and Albert R. Jonsen, "Managed Care: A House of Mirrors," *Journal of Clinical Ethics* 8, no. 3 (1997): 230–41. Likewise, the physicians stressed, not the difficulties attending denial of beneficial treatments, but rather the difficulties attending denial of non-beneficial treatments.

55. Hall, *Medical Spending Decisions*, 222 (with credit to Professor Maxwell Mehlman). Hall's theory is set forth in the book, and in two articles, "Informed Consent to Rationing Decisions," *Milbank Quarterly* 71, no. 4 (1993): 645–68, and *A Theory of Economic Informed Consent* cited in note 52 above.

56. Hall, *Medical Spending Decisions*, 129.

57. As M. Gregg Bloche notes, placing the concept of informed consent in the context of rationing introduces some radical changes: "[I]n a sense, the logic of consent has come full circle, from prophylaxis against clinical actions contrary to patients' interests to justification of professional authority to weigh the interests of others over those of the patient." M. Gregg Bloche, "Clinical Loyalties and the Social Purposes of Medicine," *JAMA* 281 (1999): 268–74, 271. Hall appears to want the moral halo that surrounds "informed consent"—versus, say, agreement to a contract—but that halo will

have to be earned. Informed consent to rationing is not a simple extension of informed consent to medical treatment.

58. Hall, *Medical Spending Decisions,* 151–52.

59. Hall, *Medical Spending Decisions,* 153.

60. Hall, *Medical Spending Decisions,* 258.

61. Laurie Zoloth-Dorfman and Susan Rubin, "The Patient as Commodity: Managed Care and the Question of Ethics," *Journal of Clinical Ethics* 6, no. 4 (1995): 339–57, 353 (emphasis added).

62. See, e.g., Steven H. Miles, "New Business for Ethics Committees," *H.E.C. Forum* 4 (1992): 97–102; Michael Felder, "An Ethics Committee for a Health Maintenance Organization: An Oxymoron? Certainly Not," *H.E.C. Forum* 4 (1992): 261–67; Michael Felder, "Can Ethics Committees Work in Managed Care Plans?" *Bioethics Forum* 12, no. 1 (1996): 10–15; Robert Lyman Potter, "An Integrated Ethics Program for Managed Care Organizations," *Trends in Health Care, Law & Ethics* 10, no. (1995): 87–90; and Joan D. Biblo, Myra J. Christopher, Linda Johnson, Robert Lyman Potter, *Ethical Issues in Managed Care: Guidelines for Clinicians and Recommendations to Accrediting Organizations* (Kansas City, Mo.: Midwest Bioethics Center, 1995); Elizabeth Heitman and Ruth Ellen Bolger, "The Healthcare Ethics Committee in the Structural Transformation of Health Care: Administrative and Organizational Ethics in Changing Times," *HEC Forum* 10, no. 2 (1998): 152–76. Tasks discussed in these sources include encouraging honest, effective and open communication, adopting and honoring statements of rights and responsibilities, educating employees, providers, and members about ethical issues and the institutional mechanisms available for addressing them, involving providers and members in developing policies and procedures to offer guidance on ethical issues, integrating ethical considerations into decision making at all levels, and ensuring that contracts are with organizations that have compatible policies, procedures and practices. Stanley Reiser, speaking to health care organizations in general and not just to managed care organizations, proposes "administrative ethics rounds" as a way of drawing attention to the ethical dimensions of the managerial role. Stanley Joel Reiser, "Administrative Case Rounds," *JAMA* 266 (1991): 2127–28.

63. Concerning proprietary practices, the assumption that secrecy promotes innovation is open to question. It is ironic that health plans and health care providers are hoarding information at the very moment when participants in other sectors of the economy are realizing the benefits of giving it away. "In other industries, vigorous competitors have abandoned efforts to segment, isolate, and safeguard knowledge in favor of open architectures that promote fluidity and information sharing." Sage, "Regulating through Information," 1792.

On confidentiality and privacy issues, see Ida Critelli Schick, "Personal Privacy and Confidentiality in an Electronic Environment," *Bioethics Forum* 12, no. 1 (1996): 25–30. The abuses mentioned include the careless failure of some clinics to delete patient identifiers from data sold to drug companies (through an intermediary), the sale of patient information (names, addresses, medical records, and income figures) to HMO recruiters by Medicaid clerks, and entry of data into electronic systems without proper safeguards against unauthorized use. In general, one may question the propriety of sharing patient data beyond the group of persons directly responsible for patient care absent consent (except as required by law), let alone selling it. One HMO reportedly saves money by informing patients of abnormal mammogram results with postcards rather than (sealed) first-class letters. Karen I. Titlow, Jonathan E. Rackoff, and Ezekial J. Emanuel, "What Will It Take to Restore Patient Trust?" *Business and Health* 17, no. 6 (1999): 61–64, 63. Another possible abuse is for a physician-hospital organization or PHO to use information it collects as a provider to benefit its health plan, e.g., using patient care data to market the plan selectively.

64. Alan R. Morse, Jr., and Allan I. Greenberg, "Letter from the Chairman and the President," in *Viewpoints: Ethics in Managed Care,* Highlights From the Harvard Pilgrim Health Care Annual Report 1997 (visited June 19, 1999) <http://www. harvardpilgrim.org/About_Us/Annual_Report/annual_letter.htm>. On the fall and rehabilitation of Harvard Pilgrim, see Laura Johannes, "Pressures on HMOs Drag Down Harvard Pilgrim," *Wall Street Journal,* 6 January 2000, A4; Liz Kowalczyk, "New Harvard Pilgrim Directors Appointed: Board to Guide HMO Out of Receivership," *Boston Globe,* 20 June 2000, C5. On some of the fallout from efforts at belt-tightening, see Liz Kowalczyk, "HMO to Cut Psychiatry Provider Payments; Some Staff Plan to Quit Harvard Pilgrim," *Boston Globe,* 18 August 2000, C1.

65. Lisa Raiola, "Questions and Answers," in *Viewpoints: Ethics in Managed Care* (visited June 19, 1999) <http://www.harvardpilgrim.org/About_Us/Annual_Report/ Q_and_A.htm>. Raiola has since departed Harvard Pilgrim.

66. Donald F. Phillips, "Erecting an Ethical Framework for Managed Care," *JAMA* 280 (1998): 2060–62.

67. On media coverage of managed care, see Chapter 2, note 16.

68. Like Kaiser, many managed care organizations include an arbitration clause in their contracts. They apparently believe that the arbitration process is less expensive than a standard court proceeding or that they will receive more favorable treatment. Arbitrators do not always favor HMOs—but the $1.2 million award in the deMeurers case does pale in comparison to initial jury awards in comparable cases.

69. Courts have held that the federal Employee Retirement Income Security Act of 1974 (ERISA) preempts state tort actions against health plans for harms that allegedly result from plan design, in cases involving employer-sponsored insurance. Employee Retirement Income Security Act of 1974, as amended, 29 U.S.C. §§ 1001–1461. The preemption provisions are even broader for employers who "self-insure," i.e., retain the insurance risk in contracting with a health plan to provide services to employees.

A recent report estimates that in 1995, 123 million people were covered by ERISA-regulated plans, of which more than 39 percent (48 million) were in self-insured plans. Craig Copeland and Bill Pierron, "Implications of ERISA for Health Benefits and the Number of Self-Funded ERISA Plans," Issue Brief, Employee Benefit Research Institute, January 1998. For a more detailed treatment of the malpractice issues, and a review of malpractice cases involving managed care organizations, see Rodwin, *Medicine, Money, and Morals,* 172–75. For more information on the use of ERISA as a defense in malpractice cases, see Wendy K. Mariner, "What Recourse? Liability for Managed-Care Decisions and the Employee Retirement Income Security Act," *New England Journal of Medicine* 343 (2000): 592–596; Margaret G. Farrell, "ERISA Preemption and Regulation of Managed Health Care," *American Journal of Law & Medicine* 23 (1997): 251–89; Wendy K. Mariner, "State Regulation of Managed Care and the Employee Retirement Income Security Act," *New England Journal of Medicine* 335 (1996): 1986–90; Alexander Morgan Capron, "Between Doctor and Patient," *Hastings Center Report* 26, no. 5 (1996): 23–24; Robert Pear, "H.M.O.'s Use a U.S. Law as a Malpractice Shield," *New York Times,* 17 November 1996, sec. 1, 16.

A possible ray of sunshine comes from *Shea v. Esensten*, cited supra. The court in *Shea* noted that ERISA imposes fiduciary obligations on plans. Among these is a duty of loyalty requiring communication of any material facts that could adversely affect a plan member's interests. The court ruled that "[w]hen an HMO's financial incentives discourage a treating doctor from providing essential health care referrals for conditions covered under the plan benefit structure [as the plaintiff alleged], the incentives must be disclosed and the failure to do so is a breach of ERISA's fiduciary duties." The fall-out from this case may be that ERISA-regulated plans, and the physicians who serve them, have firmer legal duties in the area of disclosure than plans outside ERISA. However, another federal appellate court has ruled that ERISA imposes no general duty to disclose financial incentives, although disclosure may be required in special circumstances. *Ehlmann v. Kaiser Foundation Health Plan of Texas*, 198 F.3d 552 (5th Cir. 2000). The United States Supreme Court did *not* address the disclosure issue in *Pegram v. Herdrich*, 120 S.Ct. 2143 (2000), deciding only that HMO physicians making mixed benefit-treatment decisions are not ERISA fiduciaries.

70. The posturing of the managed care industry in relation to regulation invites comment. Given the lack of consumer confidence in managed care and managed care organizations, the AAHP and other trade groups have an interest in regulation. In the public relations battle, it is helpful to point to federal and state laws, accreditation standards, and so on. At the same time, managed care organizations, like other organizations, insist that they behave well by internal will rather than external mandate, and that most regulation is unnecessary and only serves to hamper innovation. Some skepticism concerning internal will is in order. According to an article in *Hospitals & Health Networks*, the member of the President's Advisory Commission most strongly opposed to mandates vowed to implement the Consumer Bill of Rights for the 6 million enrollees in his company's plans. As of late March (four months after the release of the document), the task force assigned to the job had yet to meet, and there was no timetable for implementation. Harris Meyer, "The Right to Appeal," *Hospitals & Health Network* 72, no. 9 (1998): 23–26, 26. The latest salvo in the public relations battle has come from the "Coalition for Affordable Quality Healthcare," comprised of health plans and trade groups. See Coalition for Affordable Quality Healthcare, Progress Report, www.caqh.org/progress3.html (visited July 31, 2000); Sharon Bernstein, "Under Pressure, Health Plans Pledge Reforms," *Los Angeles Times*, 19 July 2000, A1.

71. See Jane Perkins, Kristi Olson, Lourdes Rivera and Julie Skatrud, *Making the Consumers' Voice Heard in Medicaid Managed Care: Increasing Participation, Protection and Satisfaction* (Washington, D.C.: National Health Law Program, 1996); Kristi Olson and Jane Perkins, *Recommendations for Making the Consumers' Voice Heard in Medicaid Managed Care: A Guide to Effective Consumer Involvement* (Washington, D.C.: National Health Law Program, 1999). On involving consumers/members/patients in quality improvement, see Paul D. Cleary and Susan Edgman-Levitan, "Health Care Quality: Incorporating Consumer Perspectives," *JAMA* 278 (1997): 1608–12; Allyson Ross Davies and John E. Ware, Jr., "Involving Consumers in Quality of Care Assessment," *Health Affairs* 7, no. 1 (1988): 33–48; and Susan Edgman-Levitan and Paul D. Cleary, "What Information Do Consumers Want And Need?" *Health Affairs* 15, no. 4 (1996): 42–56.

72. In the same way that the government may exert influence as the administrator of programs that managed care organizations want to participate in, purchasing cooperatives or employers that control large numbers of "covered lives" can set the agenda for

plans in their regions. Some benefits managers have used this power to force managed care organizations to offer standard benefit structures, minimizing risk selection and permitting employees to better understand coverage and make comparisons. Still, a recent poll found that 80 percent of employers consider cost the top priority when choosing health plans. Jan Greene, "Has Managed Care Lost Its Soul?" *Hospitals & Health Networks* 71, no. 10 (1997): 36–42, 42. A report devoted to the corporate pioneers is in accord. U.S. Agency for Health Care Policy and Research, *Theory and Reality of Value-Based Purchasing: Lessons From the Pioneers*, AHCPR Publication No. 98-0004, November 1997.

73. See Robert Pear, "Rulings on Medicare Rights Split White House," *New York Times*, 22 January 1999, A22.

74. In testifying before a Congressional committee concerning the consequences of HMO defections from the Medicare+Choice program, a senior official with the Health Care Financing Administration remarked that a "certain amount of market volatility must be expected when relying on the private sector to service beneficiaries." Michael M. Hash, Deputy Administrator, Health Care Financing Administration, Testimony Before the Senate Finance Committee, June 9, 1999. Quoted in "Medicare: HCFA Tells Senate Panel Medicare+Choice is Healthy," *BNA's Health Care Daily Report*, Executive Briefing, 10 June 1999.

75. For some confirmation of this, see Peter T. Kilborn, "In Managed Care, 'Consumer' Laws Benefit Doctors," *New York Times*, 16 February 1998, A1.

76. See Judith Haverman, "HMOs, Doctors Battle in State Legislatures Over Managed Care Limits," in *1996 Health Network & Alliance Sourcebook*, C141–42, C141. At least seven states have enacted any-willing provider laws that cover most providers, and 31 states have passed any-willing provider or freedom-of-choice laws restricting managed care plans from selective contracting with pharmacies. But the trend is to focus directly on preserving or enhancing the quality of care.

According to the National Conference of State Legislatures' Health Policy Tracking Service, as of July of 1999, 47 states banned gag clauses, 36 states mandated coverage for emergency care service screening and stabilization, 35 states had adopted a prudent layperson standard for reimbursement of emergency care services, 36 states provided direct access to OB/GYN services, 29 states had an independent appeals process, 28 states required disclosure of restrictive drug formularies, 22 states addressed continuity of care, and 19 states established a minimum LOS following a mastectomy. Health Policy Tracking Service, *State Managed Care Laws: A State-by-State Review* (Washington, D.C.: National Conference of State Legislatures, 1999).

77. If I were an accountant, I would be extremely irritated by comments that begin "How can you let some person with the mentality of an accountant . . . " Howard Kurtz, "Some Managed-Care Sagas Need Second Exam," *Washington Post*, 10 August 1998, A01. (The quotation is from President Clinton, whose words were apparently inspired by the story of Ricka Powers. Powers's tale of woe was sharply contested by her HMO, and the administration eventually dropped the story—but not its abuse of accountants.)

78. For example, Tennessee's TennCare program added new categories of beneficiaries and expanded benefits in the expectation of savings through increased efficiency. Evidence suggests that the program is sustained, not by the magic of managed care, but through stiffing providers. A study commissioned by the state found that TennCare

pays physicians an average of 80 to 90 percent of their costs. Further, HMOs that get into financial trouble delay payments to physicians, exacerbating the problem. Leigh Page, "TennCare at the Crossroads," *American Medical News,* 21 June 1999.

79. See Katherine Boo, "Nonprofits Struggle in a Current of Greed," *Washington Post,* 15 March 1999, A08.

80. R. Adams Dudley, Robert H. Miller, Tamir Y. Korenbrot, and Harold S. Luft, "The Impact of Financial Incentives on Quality of Health Care," *Milbank Quarterly* 76, no. 4 (1998): 649–86; Fred J. Hellinger, "The Effect of Managed Care on Quality," *Archives of Internal Medicine* 158 (1998): 833–41. See also Miles and Koepp, "Comments on the AMA Report," 308, 311, n.11, for additional citations.

81. Edward H. Yelin, Lindsey A. Criswell, and Paul G. Feigenbaum, "Health Care Utilization and Outcomes Among Persons With Rheumatoid Arthritis in Fee-for-Service and Prepaid Group Practice Settings," *JAMA* 276 (1996): 1048–53; Arnold L. Potosky, Ray M. Merrill, Gerald F. Riley, Stephen H. Taplin, William Barlow, Bruce H. Fireman, and Rachel Ballard-Barbash, "Breast Cancer Survival and Treatment in Health Maintenance Organization and Fee-for-Service Settings," *Journal of the National Cancer Institute* 89, no. 22 (1997): 1683–91. HMOs also had the edge in a comparative study of treatment of elderly patients with acute myocardial infarction conducted in Minnesota (where HMOs cannot operate unless they are not-for-profit). Stephen B. Soumerai, Thomas J. McLaughlin, Jerry H. Gurwitz, Steven Pearson, Cindy L. Christiansen, Catherine Borbas, Nora Morris, Barbara McLauglin, Xiaoming Gao, and Dennis Ross-Degnan, "Timeliness and Quality of Care for Elderly Patients With Acute Myocardial Infarction Under Health Maintenance Organization vs Fee-for-Service Insurance," *Archives of Internal Medicine* 159 (1999): 2013–20.

82. However, George Anders and others have been critical of report cards and the measures that make up the Health Plan Employer Data and Information Set or HEDIS: "'HMO report cards . . . are starting to peel back the ignorance of who cures best,'" declared *Fortune* in 1994. But in developing the HEDIS measures, HMOs such as Harvard Community Health Plan were considering what would make them look best. According to a representative of the Plan, "'We said, 'Look, we can develop some measures that will show our value. If we can do that to purchasers' satisfaction, it will give us an advantage in the marketplace.'" Anders, *Health against Wealth,* 41–42.

HEDIS 3.0 does include measures for ongoing care of people with AIDS, diabetes, and other chronic illnesses, and the Foundation for Accountability (FAcct), established by Paul Ellwood, is also working on better outcome measures. NCQA officials have taken some steps to achieve independence from the HMO industry, but Anders reports that as of mid-1996, it was still receiving 40 percent of its funding from HMOs, and HMOs controlled at least one third of the board of directors. There is another kind of industry influence: it is not much good to come up with standards if nobody will use them. One HMO surveyor says, "Our primary business is to sell to the Kaisers and Aetnas and Cignas of the world. We don't want anything in print that would get them irritated." Ibid., 258.

83. John E. Ware, Jr. et al., "Differences in 4–Year Health Outcomes for Elderly and Poor, Chronically Ill Patients Treated in HMO and Fee-for-Service Systems," *JAMA* 276 (1996): 1039–47.

84. See Joseph P. Newhouse, *Free for All? Lessons from the RAND Health Insurance Experiment* (Cambridge, Mass.: Harvard University Press, 1993).

85. Peter Shaughnessy, Robert E. Schlenker, and David F. Hittle, "Home Health Care Outcomes under Capitated and Fee-for-Service Payment," *Health Care Financing Review* 16 (1994): 187–222, 219.

86. Sheldon M. Retchin, Randall S. Brown, Shu-Chuan Jennifer Yeh, Dexter Chu, and Lorenzo Moreno, "Outcomes of Stroke Patients in Medicare Fee for Service and Managed Care," *JAMA* 278 (1997): 119–24. Forty-two percent of those enrolled in HMOs went to nursing homes after their initial hospitalization, versus 28 percent for fee-for-service. No difference was found in death rates, and quality of life was not assessed. Another study reports fewer cataract surgeries for Medicare beneficiaries in HMOs, versus fee-for-service settings, but the findings are somewhat difficult to evaluate given the lack of guidance on an appropriate level of surgeries. Caroline L. Goldzweig, Brian S. Mittman, Grace M.Carter, Tenzing Donyo, Robert H. Brook, Paul Lee, and Carol Mangione, "Variations in Cataract Extraction Rates in Medicare Prepaid and Fee-for-Service Settings," *JAMA* 277 (1997): 1765–68.

It is interesting that while women are estimated to be at 50 percent greater risk of cataract development, in the HMOs they had approximately the same rate of surgeries as men. This data may suggest that surgeries are being inappropriately performed for some men, or, more likely, inappropriately delayed or withheld for some women. See also Lars C. Erickson, David F. Torchiana, Eric C. Schneider, Jane W. Newburger, and Edward L. Hannan, "The Relationship between Managed Care Insurance and Use of Lower-Mortality Hospitals for CABG Surgery," *JAMA* 283 (2000): 1976–82 (concluding that patients in private and Medicare managed care plans in New York were significantly less likely to use lower-mortality hospitals for coronary artery bypass graft surgery than patients with private fee-for-service insurance); Jessica L. Bienstock, Karin J. Blakemore, Eric Wang, Dale Presser, Dawn Misra, and Eva K. Pressman, "Managed Care Does Not Lower Costs but May Result in Poorer Outcomes for Patients with Gestational Diabetes," *American Journal of Obstetrics and Gynecology* 177 (1997): 1035–37 (comparing outcomes at a university house staff clinic and a university-affiliated managed care organization).

87. A nationwide survey of 1,053 doctors and 768 nurses asked respondents about their experiences with and attitudes toward health plans with respect to the under 65 population. Seventy-two percent of doctors and 78 percent of nurses said managed care had decreased the quality of health care for people who are sick. Eighty-three percent of doctors and 85 percent of nurses said managed care had decreased the amount of time spent with patients. Kaiser Family Foundation/Harvard University School of Public Health, *Survey of Physicians and Nurses* (Menlo Park, Calif.: Kaiser Family Foundation, 1999). The survey was conducted between February 11 and June 5 of 1999.

The difficulty, as always, is determining the degree to which this negative assessment derives from experience with patient care versus a sense of threat to professional prerogatives or professional socialization. A 1997 survey of academic physicians and medical students found that 46.6 percent of all faculty members reported that the message they delivered to students about managed care was negative, and 55.8 percent of students and residents reported no positive influences on their attitudes toward managed care. Steven R. Simon, Richard J. D. Pan, Amy M. Sullivan, Nancy Clark-Chiarelli, Maureen T. Connelly, Antoinette S. Peters, Judith D. Singer, Thomas S. Inui, and Susan D. Block, "A Survey of Students, Residents, Faculty, and Deans at Medical Schools in the United States," *New England Journal of Medicine* 340 (1999): 928–36. (In the Kaiser survey, respondents were asked to provide stories of actual harm to patients owing to managed care practices, and these stories go some way in enhancing the credibility of the general assessments.) See also David Mechanic, Donna D. McAlpine, and Marsha Rosenthal, "Are Patients' Office Visits with Physicians Getting Shorter?" *New England Journal of Medicine* 344 (2001): 198–204.

88. Deborah A. Freund and Robert E. Hurley, "Medicaid Managed Care: Contribution to Issues of Health Reform," *Annual Review of Public Health* 16 (1995): 473–95, 487. See also John Holahan, Stephen Zuckerman, Alison Evans, and Suresh Rangarajan, "Medicaid Managed Care in Thirteen States," *Health Affairs* 17, no. 3 (1998): 43–63. The number affected continues to grow. By 1999, 17,756,603 Medicaid beneficiaries (55.59 percent) were enrolled in managed care plans. U.S. Department of Health and Human Services, "National Summary of Medicaid Managed Care Programs and Enrollment," www.hcfa.gov/medicaid/trends99.htm (visited January 29, 2001).

Also, Medicaid managed care has proved an ironic application of the rule "women and children first" (the group that meets criteria for the Aid to Families with Dependent Children or AFDC program). The difficulties affecting quality measurement for the care of low-income populations are reviewed in Sara Rosenbaum, "Protecting Children: Defining, Measuring, and Enforcing Quality in Managed Care," in *Health Care for Children: What's Right, What's Wrong, What's Next*, ed. Ruth E. K. Stein (New York: United Hospital Fund of New York, 1997), 177–98, 186–89. For a positive evaluation of New York's voluntary pilot of Medicaid Managed Care, based on patient satisfaction surveys, see Jane E. Sisk, Sheila A. Gorman, Anne Lenhard Reisinger, Sherry A. Glied, William H. DuMouchel, and Margaret M. Hynes, "Evaluation of Medicaid Managed Care: Satisfaction, Access, and Use" *JAMA* 276 (1996): 50–55.

For a policy analysis of the Oregon and Tennessee Medicaid Managed Care programs, see Marsha Gold, "Markets and Public Programs: Insights from Oregon and Tennessee," *Journal of Health Politics, Policy and Law* 22, no. 2 (1997): 633–66.

89. The "75/25 rule" requiring that at least 25 percent of enrollees in managed care plans participating in Medicaid be privately insured was more of a proxy for direct measures of quality than an attempt to diminish segregation. In any event, the rule has been rescinded. Arnold M. Epstein, "Medicaid Managed Care and High Quality: Can We Have Both?" *JAMA* 278 (1997): 1617–21, 1617. The best we can hope for is that managed care will create a solidarity of misfortune between the lower middle class (consigned to the most restrictive managed care plans by employers) and persons at the very bottom of the social ladder covered by similarly restrictive Medicaid managed care plans. Between these two lies the class of persons now in serious contention for the status of least advantaged: the "medically indigent" with too little income to purchase insurance and too much to qualify for Medicaid.

90. Freund and Hurley, "Medicaid Managed Care," 488–89. One could also mention the hardships and flat-out scandals associated with campaigns to move large numbers of Medicaid beneficiaries into managed care arrangements quickly (Medi-Cal in California in the 1960s, TennCare in Tennessee in the 1990s).

91. Epstein, "Medicaid Managed Care," 1621.

92. In at least one instance, HMO recruiters purchased patient names, addresses, medical records, and income figures from Medicaid clerks. See Schick, "Personal Privacy and Confidentiality."

93. Peter J. Cunningham, "Pressures on the Safety Net: Differences in Access to Care for Uninsured Persons By the Level of Managed Care Penetration and Uninsurance Rate in a Community," *Health Services Research* 34, no. 1 (1999): 255–70. For a

discussion of the effects of managed care on community health centers, see Helen Halpin Schauffler and Jessica Wolin, "Community Health Clinics under Managed Competition: Navigating Uncharted Waters," *Journal of Health Politics, Policy and Law* 21, no. 3 (1996): 461–88. A slightly more hopeful view of the future for community-based providers is presented in Debra J. Tipson, "Medicaid Managed Care and Community Providers: New Partnerships," *Health Affairs* 16, no. 4 (1997): 91–107.

94. Sandra J. Tanenbaum and Robert E. Hurley, "Disability and the Managed Care Frenzy: A Cautionary Note," *Health Affairs* 41, no. 4 (1995): 213–19, 213.

95. Unless another source is indicated, the information presented on CMA derives from Joseph P. Shapiro, "There When You Need It," *U.S. News and World Report*, 5 October 1998, 62–72.

96. See Mary E. Stuart and Michael Weinrich, "Beyond Managing Medicaid Costs: Restructuring Care," *Milbank Quarterly* 76, no. 2 (1998): 251–80, 269.

97. Stuart and Weinrich, "Beyond Managing Medicaid Costs," 251.

98. As of June 1999, CMA had been folded into Neighborhood Health Plan (with Master serving as chief medical officer), and Neighborhood Health Plan had been acquired by Harvard Pilgrim.

99. Oversampling assures that clinically significant issues are not "buried in evaluations of large numbers of well patients." James R. Webster and Joseph Feinglass, "Stroke Patients, 'Managed Care,' and Distributive Justice," *JAMA* 278 (1997): 161–62. A chapter in the final report issued by the President's Advisory Commission is devoted to protection of vulnerable populations. The report reviews study findings that suggest that even those African Americans and Latinos and women who enjoy access to the health care system receive less aggressive care than their white, male counterparts. Targeted performance measures might include appropriate handling of chronic illnesses such as asthma, diabetes, and hypertension that disproportionately affect disadvantaged populations.

100. William Glaser, author of the basic texts on incentives in health care, writes: "At the start of a research project, it is easy to predict that some payment systems control costs, inspire efficiency, and foster good care better than others. Such predictions actually are based on theoretical incentives rather than reality. After studying each payment system's history and after comparing countries, one has to conclude that all these hypotheses fail. Overriding the potentials of all payment systems is how they are administered by governments, payers, hospital managers, and doctors." William A. Glaser, *Paying the Hospital: The Organization, Dynamics, and Effects of Differing Financial Arrangements* (San Francisco: Jossey-Bass, 1987), 375.

CONCLUSION

1. Eliot Freidson, *Professionalism Reborn* (Chicago: University of Chicago Press, 1994), 205, 209.

2. William F. May, *The Physician's Covenant: Images of the Healer in Medical Ethics* (Philadelphia: Westminster Press, 1983), 186.

3. Some commentators have been quick to caution against presenting Minnesota as some sort of managed care nirvana. Minneapolis-St. Paul is not all that far ahead of other markets in terms of the penetration of managed care. Jan Greene, "The Minneapolis Myth," *Hospitals & Health Networks* 71, no. 3 (1997): 56–60. Minnesota is also different from other states in its tradition of social progressivism and in its long history

of engagement with prepaid health plans and group practice. For tales of the beginnings of managed care in Minnesota, see Emily Friedman, "Capitation, Integration, and Managed Care: Lessons from Early Experiments," *JAMA* 275 (1996): 957–62.

4. Jon Christianson, Roger Feldman, Jonathan P. Weiner, and Patricia Drury, "Early Experience with a New Model of Employer Group Purchasing in Minnesota," *Health Affairs* 18, no. 6 (1999): 100–14, 102.

5. Christianson et al., 103, 106. Thus far, the effects of the Choice Plus program have been limited. Participation requires a major investment on the part of an employer, hence the number of enrollees is still quite small. Further, some physicians regard the form of organization required by the program as intrusive—the bureaucrats of the managed care systems have merely been exchanged for the bureaucrats of hospital-based care systems. Physician dissatisfaction may also stem from low reimbursement rates. The program does reflect a strong commitment to risk adjustment, an important step toward eliminating the disincentive to enroll or care for sick people. See Thomas Bodenheimer and Kip Sullivan, "How Large Employers Are Shaping the Health Care Marketplace," *New England Journal of Medicine* 338 (1998): 1084–87. For a more favorable assessment of Choice Plus, and a review of some of the legal and other barriers to direct contracting, see David M. Studdert, "Direct Contracts, Data Sharing and Employee Risk Selection: New Stakes for Patient Privacy in Tomorrow's Health Insurance Markets," *American Journal of Law & Medicine* 25, nos. 2 & 3 (1999): 233–65, 236–44.

6. Participating care systems submit estimated per member per month rates (targets) for providing a standard benefit package. The employee contribution for enrollment in a particular care system is based on its target. At the end of an open enrollment period, the risk profile of the population of patients actually enrolled in a care system is analyzed, resulting in a risk-adjusted target. Risk adjustment is based on diagnosis.

Care systems are paid by the employer on a fee-for-service basis as claims are submitted, so providers bear no immediate risk, but fee schedules are linked to targets. Each quarter, the fee schedule for a particular care system is adjusted upward if actual claims for the preceding period came in under the risk-adjusted target (times three) or downward if actual claims exceeded the risk-adjusted target. Hence providers do capture some of the benefits of prevention through incremental increases in payments for other services. (A lower target made possible by decreased utilization of more expensive services may also confer a competitive advantage because it will translate into a lower employee contribution for enrollment in that care system.) Studdert, "Direct Contracts," 240–41.

7. See Milt Freudenheim, "(Loosely) Managed Health Care Is in Demand," *New York Times*, 29 September 1998, C1.

8. Although accreditation agencies have recently taken an interest in PPOs, most PPOs lack the information that is the basis for accreditation.

9. Cathy A. Schoen and Pamela Davidson, "Image and Reality: Managed Care Experiences by Type of Plan," *Bulletin of the New York Academy of Medicine* 73 (Winter Supp. 1996): 506–31, 528. Respondents were asked to rate their health plan and physician. Questions concerning plans addressed overall satisfaction, quality of service, emergency care availability, choice of doctors, ease of changing doctors, availability of advice by phone, access to specialists, reasonableness of fees, coverage of preventive care, and amount of paperwork. The survey, which was commissioned by the Commonwealth Fund and conducted by Louis Harris and associates, also found considerable variation between cities, with managed care members in Miami and Los Angeles much

more likely to rate their plans as fair or poor on a range of measures. See "A Survey of Patients in Managed Care and Fee-for-Service Settings: Survey Highlights": http://www.cmwf.org/programs/health_care/mgdcrhlt.asp (visited April 1999).

Also, where studies of processes or outcomes of care disaggregate findings in order to identify differences by organizational type, staff and group model HMOs appear to outperform the more popular IPA model HMOs. See Mark R. Wicclear, "What Can Be Learned about the Ethical Soundness of Medicare HMOs From Studies Comparing Them to Fee-for-Service Medicare?" *Journal of Ethics, Law, and Aging* 5, no. 1 (1999): 29–48, 44. A survey of physicians at three plans in the Minneapolis-St. Paul area found that those affiliated with a staff model HMO rated their plan more highly on quality and access to specialty and mental health care than physicians associated with two network model HMOs. Steven J. Borowsky, Margaret K. Davis, Christine Goertz, and Nicole Lurie, "Are All Health Plans Created Equal? The Physician's View," *JAMA* 278 (1997): 917–21. A recent analysis of HEDIS data found that staff- and group-model HMOs scored better than IPA, network, and mixed HMOs on virtually all measures of quality. David U. Himmelstein, Steffie Woolhandler, Ida Hellander, and Sidney M. Wolfe, "Quality of Care in Investor-Owned vs Not-for-Profit HMOs," *JAMA* 282 (1999): 159–63, 161.

On the other hand, a number of consumer surveys have found higher satisfaction with PPOs than managed care plans identified as "strict" based on consumer self-report of plan characteristics. See, e.g., Henry J. Kaiser Family Foundation, *National Survey of Consumer Experiences with Health Plans* (Menlo Park, Calif.: Henry J. Kaiser Family Foundation, 2000) (consumers in strict managed care plans, meaning a plan with a network *and* a gatekeeper, reported more problems than consumers with other types of health insurance); "Is an HMO for You?" *Consumer Reports* 65, no. 7 (2000): 38–41, 39 (readers of Consumer Reports were less satisfied with traditional HMOs than with HMOs with a point-of-service option or PPOs). Also, a number of studies have concluded that open-model systems, i.e., plans that do not contract with physicians on an exclusive basis, perform better on measures of patient-physician relationship than closed model systems such as group- and staff-model HMOs. For example, a study of Massachusetts state employees found that staff-model HMOs consistently underperformed other types of health plans on measures of access to care, continuity of care, comprehensiveness of care, integration of care, clinical interaction, interpersonal relationship, and trust. Dana Gelb Safran, William H. Rogers, Alvin R. Tarlov, Thomas Inui, Deborah A. Taira, Jana E. Montgomery, John E. Ware and Charles P. Slavin, "Organizational and Financial Characteristics of Health Plans: Are They Related to Primary Care Performance?" *Archives of Internal Medic*ine 160 (2000): 69–76.

10. See, e.g., Health Care Advisory Board, *Future Revenues* (Washington, D.C.: The Advisory Board Company, 1997); Harris Meyer, "Focused Factories," *Hospitals & Health Networks* 72, no. 7 (April 5, 1998): 25–30.

11. The Community Toolbox is a creation of the University of Kansas, on the Internet at ctb.lsi.ukans.edu (visited August 10, 1999). The mission of the site is "To promote community health and development by connecting people, ideas, and resources." The site includes over 3,000 downloadable pages on topics such building capacity for community change and involving people most affected by a problem. The Community Problem-Solving Guide is a detailed, step-by-step roadmap for problem-solving that proceeds from community assessment (describing the community and its vision and

identifying the problem) to in-depth analysis of the problem (identifying root causes and personal and environmental factors affecting its development) to strategic planning and intervention (identifying targets of change and how to reach them and identifying barriers, resources, and stakeholders) to evaluation and institutionalization.

12. Esther B. Fein, "For Many Physicians, E-Mail Is the High-Tech House Call," *New York Times*, 20 November 1997, A1. Of course, an e-mail message is not the appropriate vehicle for communication of a diagnosis. It is suitable for some areas of communication, and unsuitable for others.

13. "About Health Commons Institute," www.healthcommons.org/links/abouthci.html (visited August 10, 1999).

14. See David Blumenthal, "The Future of Quality Measurement and Management in a Transforming Health Care System," *JAMA* 278 (1997): 1622–25. Speculation on the effects of new information technologies on the organization of health care and medical practice closed Stanley Reiser's classic *Medicine and the Reign of Technology*. Reiser thought that new information systems might support greater centralization *and* decentralization in health care, but in his closing he emphasized the humane potential of the information revolution. Stanley Joel Reiser, *Medicine and the Reign of Technology* (Cambridge: Cambridge University Press, 1995), 226, 231.

15. For a projection of a very dark future for health care, see Peter MacPherson, "Is This Where We Want to Go?" *Hastings Center Report* 27, no. 6 (1997): 17–22.

16. Richard Smith, Howard Hiatt, and Donald Berwick, "A Shared Statement of Ethical Principles for Those Who Shape and Give Health Care: A Working Draft from the Tavistock Group," *Annals of Internal Medicine* 130 (1999): 143–47, 145. On later developments, see Frank Davidoff, "Changing the Subject: Ethical Principles for Everyone in Health Care," *Annals of Internal Medicine* 133: 386–89.

17. Himmelstein et al., "Quality of Care," 162.

18. Ken Garber, "Business Unusual," *Hospitals and Health Networks* 73, no. 2 (1999): 55–58.

19. Theodore R. Marmor, "Hype and Hyperbole: The Rhetoric and Reality of Managerial Reform in Health Care," *Journal of Health Services Research and Policy* 3, no. 1 (1998): 62–64, 64.

20. See Diana Chapman Walsh, *Corporate Physicians: Between Medicine and Management* (New Haven: Yale University Press, 1987).

21. Smith, Hiatt, and Berwick, "Shared Statement," 146.

22. The substantial numbers of physicians who report using deception to obtain coverage for services should not be a point of pride for the profession. See Kaiser Family Foundation/Harvard University School of Public Health, *Survey of Physicians and Nurses* (Menlo Park, Calif.: Kaiser Family Foundation, 1999). For an argument against the traditional "Darwinian" model of advocacy, and a promising first step toward a new model of proportional advocacy, see Steven B. Pearson, "Caring and Cost: The Challenge for Physician Advocacy," *Annals of Internal Medicine* 133: 148–53.

23. Ivan Illich used the term "specific counterproductivity" to capture the boomerang effect of technologies pursued to their logical extremes, e.g., the ways in which the expansion of modern technological medicine served to erode the capacities of individuals and communities for health and well-being. The idea is pursued in Elliot S. Fisher and H. Gilbert Welch, "Avoiding the Unintended Consequences of Growth in Medical Care: How Might More Be Worse?" *JAMA* 281 (1999): 446–53. Among other things,

Fisher and Welch suggest that technology assessment should include an analysis of how the broader population might be affected by a system change, with an eye out for unintended consequences.

24. James S. Goodwin, "Geriatrics and the Limits of Modern Medicine," *New England Journal of Medicine* 340 (1999): 1283–85. Note that one reason the elderly have rarely been found in trials is structural: Medicare payment restrictions. Also, one can imagine a trial that assesses the contribution of time, if not empathy, to outcomes. Yet even clinical trials more inclusive in terms of participation and aims would fail to capture important aspects of medicine.

25. For example, studies documenting wide local variation in utilization of health care services without apparent justification precipitated the crisis of confidence in physician judgment and supported the shift to managed care and to bureaucratic controls. Problems associated with managed care, and more particularly, capitation, have spurred research concerning risk adjustment methodologies. With advances in diagnostic adjustment, at least some of the variation in intensity of service across geographic regions is beginning to appear reasonable.

As two health services researchers remark, "The average 75-year-old man in Miami may in fact be substantially sicker than the 75-year-old man in Minneapolis." Tony Dreyfus and Richard Kronick, "Paying Plans to Care for People with Chronic Illness," in *Making Managed Care Work for the Chronically Ill*, ed. Richard Kronick and Joy de Beyer (Chicago: Health Administration Press, 1999), 27–66, 59. For an interesting analysis of the association of managed care with science and objectivity, asking, among other things, how practice variation came to be defined as a problem, see Gary S. Belkin, "The Technocratic Wish: Making Sense and Finding Power in the 'Managed' Medical Marketplace," *Journal of Health Politics, Policy and Law* 22, no. 2 (1998): 509–32.

26. Joseph P. Shapiro, "There When You Need It," *U.S. News and World Report* (October 5, 1998), 62–72.

27. Smith, Hiatt, and Berwick, "Shared Statement," 147.

28. Lisa Disch, "Publicity-Stunt Participation and Sound Bite Polemics: The Health Care Debate 1993–94," *Journal of Health Politics, Policy and Law* 27, no. 1 (1996): 3–33.

29. Darrell M. West, Diane Heith, and Chris Goodwin, "Harry and Louise Go to Washington: Political Advertising and Health Care Reform," *Journal of Health Politics, Policy and Law* 27, no. 1 (1996): 35–68, 64.

30. See Howard M. Leichter, "Oregon's Bold Experiment," *Journal of Health Politics, Policy and Law* 24, no. 1 (1999): 147–60; Lawrence Jacobs, Theodore Marmor, and Jonathan Oberlander, "The Oregon Health Plan and the Political Paradox of Rationing: What Advocates and Critics Have Claimed and What Oregon Did," *Journal of Health Politics, Policy and Law* 24, no. 1 (1999): 161–80.

31. See Chapter 5, note 81.

32. California Health Decisions, *Partners in Healthcare: Consumer Input, Consumer Impact* (Orange, Calif.: California Health Decisions, 1999), 4.

33. May, *Physician's Covenant*, 180–81.

BIBLIOGRAPHY

Addelson, Kathryn Pyne. "Some Moral Issues in Public Problems of Reproduction." *Social Problems* 37, no. 1 (1990): 1–17.

Advisory Commission on Consumer Protection and Quality in the Health Care Industry. *Consumer Bill of Rights and Responsibilities,* November 20, 1997.

———. *Quality First: Better Health Care for All Americans.* Washington, D.C.: U.S. Government Printing Office, 1998.

Alford, Robert R. *Health Care Politics.* Chicago: University of Chicago Press, 1975.

American College of Healthcare Executives. *Code of Ethics.* Chicago: American College of Healthcare Executives, 1994.

———. *Ethical Decision Making for Healthcare Executives.* Chicago: American College of Healthcare Executives, 1997.

American Medical Association. "First Code of Medical Ethics." In *Ethics in Medicine: Historical Perspectives and Contemporary Concerns,* ed. Stanley J. Reiser, Arthur J. Dyck, and William J. Curran, 26–34. Cambridge, Mass.: MIT Press, 1977.

Anders, George. *Health Against Wealth: HMOs and the Breakdown of Medical Trust.* New York: Houghton Mifflin, 1996.

Anderson, Charles W. *Pragmatic Liberalism.* Chicago: University of Chicago Press, 1990.

Annas, George. "Transferring the Ethical Hot Potato." *Hastings Center Report* 17, no. 1 (1987): 20–21.

Aquinas, Thomas. *On Law, Morality and Politics.* Edited by William P. Baumgarth and Richard J. Regan. Indianapolis: Hackett Publishing Co., 1988.

Ashley, Benedict M., and Kevin D. O'Rourke. *Health Care Ethics: A Theological Analysis.* 4th ed. Washington, D.C.: Georgetown University Press, 1997.

Avorn, Jerry, and Daniel H. Solomon. "Cultural and Economic Factors That (Mis)Shape Antibiotic Use: The Nonpharmacologic Basis of Therapeutics." *Annals of Internal Medicine* 133 (2000): 128–35.

Baggs, Judith Gedney, Sheila A. Ryan, Charles E. Phelps, J. Franklin Richeson, and Jean E. Johnson. "The Association between Interdisciplinary Collaboration and Patient Outcomes in a Medical Intensive Care Unit." *Heart & Lung* 21, no. 1 (1992): 18–24.

Barber, Benjamin R. *Strong Democracy: Participatory Politics for a New Age.* Berkeley: University of California Press, 1984.

Barr, Donald A. "The Effects of Organizational Structure on Primary Care Outcomes under Managed Care." *Annals of Internal Medicine* 122 (1995): 353–59.

Beatty, Jack. "Combating Violence." *Foundation News & Commentary* 35, no. 3 (1994): 24–29.

Beauchamp, Tom L., and James F. Childress. *Principles of Biomedical Ethics.* 4th ed. New York: Oxford University Press, 1994.

Beck, Arne, John Scott, Patrick Williams, Barbara Robertson, Deborrah Jackson,

Glenn Gade, and Pamela Cowan. "A Randomized Trial of Group Outpatient Visits for Chronically Ill Older HMO Members: The Cooperative Health Care Clinic." *Journal of the American Geriatrics Society* 45 (1997): 543–49.

Belkin, Gary S. "The Technocratic Wish: Making Sense and Finding Power in the 'Managed' Medical Marketplace." *Journal of Health Politics, Policy and Law* 22, no. 2 (1998): 509–32.

Bellah, Robert N., Richard Madsen, William M. Sullivan, Ann Swidler, and Steven M. Tipton. *The Good Society*. New York: Knopf, 1991.

Benhabib, Seyla. "Afterword: Communicative Ethics and Current Controversies in Practical Philosophy." In *The Communicative Ethics Controversy*, ed. Seyla Benhabib and Fred Dallmayr, 339–69. Cambridge, Mass.: MIT Press, 1990.

———. "The Generalized and the Concrete Other." In *Women and Moral Theory*, ed. Eva Feder Kittay and Diana T. Meyers, 154–77. Totowa, N.J.: Rowman & Littlefield, 1987.

———. "The Methodological Illusions of Modern Political Theory: The Case of Rawls and Habermas." *Neue Hefte Für Philosophie* 21 (1982): 47–74.

———. *Situating the Self*. Cambridge: Polity Press, 1992.

Benjamin, Jessica. *The Bonds of Love*. New York: Pantheon Books, 1988.

Bentham, Jeremy. *An Introduction to the Principles of Morals and Legislation* (excerpts). In *Utilitarianism and Other Essays*, ed. Alan Ryan, 65–111. Hammondshire, England: Penguin Books, 1987.

Berenson, Robert A. "A Physician's View of Managed Care." *Health Affairs* 10, no. 4 (1991): 106–19.

Beresford, Eric B. "Uncertainty and the Shaping of Medical Decisions." *Hastings Center Report* 21, no. 4 (1991): 6–11.

Bernstein, Richard J. *Philosophical Profiles: Essays in a Pragmatic Mode*. Cambridge: Polity Press, 1986.

Berwick, Donald M. "Payment By Capitation and the Quality of Care." *New England Journal of Medicine* 335 (1996): 1227–31.

Biblo, Joan D., Myra J. Christopher, Linda Johnson, and Robert Lyman Potter. *Ethical Issues in Managed Care: Guidelines for Clinicians and Recommendations to Accrediting Organizations*. Kansas City, Mo.: Midwest Bioethics Center, 1995.

Bienstock, Jessica L., Karin J. Blakemore, Eric Wang, Dale Presser, Dawn Misra, and Eva K. Pressman. "Managed Care Does Not Lower Costs but May Result in Poorer Outcomes for Patients with Gestational Diabetes." *American Journal of Obstetrics and Gynecology* 177 (1997): 1035–37.

Bloche, M. Gregg. "Clinical Loyalties and the Social Purposes of Medicine." *JAMA* 281 (1999): 268–74.

———. "Fidelity and Deceit at the Bedside." *JAMA* 283 (2000): 1881–84.

Blumenthal, David. "The Future of Quality Measurement and Management in a Transforming Health Care System." *JAMA* 278 (1997): 1622–25.

Blumenthal, David, and Arnold M. Epstein. "The Role of Physicians in the Future of Quality Management." *New England Journal of Medicine* 335 (1996): 1328–31.

Bodenheimer, Thomas. "Selective Chaos." *Health Affairs* 19, no. 4 (2000): 200–5.

Bodenheimer, Thomas S., and Kevin Grumbach. "Capitation or Decapitation: Keeping Your Head in Changing Times." *JAMA* 276 (1996): 1025–31.

Bodenheimer, Thomas, and Kip Sullivan. "How Large Employers Are Shaping the Health Care Marketplace." *New England Journal of Medicine* 338 (1998): 1084–87.

Bibliography

Bodenheimer, Thomas, and Lawrence Casalino. "Executives with White Coats: The Work and World View of Managed-Care Medical Directors." *New England Journal of Medicine* 341 (1999): 1945–48.

Bogardus, Stanley T., Jr., Eric Holmboe, and James F. Jekel, "Perils, Pitfalls, and Possibilities in Talking about Medical Risk." *JAMA* 281 (1999): 1037–41.

Borowsky, Steven J., Margaret K. Davis, Christine Goertz, and Nicole Lurie. "Are All Health Plans Created Equal? The Physician's View." *JAMA* 278 (1997): 917–21.

Boston Women's Health Book Collective. *The New Our Bodies, Ourselves.* New York: Simon & Schuster, 1992.

Boudon, Raymond. *The Unintended Consequences of Social Action.* New York: St. Martin's Press, 1982.

Boyle, Philip J., and Daniel Callahan, eds. *What Price Mental Health?: The Ethics and Politics of Setting Priorities.* Washington, D.C.: Georgetown University Press, 1995.

Brewer, Kathryn Balstad. "Management as a Practice: A Response to Alasdair MacIntyre." *Journal of Business Ethics* 16, no. 8 (1997): 825–33.

Brodeur, Dennis. "Health Care Institutional Ethics: Broader Than Clinical Ethics." In *Health Care Ethics: Critical Issues,* ed. John F. Monagle and David C. Thomasma, 358–65. Gaithersburg, Md.: Aspen Publishers, 1994.

Brodie, Mollyann, Lee Ann Brady, and Drew E. Altman. "Media Coverage of Managed Care: Is There a Negative Bias?" *Health Affairs* 17, no. 1 (1998): 9–34.

Brody, Howard. *The Healer's Power.* New Haven, Conn.: Yale University Press, 1992.

Brown, Lawrence D. *Politics and Health Care Organization: HMOs as Federal Policy.* Washington, D.C.: The Brookings Institution, 1983.

Brownlea, Arthur. "Participation: Myths, Realities and Prognosis." *Social Science and Medicine* 25, no. 6 (1987): 605–14.

Bulger, Roger J. "Covenant, Leadership, and Value Formation in Academic Health Centers." In *Integrity in Health Care Institutions,* ed. Ruth Ellen Bulger and Stanley Joel Reiser, 3–17. Iowa City: University of Iowa Press, 1990.

Burns, Lawton R., John Cacciamani, James Clement, and Welman Aquino. "The Fall of the House of AHERF: The Allegheny Bankruptcy." *Health Affairs* 19, no. 1 (2000): 7–41.

California Health Decisions. *Partners in Healthcare: Consumer Input, Consumer Impact.* Orange, Calif.: California Health Decisions, 1999.

Callahan, Joan C. "Professions, Institutions, and Moral Risk." In *Professional Ethics and Social Responsibility,* ed. Daniel E. Wueste, 243–70. London: Rowman & Littlefield, 1994.

Campbell, James. *Understanding John Dewey: Nature and Cooperative Intelligence.* Chicago: Open Court Publishing Co., 1995.

Capron, Alexander Morgan. "Between Doctor and Patient." *Hastings Center Report* 26, no. 5 (1996): 23–24.

———. "Oregon's Disability: Principles or Politics?" *Hastings Center Report* 22, no. 6 (1992): 18–20.

Cerne, Frank. "Cash Kings." *Hospitals & Health Networks* 69, no. 7 (1995): 51–54.

Chambliss, Daniel F. *Beyond Caring: Hospitals, Nurses, and the Social Organization of Ethics.* Chicago: University of Chicago Press, 1996.

Charles, Cathy and Suzanne DeMaio. "Lay Participation in Health Care Decision Making: A Conceptual Framework." *Journal of Health Politics, Policy and Law* 18, no. 4 (1993): 881–904.

Bibliography

Christianson, Jon, Roger Feldman, Jonathan P. Weiner, and Patricia Drury. "Early Experience with a New Model of Employer Group Purchasing in Minnesota." *Health Affairs* 18, no. 6 (1999): 100–14.

Coddington, Dean C., Keith D. Moore, and Elizabeth A. Fischer. *Making Integrated Health Care Work.* Englewood, Colo.: Center for Research in Ambulatory Health Care Administration, 1996.

Congressional Budget Office. *Trends in Health Care Spending by the Private Sector.* Washington, D.C.: Congressional Budget Office, 1997.

Connor, Eileen, and Fitzhugh Mullan, eds. *Community Oriented Primary Care: New Directions for Health Policy.* Washington, D.C.: National Academy Press, 1983.

Conrad, Douglas A., Charles Maynard, Allen Cheadle, Scott Ramsey, Miriam Marcus-Smith, Howard Kirz, Carolyn A. Madden, Diane Martin, Edward B. Perrin, Thomas Wickizer, Brenda Zierler, Austin Ross, Jay Noren, and Su-Ying Liang. "Primary Care Physician Compensation Method in Medical Groups." *JAMA* 279 (1998): 853–58.

Copeland, Craig, and Bill Pierron. "Implications of ERISA for Health Benefits and the Number of Self-Funded ERISA Plans." Issue Brief, Employee Benefit Research Institute, January 1998.

Council on Ethical and Judicial Affairs, American Medical Association. "Ethical Issues in Managed Care." *JAMA* 273 (1995): 330–35.

Crowley, Walt. *To Serve the Greatest Number: A History of Group Cooperative of Puget Sound.* Seattle: University of Washington Press, 1996.

Cunningham, Peter J. "Pressures on the Safety Net: Differences in Access to Care for Uninsured Persons by the Level of Managed Care Penetration and Uninsurance Rate in a Community." *Health Services Research* 34, no. 1 (1999): 255–70.

Daly, Herman E., and John B. Cobb, Jr. *For the Common Good.* Boston: Beacon Press, 1989.

Daniels, Norman, Donald W. Light, and Ronald L. Caplan. *Benchmarks of Fairness for Health Care Reform.* New York: Oxford University Press, 1996.

Daniels, Norman, and James Sabin. "Last Chance Therapies and Managed Care: Pluralism, Fair Procedures, and Legitimacy." *Hastings Center Report* 28, no. 2 (1998): 27–41.

———. "Limits to Health Care: Fair Procedures, Democratic Deliberation, and the Legitimacy Problem for Insurers." *Philosophy & Public Affairs* 26, no. 4 (1997): 303–50.

Davidoff, Frank. "Changing the Subject: Ethical Principles for Everyone in Health Care." *Annals of Internal Medicine* 133: 148–53.

Davies, Allyson Ross, and John E. Ware, Jr. "Involving Consumers in Quality of Care Assessment." *Health Affairs* 7, no. 1 (1988): 33–48.

De Sousa, Ronald. *The Rationality of Emotion.* Cambridge, Mass.: MIT Press, 1987.

Dewey, John. *Freedom and Culture.* New York: G. P. Putnam, 1939.

———. *The Later Works: 1925–1953,* ed. Jo Ann Boydston. 17 vols. Carbondale: Southern Illinois University Press, 1981–90.

———. *The Middle Works: 1899–1924,* ed. Jo Ann Boydston. 15 vols. Carbondale: Southern Illinois University Press, 1976–83.

———. *The Public and Its Problems.* New York: Henry Holt and Company, 1927. Reprint, Athens, Ohio: Swallow Press, 1980.

Dewey, John, and James Hayden Tufts. *Ethics.* New York: Henry Holt, 1909.

DiMaggio, Paul J., and Walter W. Powell. "The Iron Cage Revisited: Institutional Isomorphism and Collective Rationality in Organizational Fields." *American Sociological Review* 48 (1983): 147–60.

Disch, Lisa. "Publicity-Stunt Participation and Sound Bite Polemics: The Health Care Debate 1993–94." *Journal of Health Politics, Policy and Law* 27, no. 1 (1996): 3–33.

Dobson, John. "MacIntyre's Position on Business: A Response to Wicks." *Business Ethics Quarterly* 7, no. 4 (1997): 125–32.

Dougherty, Charles J. *Back to Reform: Values, Markets, and the Health Care System.* New York: Oxford University Press, 1996.

Dreyfus, Hubert L., and Stuart E. Dreyfus. "From Socrates to Expert Systems: The Limits of Calculative Rationality." In *Interpretive Social Science: A Second Look,* ed. Paul Rabinow and William M. Sullivan, 327–50. Berkeley: University of California Press, 1987.

Dreyfus, Tony, and Richard Kronick. "Paying Plans to Care for People with Chronic Illness." In *Making Managed Care Work for the Chronically Ill,* ed. Richard Kronick and Joy de Beyer, 27–66. Chicago: Health Administration Press, 1999.

Dudley, R. Adams, Robert H. Miller, Tamir Y. Korenbrot, and Harold S. Luft. "The Impact of Financial Incentives on Quality of Health Care." *Milbank Quarterly* 76, no. 4 (1998): 649–86.

Eddy, David M. "Applying Cost-effectiveness Analysis: The Inside Story." *JAMA* 268 (1992): 2575–82.

———. "Broadening the Responsibilities of Practitioners: The Team Approach." *JAMA* 269 (1993): 1849–55.

———. "Principles for Making Difficult Decisions in Difficult Times." *JAMA* 271 (1994): 1792–98.

Edgman-Levitan, Susan, and Paul D. Cleary. "What Information Do Consumers Want And Need?" *Health Affairs* 15, no. 4 (1996): 42–56.

Elhauge, Einer. *Allocating Health Care Morally.* 82 Calif. L. Rev. 1449 (1994).

Emanuel, Ezekiel J. *The Ends of Human Life.* Cambridge, Mass.: Harvard University Press, 1991.

———. "Medical Ethics in the Era of Managed Care: The Need for Institutional Structures Instead of Principles for Individual Cases." *Journal of Clinical Ethics* 6, no. 4 (1995): 335–38.

Emanuel, Ezekiel J., and Nancy Neveloff Dubler. "Preserving the Physician-Patient Relationship in the Era of Managed Care." *JAMA* 273, no. 4 (1995): 323–29.

Emanuel, Ezekiel J., and Linda L. Emanuel. "Preserving Community in Health Care." *Journal of Health Politics, Policy and Law* 22 (1997): 147–84.

Emergency Care Research Institute. *High Dose Chemotherapy with Autologous Bone Marrow Transplantation and/or Blood Cell Transplantation for the Treatment of Metastatic Breast Cancer.* Technology Assessment Custom Report Level 2. Plymouth Meeting, Pa.: ECRI, March 1994.

Engelhardt, H. Tristram, Jr. *The Foundations of Bioethics.* 2nd ed. New York: Oxford University Press, 1996.

Engelhardt, H. Tristram, Jr. and Michael A. Rie. "Morality for the Medical-Industrial Complex: A Code of Ethics for the Mass Marketing of Health Care." *New England Journal of Medicine* 319 (1988): 1086–89.

Epstein, Arnold M. "Medicaid Managed Care and High Quality: Can We Have Both?" *JAMA* 278 (1997): 1617–21.

Erikson, Erik H. *Identity: Youth and Crisis.* New York: W. W. Norton & Co., 1963.

Erickson, Lars C., David F. Torchiana, Eric C. Schneider, Jane W. Newburger, and Edward L. Hannan. "The Relationship between Managed Care Insurance and Use of Lower-Mortality Hospitals for CABG Surgery." *JAMA* 283 (2000): 1976–82.

Etheredge, Lynn, Stanley Jonz, and Lawrence Lewin, "What Is Driving Health System Change?" *Health Affairs* 15, no. 4 (1996): 93–104.

Fagin, Claire M. "Collaboration between Nurses and Physicians: No Longer a Choice." *Academic Medicine* 67, no. 5 (1992): 295–303.

Farrell, Margaret G. "ERISA Preemption and Regulation of Managed Health Care." *American Journal of Law & Medicine* 23 (1997): 251–89.

Felder, Michael. "Can Ethics Committees Work in Managed Care Plans?" *Bioethics Forum* 12, no. 1 (1996): 10–15.

———. "An Ethics Committee for a Health Maintenance Organization: An Oxymoron? Certainly Not." *H.E.C. Forum* 4 (1992): 261–67.

Fins, Joseph J., Franklin G. Miller, and Matthew D. Bacchetta. "Clinical Pragmatism: Bridging Theory and Practice." *Kennedy Institute of Ethics Journal,* 8, no. 1 (1998): 37–42.

Fisher, Elliot S., and H.Gilbert Welch,. "Avoiding the Unintended Consequences of Growth in Medical Care: How Might More Be Worse?" *JAMA* 281 (1999): 446–53.

Flanagan, Owen. *Varieties of Moral Personality.* Cambridge, Mass.: Harvard University Press, 1991.

Fleck, Leonard M. *Just Health Care Rationing: A Democratic Decisionmaking Approach.* 140 University of Pennsylvania Law Review 1597 (1992).

Frankena, William K. *Ethics.* 2nd ed. Englewood Cliffs: Prentice-Hall, 1973.

Freidson, Eliot. *Doctoring Together.* New York: Elsevier, 1975.

———. *Medical Work in America.* New Haven: Yale University Press, 1989.

———. *Professionalism Reborn.* Chicago: University of Chicago Press, 1994.

Freire, Paulo. *Pedagogy of Hope: Reliving Pedagogy of the Oppressed.* Trans. Robert R. Barr. New York: Continuum, 1994.

Freund, Deborah A., and Robert E. Hurley. "Medicaid Managed Care: Contribution to Issues of Health Reform." *Annual Review of Public Health* 16 (1995): 473–95.

Friedland, Roger, and Robert R. Alford. "Bringing Society Back In: Symbols, Practices, and Institutional Contradictions." In *The New Institutionalism in Organizational Analysis,* ed. Walter W. Powell and Paul J. DiMaggio, 232–63. Chicago: University of Chicago Press, 1991.

Friedman, Emily. "Capitation, Integration, and Managed Care: Lessons from Early Experiments." *JAMA* 275 (1996): 957–62.

———. "A Matter of Value: Profits and Losses in Healthcare." *Health Progress* 77, no. 3 (1996): 28–34, 48.

Friedman, Milton. "The Social Responsibility of Business Is to Increase Its Profits." *New York Times Magazine,* 13 September 1970, 122–26.

Fuchs, Victor R. "Managed Care and the Merger Mania." *JAMA* 277 (1997): 920–21.

Garg, Pushkal P., Kevin D. Frick, Marie Diener-West, and Neil R. Powe. "Effects of the Ownership of Dialysis Facilities on Patients' Survival and Referral for Transplantation." *New England Journal of Medicine* 341 (1999): 1653–60.

Gervais, Karen G., Reinhard Priester, Dorothy E. Vawter, Kimberly K. Otte, and Mary M. Solberg, ed. *Ethical Challenges in Managed Care.* Washington, D.C.: Georgetown University Press, 1999.

Bibliography

Giacomini, Mita, Harold S. Luft, and James C. Robinson. "Risk Adjusting Community-Rated Health Plan Premiums: A Survey of Risk Assessment Literature and Policy Applications." *Annual Review of Public Health* 16 (1995): 401–30.

Gibbs, Deborah A., Judith A. Sangl, and Barri Burrus. "Consumer Perspectives on Information Needs for Health Plan Choice." *Health Care Financing Review* 18, no. 1 (1996): 55–73.

Giddens, Anthony. *Central Problems in Social Theory.* Berkeley: University of California Press, 1979.

Ginzburg, Eli. "Managed Care and the Competitive Market in Health Care: What They Can and Cannot Do." *JAMA* 277 (1997): 1812–13.

Glaser, William A. *Paying the Hospital: The Organization, Dynamics, and Effects of Differing Financial Arrangements.* San Francisco: Jossey-Bass, 1987.

Glassman, Peter A., Peter D. Jacobson, and Steven Asch. "Medical Necessity and Defined Coverage Benefits in the Oregon Health Plan." *American Journal of Public Health* 87 (1997): 1053–58.

Gold, Marsha. "Markets and Public Programs: Insights from Oregon and Tennessee." *Journal of Health Politics, Policy and Law* 22, no. 2 (1997): 633–66.

Gold, Marsha R., Robert Hurley, Timothy Lake, Todd Ensor, and Robert Berenson. "A National Survey of the Arrangements Managed-Care Plans Make with Physicians." *New England Journal of Medicine* 333 (1995): 1678–83.

Gold, Marsha R., Louise B. Russell, Joanna E. Siegel, and Milton C. Weinstein, ed. *Cost-Effectiveness in Health and Medicine.* New York: Oxford University Press, 1996.

Goldzweig, Caroline L., Brian S. Mittman, Grace M. Carter, Tenzing Donyo, Robert H. Brook, Paul Lee, and Carol Mangione. "Variations in Cataract Extraction Rates in Medicare Prepaid and Fee-for-Service Settings." *JAMA* 277 (1997): 1765–68.

Goodpaster, Kenneth E., and John B. Matthews, Jr. "Can a Corporation Have a Conscience?" In Kenneth E. Goodpaster. *Ethics in Management.* Boston: HBS Case Services, 1984, 145–54. Originally published in *Harvard Business Review* (January–February 1982).

Goodwin, James S. "Geriatrics and the Limits of Modern Medicine." *New England Journal of Medicine* 340 (1999): 1283–85.

Goold, Susan D. "Allocating Health Care: Cost-Utility Analysis, Informed Democratic Decision Making, or the Veil of Ignorance." *Journal of Health Politics, Policy and Law* 21, no. 1 (1996): 69–98.

Goold, Susan D., and Howard Brody. "Rationing Decisions in Managed Care Settings: An Ethical Analysis." In *Health Care Crisis? The Search for Answers,* ed. Robert I. Misbin, Bruce Jennings, David Orentlicher, and Marvin Dewar, 135–64. Frederick, Md.: UPG, 1995.

Gray, Bradford H. *The Profit Motive and Patient Care: The Changing Accountability of Doctors and Hospitals.* Cambridge, Mass.: Harvard University Press, 1991.

Gray, Bradford H., ed. *For-Profit Enterprise in Health Care.* Washington, D.C.: National Academy Press, 1986.

Greene, Jan. "Has Managed Care Lost Its Soul?" *Hospitals & Health Networks* 71, no. 10 (1997): 36–42.

———. "The Minneapolis Myth." *Hospitals & Health Networks* 71, no. 3 (1997): 56–60.

Greenfield, Sheldon, Sherrie Kaplan, and John E. Ware. "Expanding Patient Involvement in Care: Effects on Patient Outcomes." *Annals of Internal Medicine* 102 (1985): 520–28.

———. "Controlling Costs: The Case of Kaiser." *JAMA* 274 (1995): 1135.

Grumbach, Kevin, Dennis Osmond, Karen Vranizan, Deborah Jaffee, and Andrew Bindman. "Primary Care Physicians' Experience of Financial Incentives in Managed-Care Systems." *New England Journal of Medicine* 339 (1998): 1516–21.

Grumbach, Kevin, Joe V. Selby, Cheryl Damberg, Andrew B. Bindman, Charles Quesenberry, Jr., Alison Truman, and Connie Uratsu. "Resolving the Gatekeeper Conundrum: What Patients Value in Primary Care and Referrals to Specialists." *JAMA* 282 (1999): 261–66.

Gunn, Giles. "Pragmatism, Democracy, and the Imagination: Rethinking the Deweyan Legacy." In *Pragmatism: From Progressivism to Postmodernism*, ed. David Depew, 298–313. Westport: Praeger, 1995.

Gutting, Gary. *Pragmatic Liberalism and the Critique of Modernity*. New York: Cambridge University Press, 1999.

Hagland, Mark. "Dangling Modifiers." *Hospitals & Health Networks* 71, no. 7 (1997): 70–74.

Halévy, Elie. *The Growth of Philosophic Radicalism*. Translated by May Morris. New York: Macmillan, 1928.

Hall, Mark A. "Informed Consent to Rationing Decisions." *Milbank Quarterly* 71, no. 4 (1993): 645–68.

———. *Making Medical Spending Decision: The Law, Ethics, and Economics of Rationing Mechanisms*. New York: Oxford University Press, 1997.

———. *A Theory of Economic Informed Consent*. Georgia Law Review 31 (1997): 511–86.

Hall, Robert M. *An Introduction to Healthcare Organizational Ethics*. New York: Oxford University Press, 2000.

Halm, Ethan A., Nancyanne Causino, and David Blumenthal. "Is Gatekeeping Better Than Traditional Care? A Survey of Physicians' Attitudes." *JAMA* 278 (1997): 1677–81.

Handy, Charles. "Balancing Corporate Power: A New Federalist Paper." *Harvard Business Review* 70 (November–December 1992): 59–72.

Hasan, Malik M. "Let's End the Nonprofit Charade." *New England Journal of Medicine* 334 (1996): 1055–57.

Haste, Helen. "Morality, Self, and Sociohistorical Context: The Role of Lay Social Theory." In *The Moral Self*, ed. Gil G. Noam and Thomas E. Wren, 175–208. Cambridge, Mass.: MIT Press, 1993.

Hatch, John W., and Eugenia Eng. "Community Participation and Control: or Control of Community Participation." In Victor W. Sidel and Ruth Sidel, eds., *Reforming Medicine: Lessons of the Last Quarter Century*, 223–44. New York: Pantheon Books, 1984.

Haughton, James G. "Determinants of the Culture and Personality of Institutions." In *Integrity in Health Care Institutions*, ed. Ruth Ellen Bulger and Stanley Joel Reiser, 141–47. Iowa City: University of Iowa Press, 1990.

Health Care Advisory Board. *Future Revenues*. Washington, D.C.: The Advisory Board Company, 1997.

Health Policy Tracking Service. *State Managed Care Laws: A State-by-State Review*. Washington, D.C.: National Conference of State Legislatures, 1999.

Hegarty, Mary Loyola. *Serving With Gladness: The Origin and History of the Congregation of the Sisters of Charity of the Incarnate Word, Houston, Texas*. Milwaukee: Bruce Publishing Co., 1967.

Heitman, Elizabeth, and Ruth Ellen Bolger. "The Healthcare Ethics Committee in the Structural Transformation of Health Care: Administrative and Organizational Ethics in Changing Times." *HEC Forum* 10, no. 2 (1998): 152–76.

Hellinger, Fred J. "The Effect of Managed Care on Quality." *Archives of Internal Medicine* 158 (1998): 833–41.

Henry J. Kaiser Family Foundation. *For-Profit Health Care Companies: Trends and Issues.* Menlo Park, Calif.: Henry J. Kaiser Family Foundation, 1998.

Henry J. Kaiser Family Foundation. *National Survey of Consumer Experiences with Health Plans.* Menlo Park, Calif.: Kaiser Family Foundation, 2000.

———. *Kaiser/Harvard National Survey of Americans' Views of Managed Care.* Menlo Park, Calif.: Henry J. Kaiser Family Foundation, 1997.

Hillman, Alan L. "Health Maintenance Organizations, Financial Incentives, and Physician's Judgments." *Annals of Internal Medicine* 112 (1990): 891–93.

———. "Managing the Physician: Rules Versus Incentives." *Health Affairs* 10, no. 4 (1991): 138–46.

———. "Mediators of Patient Trust." *JAMA* 280 (1998): 1703–4.

Hillman, Alan L., Mark V. Pauly, and Joseph J. Kerstein. "How Do Financial Incentives Affect Physicians' Clinical Decisions and the Financial Performance of Health Maintenance Organizations?" *New England Journal of Medicine* 321 (1989): 86–92.

Himmelstein, David U., Steffie Woolhandler, Ida Hellander, and Sidney M. Wolfe. "Quality of Care in Investor-Owned vs Not-for-Profit HMOs." *JAMA* 282 (1999): 159–63.

Hirschman, Albert O. *The Passions and the Interests: Political Arguments for Capitalism before Its Triumph.* Princeton, N.J.: Princeton University Press, 1977.

Hirst, Paul. *Associative Democracy: New Forms of Economic and Social Governance.* Amherst: University of Massachusetts Press, 1994.

Holahan, John, Stephen Zuckerman, Alison Evans, and Suresh Rangarajan. "Medicaid Managed Care in Thirteen States." *Health Affairs* 17, no. 3 (1998): 43–63.

Horton, Richard. "After Bezwoda." *The Lancet* 355 (2000): 942–43.

Huff, Charlotte. "Back-to-School Bonus." *Hospitals & Health Networks* 72, no. 20 (1998): 20.

Iglehart, John K. "Changing Course in Turbulent Times: An Interview with David Lawrence." *Health Affairs* 13, no. 5 (1994): 65–77.

———. "Listening In On the Duke University Private Sector Conference." *New England Journal of Medicine* 336 (1997): 1827–31.

———. "Managed Care." *New England Journal of Medicine* 327 (1992): 742–47.

Illich, Ivan. *Medical Nemesis: The Expropriation of Health.* New York: Pantheon Books, 1982.

Illingworth, Patricia. "Bluffing, Puffing and Spinning in Managed-Care Organizations." *Journal of Medicine and Philosophy* 25, no. 1 (2000): 62–76.

Isaacs, Stephen L. "Consumers' Information Needs: Results of a National Survey." *Health Affairs* 15, no. 4 (1996): 31–41.

Jackall, Robert. *Moral Mazes: The World of Corporate Managers.* New York: Oxford University Press, 1988.

Jackson, Debra, and Maree Raftos. "In Uncharted Waters: Confronting the Culture of Silence in a Residential Care Institution." *International Journal of Nursing Practice* 3, no. 1 (1997): 34–39.

Jameton, Andrew. "Dilemmas of Moral Distress: Moral Responsibility and Nursing

Practice." *AWHONNS Clinical Issues in Perinatal and Women's Health Nursing* 4, no. 4 (1993): 542–51.

Jansen, Lynn A. "Assessing Clinical Pragmatism." *Kennedy Institute of Ethics Journal* 8, no. 1 (1998): 23–36.

Jecker, Nancy S., and Albert R. Jonsen. "Managed Care: A House of Mirrors." *Journal of Clinical Ethics* 8, no. 3 (1997): 230–41.

Joas, Hans. *Pragmatism and Social Theory*. Chicago: University of Chicago Press, 1993.

Joint Commission on the Accreditation of Heathcare Organizations. *1996 Comprehensive Accreditation Manual for Hospitals*. Oakbrook Terrace, Ill.: JCAHO, 1995.

Jollis, James G., Elizabeth R. DeLong, Eric D. Peterson, Lawrence H. Muhlbaier, Donald F. Fortin, Robert M. Califf, and Daniel B. Mark. "Outcome of Acute Myocardial Infarction According to the Specialty of the Admitting Physician." *New England Journal of Medicine* 335 (1996): 1880–87.

Jonsen, Albert R. "Barbarians at the Gates: Medicine, Money, and Morality." *Ophthalmology* 99 (1992): 162–64.

———. *The New Medicine and the Old Ethics*. Cambridge, Mass.: Harvard University Press, 1990.

Kaiser Family Foundation/Harvard University School of Public Health. *Survey of Physicians and Nurses*. Menlo Park, Calif.: Kaiser Family Foundation, 1999.

Kao, Audiey C., Diane C. Green, Alan M. Zaslavsky, Jeffrey P. Koplan, and Paul D. Cleary. "The Relationship Between Method of Physician Payment and Patient Trust." *JAMA* 280 (1998): 1708–14.

Kapur, Kanika, Geoffrey F. Joyce, Krista A. Van Vorst, and Jose J. Escarce. "Expenditures for Physician Services under Alternative Models of Managed Care." *Medical Care Research and Review* 57, no. 2 (2000): 161–81.

Kass, Leon R. "Practicing Ethics: Where's the Action?" *Hastings Center Report* 20, no. 1 (1990): 5–12.

Katz, Jay. *The Silent World of Doctor and Patient*. New York: Free Press, 1984.

Kaufman-Osborn, Timothy V. *Politics/Sense/Experience: A Pragmatic Inquiry into the Promise of Democracy*. Ithaca, N.Y.: Cornell University Press, 1991.

Kelly, Susan E., and Barbara A. Koenig. "'Rescue' Technologies following High-Dose Chemotherapy for Breast Cancer: How Social Context Shapes the Assessment of Innovative, Aggressive, and Lifesaving Medical Technologies." In *Getting Doctors to Listen: Ethics and Outcomes Data in Context*, ed. Philip J. Boyle, 127–52. Washington, D.C.: Georgetown University Press, 1998.

Kelman, Steven. "Cost-Benefit Analysis: An Ethical Critique." *Regulation* 5, no. 1 (1981): 33–40.

Kenkel, Donald, Mark Berger, and Glenn Blomquist. "Contingent Valuation of Health." In *Valuing Health for Policy: An Economic Approach*, ed. George Tolley, Donald Kenkel, and Robert Fabian, 72–104. Chicago: University of Chicago Press, 1994.

Kitahata, Mari M., Thomas D. Koepsell, Richard A. Deyo, Clare L. Maxwell, Wayne T. Dodge, and Edward H. Wagner. "Physicians' Experience with the Acquired Immunodeficiency Syndrome as a Factor in Patients' Survival." *New England Journal of Medicine* 334 (1996): 701–6.

Kofman, Fred and Peter M. Senge. "Communities of Commitment: The Heart of Learning Organizations." *Organizational Dynamics* 22, no. 2 (1993): 5–23.

Kohn, Linda T., Janet M. Corrigan, and Molla S. Donaldson, eds. *To Err Is Human: Building a Safer Health System*. Washington, D.C.: National Academy Press, 2000.

Kretzmann, John P., and John L. McKnight. *Building Communities from the Inside Out: A Path Toward Finding and Mobilizing a Community's Assets.* Evanston, Ill.: Institute for Policy Research, 1993.

Kuttner, Robert. "Columbia/HCA and the Resurgence of the For-Profit Hospital Business." *New England Journal of Medicine* 335 (1996): 446–51.

———. "The Corporation in America: Is It Socially Redeemable?" *Dissent* 40, no. 1 (1993): 35–49.

———. "Must Good HMOs Go Bad?" (Parts I & II) *New England Journal of Medicine* 338 (1998): 1558–63, 1635–39.

Larson, Erik. "The Soul of an HMO." *Time,* 22 January 1996, 44–52.

Lasch, Christopher. *The True and Only Heaven: Progress and Its Critics.* New York: Norton, 1991.

Lassen, April A., Donna M. Fosbinder, Stephen Minton, and M. Mureno Robins. "Nurse/Physician Collaborative Practice: Improving Health Care Quality While Decreasing Cost." *Nursing Economics* 15, no. 2 (1997): 87–91, 104.

Latham, Stephen R. "Regulation of Managed Care Incentive Payments to Physicians." *American Journal of Law & Medicine* 22, no. 4 (1996): 399–432.

Leape, Lucian L. "Error in Medicine." *JAMA* 272 (1994): 1851–57.

Leape, Lucien L., David D. Woods, Martin J. Hatlie, Kenneth W. Kizer, Steven A. Schroeder, and George D. Lundberg. "Promoting Patient Safety by Preventing Medical Error." *JAMA* 280 (1998): 1444–47.

LeGrand, Julian. "Equity versus Efficiency: The Elusive Trade-Off." *Ethics* 100, no. 3 (1990): 554–68.

Leiser, Burton M. "The Rabbinic Tradition and Corporate Morality." In *The Judeo-Christian Vision and the Modern Business Corporation,* ed. Oliver Williams and John Houck, 141–58. Notre Dame, Ind.: University of Notre Dame Press, 1982.

Lewinsohn-Zamir, Daphna. *Consumer Preferences, Citizen Preferences, and the Provision of Public Goods.* 108 Yale Law Journal 377 (1998).

Lewis, Randall J. Letter to the Editor. *New England Journal of Medicine* 333 (1995): 1220.

Light, Donald W. "Escaping the Traps of Postwar Western Medicine." *European Journal of Public Health* 3 (1993): 281–89.

———. "Reforming America's Health System: Origins and Dilemmas." Transcript of lectures delivered Nov. 14–18, 1994 at the University of Texas-Houston Health Science Center (HPI Discussion Paper no. 7). Houston, Tex.: Health Policy Institute, University of Texas-Houston Health Science Center, 1996.

Lindorff, Dave. *Marketplace Medicine: The Rise of For-Profit Hospital Chains.* New York: Bantam Books, 1992.

Linzer, Mark et al. "Managed Care, Time Pressure, and Physician Job Satisfaction: Results from the Physician Worklife Study." *Journal of General Internal Medicine* 15 (2000): 441–50.

Lumsdon, Kevin. "Working Smarter, Not Harder." *Hospitals & Health Networks* 69, no. 21 (1995): 27–31.

MacIntyre, Alasdair. *After Virtue: A Study in Moral Theory.* 2nd ed. Notre Dame, Ind.: University of Notre Dame Press, 1984.

———. "The End of Ideology and the End of the End of Ideology." In *Against the Self-Images of the Age: Essays on Ideology and Philosophy.* New York: Schocken Books, 1971.

———. "Why are the Problems of Business Ethics Insoluble?" In *Moral Responsibility and the Professions,* ed. Bernard Baumrin and Benjamin Freedman, 350–59. New York: Haven Publications, 1983.

Macklin, Ruth. *Enemies of Patients.* New York: Oxford University Press, 1993.

———. "The Ethics of Managed Care." *Trends in Health Care, Law & Ethics* 10, no. 1/2 (1995): 63–66.

MacPherson, Peter. "Is This Where We Want to Go?" *Hastings Center Report* 27, no. 6 (1997): 17–22.

Mahowald, Mary Briody. *An Idealistic Pragmatism.* The Hague: Martinus Nijhoff, 1972.

———. "On Treatment of Myopia: Feminist Standpoint Theory and Bioethics." In *Feminism & Bioethics: Beyond Reproduction,* ed. Susan M. Wolf, 95–115. New York: Oxford University Press, 1996.

Malone, Thomas W. "Is Empowerment Just a Fad? Control, Decision Making, and IT." *Sloan Management Review* 38, no. 2 (1997): 23–35.

Mariner, Wendy K. "Business vs. Medical Ethics: Conflicting Standards for Managed Care." *Journal of Law, Medicine & Ethics* 23, no. 3 (1995): 236–46.

———. "Standards of Care and Standard Form Contracts: Distinguishing Patient Rights and Consumer Rights in Managed Care." *Journal of Contemporary Health Law and Policy* 15, no. 1 (1998): 1–55.

———. "State Regulation of Managed Care and the Employee Retirement Income Security Act." *New England Journal of Medicine* 335 (1996): 1986–90.

———. "What Recourse? Liability for Managed-Care Decisions and the Employee Retirement Income Security Act." *New England Journal of Medicine* 343 (2000): 592–96.

Marmor, Theodore R. "Hype and Hyperbole: The Rhetoric and Reality of Managerial Reform in Health Care." *Journal of Health Services Research and Policy* 3, no. 1 (1998): 62–64.

Marquis, M. Susan. "Consumers' Knowledge about Their Health Insurance Coverage." *Health Care Financing Review* 5 (1983): 65–80.

Marshall, Martin N., Paul G. Shekelle, Sheila Leatherman, and Robert H. Brook. "The Public Release of Performance Data." *JAMA* 283 (2000): 1866–74.

Marx, Karl. *Capital.* Vol. 2. London: Swan, Sonnenschein, Lowrey & Co., 1887.

May, William F. "Code, Covenant, Contract, or Philanthropy?" *Hastings Center Report* 5, no. 6 (1975): 29–38.

———. "Money and the Medical Profession." *Kennedy Institute of Ethics Journal* 7, no. 1 (1997): 1–13.

———. *The Physician's Covenant: Images of the Healer in Medical Ethics.* Philadelphia: Westminster Press, 1983.

———. "The Virtues in a Professional Setting." *Soundings* 67, no. 3 (1984): 245–66.

McArthur, John H. and Francis D. Moore. "The Two Cultures and the Health Care Revolution: Commerce and Professionalism in Medical Care." *JAMA* 277 (1997): 985–89.

McCann, Dennis P. "Toward a Theology of the Corporation: A Second Chance for Catholic Social Teaching." In *Catholic Social Thought and the New World Order,* ed. Oliver F. Williams and John W. Houck, 329–50. Notre Dame, Ind.: University of Notre Dame Press, 1993.

McGee, Glenn. *The Perfect Baby: A Pragmatic Approach to Genetics.* New York: Rowman & Littlefield, 1997.

Bibliography

McGee, Glenn, ed. *Pragmatic Bioethics*. Nashville, Tenn.: Vanderbilt University Press, 1999.

McKnight, John. *The Careless Society: Community and Its Counterfeits*. New York: Basic Books, 1995.

Mechanic, David. "Managed Care as a Target of Distrust." *JAMA* 277 (1997): 1810–11.

———. "Rationing of Medical Care and the Preservation of Clinical Judgment." *Journal of Family Practice* 11 (1980): 431–33.

———. "Trust and Informed Consent to Rationing." *Milbank Quarterly* 72, no. 2 (1994): 217–23.

Mechanic, David, Donna D. McAlpine, and Marsha Rosenthal. "Are Patients' Office Visits with Physicians Getting Shorter?" *New England Journal of Medicine* 344 (2001): 198–204.

Mechanic, David, and Mark Schlesinger. "The Impact of Managed Care on Patients' Trust in Medical Care and Their Physicians." *JAMA* 275 (1996): 1693–97.

Melhado, Evan M. "Economic Theory, Economists, and the Formulation of Health Policy." *Journal of Health Politics, Policy and Law* 25, no. 1 (2000): 233–54.

Menzel, Paul, Marsha R. Gold, Erik Nord, Jose-Louis Pinto-Prades, Jeff Richardson, and Peter Ubel. "Toward a Broader View of Values in Cost-Effectiveness Analysis of Health." *Hastings Center Report* 29, no. 3 (1999): 7–15.

Merton, Robert K. *Mass Persuasion: The Social Psychology of a War Bond Drive*. New York: Harper, 1946.

Meyer, Harris. "Focused Factories." *Hospitals & Health Networks*, 72, no. 7 (April 5, 1998): 25–30.

———. "The Right to Appeal." *Hospitals & Health Network* 72, no. 9 (1998): 23–26.

Michels, Robert. *Political Parties*. Glencoe, Ill.: Free Press, 1949.

Miles, Steven H. "New Business for Ethics Committees." *H.E.C. Forum* 4, no. 2 (1992): 97–102.

Miles, Steven H., and Robert Koepp. "Comments on the AMA Report 'Ethical Issues in Managed Care.'" *Journal of Clinical Ethics* 6, no. 4 (1995): 306–11.

Miles, Steven H., and Ruth A. Mickelsen. "Introduction: Managed Care: New Institutions and Time-Honored Values." *Journal of Law, Medicine & Ethics* 23, no. 3 (1995): 221–22.

Millenson, Michael L. *Demanding Medical Excellence: Doctors and Accountability in the Information Age*. Chicago: University of Chicago Press, 1997.

Miller, Franklin G., Joseph J. Fins, and Matthew D. Bacchetta. "Clinical Pragmatism: John Dewey and Clinical Ethics." *Journal of Contemporary Health Law and Policy* 13, no. 1 (1996): 27–51.

Miller, Tracy E., and Carol R. Horowitz. "Disclosing Doctors' Incentives: Will Consumers Understand and Value the Information." *Health Affairs* 19, no. 4 (2000): 149–55.

Miller, Tracy E., and William M. Sage. "Disclosing Physician Financial Incentives." *JAMA* 281 (1999): 1424–30.

Milner, Murray, Jr. *Unequal Care*. New York: Columbia University Press, 1980.

Montoya, Isaac D., and Alan J. Richard. "A Comparative Study of Codes of Ethics in Health Care Facilities and Energy Companies." *Journal of Business Ethics* 13, no. 9 (1994): 713–17.

Moody-Adams, Michele. "On the Old Saw That Character Is Destiny." In *Identity,*

Character, and Morality: Essays in Moral Psychology, ed. Owen Flanagan and Amélie Oksenberg Rorty, 111–31. Cambridge, Mass.: MIT Press, 1990.

Morreim, E. Haavi. *Balancing Act: The New Medical Ethics of Medicine's New Economics.* Dordrecht: Kluwer Academic Publishers, 1991.

———. "Moral Justice and Legal Justice in Managed Care: The Ascent of Contributive Justice." *Journal of Law, Medicine & Ethics* 23, no. 3 (1995): 247–65.

———. "To Tell the Truth: Disclosing the Incentives and Limits of Managed Care." *American Journal of Managed Care* 3 (1997): 35–43.

Mullan, Fitzhugh. "Sam Ho, MD: Idealist, Innovator, Entrepreneur, in Conversation with Fitzhugh Mullan, MD." *JAMA* 281 (1999): 947–51.

Mycek, Sheri. "Triage for Trouble Spots." *Hospitals & Health Networks* 72, no. 7 (1998): 40–41.

Nagel, Jack H. *Combining Deliberation and Fair Representation in Community Health Decisions.* 140 University of Pennsylvania Law Review 1965 (1992).

National Conference of Catholic Bishops. "Pastoral Letter on Health and Health Care." *Origins* 11, no. 25 (1981): 400–2.

Nelson, James Lindemann. "Moral Teachings from Unexpected Quarters." *Hastings Center Report* 30, no. 1 (2000): 12–17.

Newhouse, Joseph P. *Free for All? Lessons from the RAND Health Insurance Experiment.* Cambridge, Mass.: Harvard University Press, 1993.

Niebuhr, Reinhold. "The Christian Faith and the Economic Life of Liberal Society." In *Faith and Politics,* ed. Ronald H. Stone, 139–64. New York: George Braziller, 1968.

———. "Man's Selfhood in Its Self-Seeking and Self-Giving." In *Man's Nature and His Communities.* New York: Scribner's, 1965.

———. *Moral Man and Immoral Society.* New York: Scribner's, 1944.

The 1996 Health Network & Alliance Sourcebook. Washington, D.C.: Faulkner & Gray's Healthcare Information Center, 1996.

Nozick, Robert. *Anarchy, State, and Utopia.* New York: Basic Books, 1974.

———. *The Examined Life: Philosophical Meditations.* New York: Simon and Schuster, 1989.

Nussbaum, Martha C. *The Fragility of Goodness: Luck and Ethics in Greek Tragedy and Philosophy.* Cambridge: Cambridge University Press, 1986.

Nwachukwu, Saviour L. S., and Scott J. Vitell, Jr. "The Influence of Corporate Culture in Managerial Ethical Judgments." *Journal of Business Ethics* 16, no. 8 (1997): 757–76.

Olson, Kristi, and Jane Perkins. *Recommendations for Making the Consumers' Voice Heard in Medicaid Managed Care: A Guide to Effective Consumer Involvement.* Washington, D.C.: National Health Law Program, 1999.

O'Neill, Onora. *Towards Justice and Virtue.* Cambridge: Cambridge University Press, 1996.

Orlowski, James P., and Leon Wateska. "The Effects of Pharmaceutical Firm Enticements on Physician Prescribing Patterns." *Chest* 102, no. 1 (1992): 270–73.

O'Rourke, Kevin D., and Philip Boyle. *Medical Ethics: Sources of Catholic Teaching.* 2nd ed. Washington, D.C.: Georgetown University Press, 1993.

Paine, Lynn Sharp. "Managing for Organizational Integrity." *Harvard Business Review* 72 (March–April 1994): 106–17.

Pauly, Mark V. *Medical Care at Public Expense: A Study in Applied Welfare Economics.* New York: Praeger, 1971.

Pearson, Steven D. "Caring and Cost: The Challenge for Physician Advocacy." *Annals of Internal Medicine* 133: 148–53.

Pearson, Steven D., James E. Sabin, and Ezekial J. Emanuel. "Ethical Guidelines for Physician Compensation Based on Capitation." *New England Journal of Medicine* 339 (1998): 689–93.

Pellegrino, Edmund D., and David Thomasma. *A Philosophical Basis of Medical Practice.* New York: Oxford University Press, 1981.

Pentz, Rebecca D. "Beyond Case Consultation: An Expanded Model for Organizational Ethics." *Journal of Clinical Ethics* 10, no. 1 (1999): 34–41.

Peppin, John F. "Business Ethics and Health Care: The Re-emerging Institution-Patient Relationship." *Journal of Medicine and Philosophy* 24, no. 5 (1999): 535–50.

Perkins, Jane, Kristi Olson, Lourdes Rivera, and Julie Skatrud. *Making the Consumers' Voice Heard in Medicaid Managed Care: Increasing Participation, Protection and Satisfaction.* Washington, D.C.: National Health Law Program, 1996.

Perrow, Charles. *Complex Organizations: A Critical Essay.* 3rd ed. New York: Random House, 1986.

Peters, William P., and Mark C. Rogers. "Variation in Approval by Insurance Companies of Coverage for Autologous Bone Marrow Transplantation for Breast Cancer." *New England Journal of Medicine* 330 (1994): 473–477.

Pfeffer, Jeffrey. "Six Dangerous Myths about Pay." *Harvard Business Review* 76, no. 3 (1998): 109–19.

Pont, Edward A. "The Culture of Physician Autonomy; 1900 to the Present." *Cambridge Quarterly of Healthcare Ethics* 9, no. 1 (2000): 98–119.

Porter, Jean. *Moral Action and Christian Ethics.* Cambridge: Cambridge University Press, 1995.

Porter, Roger J. "Conflicts of Interest in Research: The Fundamentals." In *Biomedical Research: Collaboration and Conflict of Interest,* ed. Roger J. Porter and Thomas E. Malone, 121–34. Baltimore: Johns Hopkins University Press, 1992.

Potosky, Arnold L., Ray M. Merrill, Gerald F. Riley, Stephen H. Taplin, William Barlow, Bruce H. Fireman, and Rachel Ballard-Barbash. "Breast Cancer Survival and Treatment in Health Maintenance Organization and Fee-for-Service Settings." *Journal of the National Cancer Institute* 89, no. 22 (1997): 1683–91.

Potter, Robert Lyman. "An Integrated Ethics Program for Managed Care Organizations." *Trends in Health Care, Law & Ethics* 10, no. 1/2 (1995): 87–90.

Povar, Gail, and Jonathan Moreno. "Hippocrates and the Health Maintenance Organization." *Annals of Internal Medicine* 109 (1988): 419–24.

Quinn, J. Kevin, J. David Reed, M. Neil Browne, and Wesley J. Hiers. "Honesty, Individualism, and Pragmatic Business Ethics: Implications for Corporate Hierarchy." *Journal of Business Ethics* 16 (1997): 1419–30.

Rabkin, Mitchell T. "The Hospital-Academic Health Center Interface: The Community of Practice and the Community of Learning." In *Integrity in Health Care Institutions,* ed. Ruth Ellen Bulger and Stanley Joel Reiser, 130–40. Iowa City: University of Iowa Press, 1990.

Rabkin, Mitchell T., and Laura Avakian. "Participatory Management at Boston's Beth Israel Hospital." *Academic Medicine* 67, no. 5 (1992): 289–294.

Rawls, John. *A Theory of Justice.* Cambridge: Belknap Press, 1971.

———. "Two Concepts of Rules." *Philosophical Review* 64, no. 1 (1995): 3–32.

Regan, Alycia C. "Regulating the Business of Medicine: Models for Integrating Ethics and Managed Care." *Columbia Journal of Law and Social Problems* 30 (1997): 635–84.

Reinhardt, Uwe E. "The Rise and Fall of the Physician Practice Management Industry." *Health Affairs* 19, no. 1 (2000): 42–55.

———. "Wanted: A Clearly Articulated Social Ethics for American Health Care." *JAMA* 278 (1997): 1446–47.

Reiser, Stanley Joel. "Administrative Case Rounds." *JAMA* 266 (1991): 2127–28.

———. "Complicated Interactions." *Hastings Center Report* 24, no. 3 (1994): 48.

———. "The Era of the Patient: Using the Experience of Illness in Shaping the Missions of Health Care." *JAMA* 269 (1993): 1012–17.

———. "The Ethical Life of Health Care Organizations." *Hastings Center Report* 24, no. 6 (1994): 28–35.

———. *Medicine and the Reign of Technology.* Cambridge: Cambridge University Press, 1995.

Relman, Arnold S., and Uwe Reinhardt. "An Exchange on For-Profit Health Care." In *For-Profit Enterprise in Health Care*, ed. Bradford H. Gray, 209–23. Washington, D.C.: National Academy Press, 1986.

Retchin, Sheldon M., Randall S. Brown, Shu-Chuan Jennifer Yeh, Dexter Chu, and Lorenzo Moreno. "Outcomes of Stroke Patients in Medicare Fee for Service and Managed Care." *JAMA* 278 (1997): 119–24.

Rhodes, Rosamond, and James J. Strain. "Trust and Transforming Medical Institutions." *Cambridge Quarterly of Healthcare Ethics* 9, no. 2 (2000): 205–17.

Robinson, James C. "The Dynamics and Limits of Corporate Growth in Health Care." *Health Affairs* 15, no. 2 (1996): 155–69.

———. "Use and Abuse of the Medical Loss Ratio to Measure Health Plan Performance." *Health Affairs* 16, no. 4 (1997): 176–87.

Rochefort, David. "The Role of Anecdotes in Regulating Managed Care." *Health Affairs* 17, no. 6 (1998): 142–49.

Rocky Mountain Center for Healthcare Ethics. *Code of Ethics for Managed Care in Colorado: Working Document.* Denver, Colo.: Rocky Mountain Center for Healthcare Ethics, 1997.

Rodwin, Marc A. "Conflicts in Managed Care." *New England Journal of Medicine* 332 (1995): 604–607.

———. *Medicine, Money and Morals: Physicians' Conflicts of Interest.* New York: Oxford University Press, 1993.

Rosenbaum, Sara. "Protecting Children: Defining, Measuring, and Enforcing Quality in Managed Care." In *Health Care for Children: What's Right, What's Wrong, What's Next*, ed. Ruth E. K. Stein, 177–198. New York: United Hospital Fund of New York, 1997.

Rosenberg, Charles E. *The Care of Strangers: The Rise of America's Hospital System.* New York: Basic Books, 1987.

Rosner, David. *A Once Charitable Enterprise: Hospitals and Health Care in Brooklyn and New York, 1885–1915.* Cambridge: Cambridge University Press, 1982.

Rothman, David J. "Medical Professionalism: Focusing on the Real Issues." *New England Journal of Medicine* 342 (2000): 1284–86.

Ryan, Alan. *John Dewey and the High Tide of American Liberalism.* New York: W. W. Norton & Company, 1995.

Sabin, James E. and Carlos Neu. "Real World Resource Allocation: The Concept of 'Good-Enough' Psychotherapy." *Bioethics Forum* 12, no. 1 (1996): 3–9.

Safran, Dana Gelb, William H. Rogers, Alvin R. Tarlov, Thomas Inui, Deborah A. Taira, Jana E. Montgomery, John E. Ware and Charles P. Slavin. "Organizational and Financial Characteristics of Health Plans: Are They Related to Primary Care Performance?" *Archives of Internal Medicine* 160 (2000): 69–76.

Sage, William M. "Regulating through Information: Disclosure Laws and American Health Care." 99 Columbia Law Review 1701 (1999).

St. Peter, Robert F., Marie C. Reed, Peter Kemper, and David Blumenthal. "Changes in the Scope of Care Provided by Primary Care Physicians." *New England Journal of Medicine* 341 (1999): 1980–85.

Schauffler, Helen Halpin and Jessica Wolin. "Community Health Clinics under Managed Competition: Navigating Uncharted Waters." *Journal of Health Politics, Policy and Law* 21, no. 3 (1996): 461–88.

Schick, Ida Critelli. "Personal Privacy and Confidentiality in an Electronic Environment." *Bioethics Forum* 12, no. 1 (1996): 25–30.

Schlesinger, Mark. "Countervailing Agency: A Strategy of Principled Regulation under Managed Competition." *Milbank Quarterly* 75, no. 1 (1997): 35–87.

———. "Paradigms Lost: The Persisting Search for Community in U.S. Health Policy." *Journal of Health Politics, Policy and Law* 22, no. 4 (1997): 937–92.

Schlesinger, Mark, Bradford Gray, Gerard Carrino, Mary Duncan, Michael Gusmano, Vincent Antonelli, and Jennifer Stuber, "A Broader Vision for Managed Care, Part 2: A Typology of Community Benefits." *Health Affairs* 17, no. 5 (1998): 26–49.

Schneider, Carl E. *The Practice of Autonomy: Patients, Doctors, and Medical Decisions.* New York: Oxford University Press, 1998.

Schoen, Cathy A., and Pamela Davidson. "Image and Reality: Managed Care Experiences by Type of Plan." *Bulletin of the New York Academy of Medicine* 73 (Winter Supp. 1996): 506–31.

Schriger, David L., Larry J. Baraff, William H. Rogers, and Shan Cretin. "Implementation of Clinical Guidelines Using a Computer Charting System: Effects on the Initial Care of Healthcare Workers Exposed to Body Fluids." *JAMA* 278 (1997): 1585–90.

Scott, Richard. *Organizations: Rational, Natural, and Open Systems.* 3rd ed. Englewood Cliffs, N.J.: Prentice-Hall, 1992.

Scott, Robert A., Linda H. Aiken, David Mechanic, and Julius Moravcsik. "Organizational Aspects of Caring." *Milbank Quarterly* 73, no. 1 (1995): 77–93.

Scovern, Henry. "Hired Help: A Physician's Experiences in a For-Profit Staff-Model HMO." *New England Journal of Medicine* 319, no. 12 (1988): 787–90.

Selznick, Philip. *The Moral Commonwealth: Social Theory and the Promise of Community.* Berkeley: University of California Press, 1992.

———. *TVA and the Grass Roots: A Study in the Sociology of Formal Organization.* New York: Harper Torchbooks, 1966. Originally published in 1949 by the University of California Press.

Serb, Chris. "More Than Medicine." *Health & Hospital Networks* 73, no. 8 (1999): A-4–A-5.

Shadid, Michael A. *Crusading Doctor: My Fight for Cooperative Medicine.* Boston: Meador Pub. Co., 1956. Reprint, Norman, Okla. and London: University of Oklahoma Press, 1992.

Shapiro, Joseph P. "There When You Need It." *U.S. News and World Report*, 5 October 1998, 62–72.

Shapiro, Robyn S., Kristen A. Tym, Jeffrey L. Gudmundson, Arthur R. Derse, and John P. Klein. "Managed Care: Effects on the Physician-Patient Relationship." *Cambridge Quarterly of Healthcare Ethics* 9, no. 1 (2000): 71–81.

Shaughnessy, Peter, Robert E. Schlenker, and David F. Hittle. "Home Health Care Outcomes Under Capitated and Fee-for-Service Payment." *Health Care Financing Review* 16 (1994): 187–222.

Sheils, John, and Paul Hogan. "Cost of Tax-Exempt Health Benefits in 1998." *Health Affairs* 18, no. 2 (1999): 176–79.

Shortell, Stephen M., Robin R. Gillies, David A. Anderson, Karen Morgan Erickson, and John B. Mitchell. *Remaking Health Care in America: Building Organized Delivery Systems.* San Francisco: Jossey-Bass, 1996.

Silberner, Joanne. "Competition Threatens Survival of Catholic Hospitals." National Public Radio Morning Edition (March 12, 1996), 16–18 (transcript).

Simon, Steven R., Richard J. D. Pan, Amy M. Sullivan, Nancy Clark-Chiarelli, Maureen T. Connelly, Antoinette S. Peters, Judith D. Singer, Thomas S. Inui, and Susan D. Block. "A Survey of Students, Residents, Faculty, and Deans at Medical Schools in the United States." *New England Journal of Medicine* 340 (1999): 928–36.

Singer, Lawrence E. "The Conversion Conundrum: The State and Federal Response to Hospitals' Changes in Charitable Status." *American Journal of Law & Medicine* 23 (1997): 221–50.

Sisk, Jane E., Sheila A. Gorman, Anne Lenhard Reisinger, Sherry A. Glied, William H. DuMouchel, and Margaret M. Hynes. "Evaluation of Medicaid Managed Care: Satisfaction, Access, and Use." *JAMA* 276 (1996): 50–55.

Smith, Adam. *The Wealth of Nations,* ed. Edwin Cannan. Chicago: University of Chicago Press, 1976.

Smith, John E. "The Value of Community: Dewey and Royce." *Southern Journal of Philosophy* 12, no. 4 (1974): 469–79.

Smith, Richard, Howard Hiatt, and Donald Berwick. "A Shared Statement of Ethical Principles for Those Who Shape and Give Health Care: A Working Draft from the Tavistock Group." *Annals of Internal Medicine* 130 (1999): 143–47.

Solomon, Robert C. *Ethics and Excellence: Cooperation and Integrity in Business.* New York: Oxford University Press, 1992.

———. *A Passion for Justice: Emotions and the Origins of the Social Contract.* New York: Addison-Wesley Publishing, 1990.

———. *The Passions.* New York: Anchor Press/Doubleday, 1976.

Soumerai, Stephen B., Thomas J. McLaughlin, Jerry H. Gurwitz, Steven Pearson, Cindy L. Christiansen, Catherine Borbas, Nora Morris, Barbara McLauglin, Xiaoming Gao, and Dennis Ross-Degnan. "Timeliness and Quality of Care for Elderly Patients With Acute Myocardial Infarction Under Health Maintenance Organization vs Fee-for-Service Insurance." *Archives of Internal Medicine* 159 (1999): 2013–20.

Spencer, Edward M., Ann E. Mills, Mary V. Rorty, and Patricia H. Werhane. *Organization Ethics in Health Care.* New York: Oxford University Press, 2000.

Stackhouse, Max. "Jesus and Economics: A Century of Reflection." In *The Bible in American Law, Politics, and Political Rhetoric,* ed. James Turner Johnson. Philadelphia: Fortress Press, 1985, 107–51.

Stadtmauer, Edward A., et al. "Conventional-Dose Chemotherapy Compared with

High-Dose Chemotherapy Plus Autologous Hematopoietic Stem-Cell Transplantation for Metastatic Breast Cancer." *New England Journal of Medicine* 342 (2000): 1069–76.

Starr, Paul. *The Social Transformation of American Medicine*. New York: Basic Books, 1982.

Stassen, Glen. "Michael Walzer's Situated Justice." *Journal of Religious Ethics* 22, no. 2 (1994): 375–99.

Stephenson, Joan. "Bone Marrow/Stem Cells: No Edge in Breast Cancer." *JAMA* 281 (1999): 1576–78.

———. "Opinions Divided on High-Dose Chemotherapy for Breast Cancer." *JAMA* 282 (1999): 119.

———. "Researchers Struggle with Trials of Stem-Cell Transplants for Breast Cancer." *JAMA* 277 (1997): 1827–29.

Stevens, Rosemary. *In Sickness and in Wealth: American Hospitals in the Twentieth Century*. New York: Basic Books, 1989.

Stone, Christopher D. "Corporate Accountability in Law and Morals." In *The Judeo-Christian Vision and the Modern Corporation*, ed. Oliver F. Williams and John W. Houck, 264–91. Notre Dame, Ind.: University of Notre Dame Press, 1982.

Stone, Deborah A. "The Doctor as Businessman: The Changing Politics of a Cultural Icon." *Journal of Health Politics, Policy and Law* 22, no. 2 (1997): 533–56.

Stout, James W., Lisa C. White, La Tonya Rogers, Teresa McRorie, Barbara Morray, Marijo Miller-Ratcliffe, and Gregory J. Redding. "The Asthma Outreach Project: A Promising Approach to Comprehensive Asthma Management." *Journal of Asthma* 35, no. 1 (1998): 119–127.

Stout, Jeffrey. *Ethics after Babel: The Languages of Morals and Their Discontents*. Boston: Beacon Press, 1988.

Street, Richard L., and Becky Voigt. "Patient Participation in Deciding Breast Cancer Treatment and Subsequent Quality of Life." *Medical Decision Making* 17 (1997): 298–306.

Stuart, Mary E., and Michael Weinrich. "Beyond Managing Medicaid Costs: Restructuring Care." *Milbank Quarterly* 76, no. 2 (1998).

Studdert, David M. "Direct Contracts, Data Sharing and Employee Risk Selection: New Stakes for Patient Privacy in Tomorrow's Health Insurance Markets." *American Journal of Law & Medicine* 25, nos. 2 & 3 (1999): 233–65.

Sugar, Sam J. Letter to the Editor. *New England Journal of Medicine* 333 (1995): 1220.

Sullivan, William M. *Work and Integrity: The Crisis and Promise of Professionalism in America*. New York: HarperCollins, 1995.

Sutton, Francis X., Seymour R. Harris, Carl Kaysen, and James Tobin. *The American Business Creed*. Cambridge, Mass.: Harvard University Press, 1956.

Swartz, Katherine and Troyen A. Brennan. "Integrated Health Care, Capitated Payment, and Quality: The Role of Regulation." *Annals of Internal Medicine* 124, no. 4 (1996): 442–448.

Taira, Deborah A., Dana Gelb Safran, Todd B. Seto, William H. Rogers, and Alvin R. Tarlov. "The Relationship between Patient Income and Physician Discussion of Health Risk Behaviors." *JAMA* 278, no. 17 (1997): 1412–17.

Tanenbaum, Sandra J., and Robert E. Hurley. "Disability and the Managed Care Frenzy: A Cautionary Note." *Health Affairs* 41, no. 4 (1995): 213–19.

Tawney, R. H. *The Acquisitive Society*. New York: Harcourt, Brace & World, 1948.

284

Thompson, Dennis F. "Hospital Ethics." *Cambridge Quarterly of Healthcare Ethics* 1, no. 3 (1992): 203–15.

Thompson, Joseph W., James Bost, Faruque Ahmed, Carrie E. Ingells, and Cary Sennett. "The NCQA's Quality Congress: Evaluating Managed Care in the United States." *Health Affairs* 17, no. 1 (1998): 152–58.

Tipson, Debra J. "Medicaid Managed Care and Community Providers: New Partnerships." *Health Affairs* 16, no. 4 (1997): 91–107.

Titlow, Karen I., Jonathan E. Rackoff, and Ezekial J. Emanuel. "What Will It Take to Restore Patient Trust?" *Business and Health* 17, no. 6 (1999): 61–64.

Tollefsen, Christopher. "What Would John Dewey Do? The Promises and Perils of Pragmatic Bioethics." *Journal of Medicine and Philosophy* 25, no. 1 (2000): 77–106.

Tolley, George, Donald Kenkel, and Robert Fabian. "State-of-the-Art Health Values." In *Valuing Health for Policy: An Economic Approach*, ed. George Tolley, Donald Kenkel, and Robert Fabian, 323–44. Chicago: University of Chicago Press, 1994.

Tolley, George, Donald Kenkel, Robert Fabian, and David Webster. "The Use of Health Values in Policy." In *Valuing Health for Policy: An Economic Approach*, ed. George Tolley, Donald Kenkel, and Robert Fabian, 345–91. Chicago: University of Chicago Press, 1994.

Toulmin, Stephen. "Medical Institutions and Their Moral Constraints." In *Integrity in Health Care Institutions*, ed. Ruth Ellen Bulger and Stanley Joel Reiser, 21–32. Iowa City: University of Iowa Press, 1990.

Trotter, Griffin. *The Loyal Physician: Roycean Ethics and the Practice of Medicine*. Nashville, Tenn.: Vanderbilt University Press, 1997.

Trubac, Edward R. "Economic Guidelines for Corporate Decision-Making." In *The Judeo-Christian Vision and the Modern Corporation*, ed. Oliver F. Williams and John W. Houck, 33–54. Notre Dame, Ind.: University of Notre Dame Press, 1982.

Ubel, Peter A. *Pricing Life: Why It's Time for Health Care Rationing*. Cambridge, Mass.: MIT Press, 2000.

Ubel, Peter A., Michael L. DeKay, Jonathan Baron, and David A. Asch. "Cost-Effectiveness Analysis in a Setting of Budget Constraints." *New England Journal of Medicine* 334 (1996): 1174–77.

U.S. Agency for Health Care Policy and Research. *Theory and Reality of Value-based Purchasing: Lessons from the Pioneers*. AHCPR Publication No. 98-0004, November 1997.

Veatch, Robert M. "Allocating Health Resources Ethically: New Roles for Administrators and Clinicians." *Frontiers of Health Services Management* 8, no. 1 (1991): 3–29.

———. *A Theory of Medical Ethics*. New York: Basic Books, 1981.

———. "Who Should Manage Care? The Case for Patients." *Kennedy Institute of Ethics Journal* 7, no. 4 (1997): 391–401.

Wagner, Edward H., Brian T. Austin, and Michael Von Korff. "Organizing Care for Patients with Chronic Illness." *Milbank Quarterly* 74, no. 4 (1996): 522–44.

Wallich, Paul. "Not So Blind After All: Randomized Trials—the Linchpin of Medicine—May Often Be Rigged." *Scientific American* 274 (May 1996): 20–22.

Walsh, Diana Chapman. *Corporate Physicians: Between Medicine and Management*. New Haven: Yale University Press, 1987.

Walzer, Michael. "The Idea of Civil Society." *Dissent* 38 (1991): 293–304.

———. *Spheres of Justice: A Defense of Pluralism and Equality*. Princeton: Princeton University Press, 1983.

285

Bibliography

Ware, John E., Jr., Martha Bayliss, William H. Rogers, Mark Kosinski, and Alvin R. Tarlov. "Differences in 4-Year Health Outcomes for Elderly and Poor, Chronically Ill Patients Treated in HMO and Fee-for-Service Systems." *JAMA* 276 (1996): 1039–47.

Waymack, Mark. "Health Care as a Business: The Ethic of Hippocrates Versus the Ethic of Managed Care." *Business & Professional Ethics Journal* 9, no. 3/4 (1990): 69–78.

Wazana, Ashley. "Physicians and the Pharmaceutical Industry: Is a Gift Ever Just a Gift?" *JAMA* 283 (2000): 373–80.

Webster, James R. and Joseph Feinglass. "Stroke Patients, 'Managed Care,' and Distributive Justice." *JAMA* 278 (1997): 161–162.

Weiner, Herman. "The Permanente Medical Groups: Organization and Responsibilities." In *The Kaiser-Permanente Medical Care Program*, ed. Anne R. Somers, 91–96. New York: Commonwealth Fund, 1971.

Weingarten, Scott. "Practice Guidelines and Prediction Rules Should Be Subject to Careful Clinical Testing." *JAMA* 277 (1997): 1977–1978.

West, Darrell M., Diane Heith, and Chris Goodwin. "Harry and Louise Go to Washington: Political Advertising and Health Care Reform." *Journal of Health Politics, Policy and Law* 27, no. 1 (1996): 35–68.

Westbrook, Robert B. *John Dewey and American Democracy.* Ithaca, N.Y.: Cornell University Press, 1991.

White, James Boyd. "How Should We Talk about Corporations? The Languages of Economics and Citizenship." *Yale Law Journal* 94 (1985): 1416–25.

Wicclear, Mark R. "What Can Be Learned about the Ethical Soundness of Medicare HMOs from Studies Comparing Them to Fee-for-Service Medicare?" *Journal of Ethics, Law, and Aging* 5, no. 1 (1999): 29–48.

Willard, Fred. Letter to the Editor. *New England Journal of Medicine* 333 (1995): 1221.

Wolf, Susan M. "Health Care Reform and the Future of Physician Ethics." *Hastings Center Report* 24, no. 2 (1994): 28–41.

———. "Shifting Paradigms in Bioethics and Health Law: The Rise of a New Pragmatism." *American Journal of Law & Medicine* 20, no. 4 (1994): 395–415.

Wolfe, Alan. *Whose Keeper? Social Science and Moral Obligation.* Berkeley, Calif.: University of California Press, 1989.

Wong, Kenman L. *Medicine and the Marketplace: The Moral Dimensions of Managed Care.* Notre Dame, Ind.: University of Notre Dame Press, 1998.

Woodstock Theological Center. *Ethical Considerations in the Business Aspects of Health Care.* Washington, D.C.: Georgetown University Press, 1995.

Wyschogrod, Edith. "The Logic of Artifactual Existents: John Dewey and Claude Lévi-Strauss." In *John Dewey: Critical Assessments*, ed. J. E. Tiles. Vol. 4, 158–73. London: Routledge, 1992.

Yelin, Edward H., Lindsey A. Criswell, and Paul G. Feigenbaum. "Health Care Utilization and Outcomes among Persons with Rheumatoid Arthritis in Fee-for-Service and Prepaid Group Practice Settings." *JAMA* 276 (1996): 1048–53.

Zendle, Les. "Controlling Costs: The Case of Kaiser." *JAMA* 274 (1995): 1135.

Zoloth-Dorfman, Laurie and Susan Rubin. "The Patient as Commodity: Managed Care and the Question of Ethics." *Journal of Clinical Ethics* 6, no. 4 (1995): 339–57.

Zussman, Robert. "The Contributions of Sociology to Medical Ethics." *Hastings Center Report* 30, no. 1 (2000): 7–11.

INDEX

MARY R. ANDERLIK, Associate Professor, School of Medicine, and Research Scholar, Institute for Bioethics, Health Policy and Law, University of Louisville, has an A.B. from Bryn Mawr College, a J.D. from Yale Law School, and a Ph.D. from Rice University. She spent a number of years as an associate in the Banking and Commercial Transactions group at Sidley & Austin. Prior to joining the Institute, she held a postdoctoral fellowship in Clinical Ethics at the University of Texas M.D. Anderson Cancer Center. At the Institute, Dr. Anderlik works on projects in the areas of managed care, disability, genetics, and privacy.